T0122394

Health Information Science

Series editor

Yanchun Zhang

More information about this series at http://www.springer.com/series/11944

Xiao-Xia Yin · Sillas Hadjiloucas
Yanchun Zhang

Pattern Classification of Medical Images: Computer Aided Diagnosis

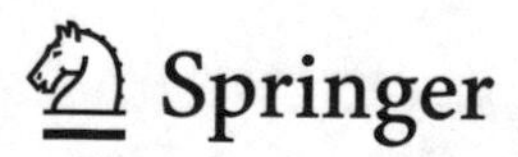
Springer

Xiao-Xia Yin
Victoria University
Melbourne, VIC
Australia

Yanchun Zhang
Victoria University
Melbourne, VIC
Australia

Sillas Hadjiloucas
Biomedical Engineering, School of Biological Sciences
University of Reading
Reading
UK

ISSN 2366-0988 ISSN 2366-0996 (electronic)
Health Information Science
ISBN 978-3-319-86061-9 ISBN 978-3-319-57027-3 (eBook)
DOI 10.1007/978-3-319-57027-3

Softcover reprint of the hardcover 1st edition 2017

Printed on acid-free paper

This Springer imprint is published by Springer Nature
The registered company is Springer International Publishing AG
The registered company address is: Gewerbestrasse 11, 6330 Cham, Switzerland

Preface

This book discusses recent advances in biomedical sensing as well as image analysis and processing techniques so as to develop a unified framework for computer-aided disease diagnosis. One of the aims is to discuss different approaches that will enable us to efficiently and reliably identify different features that are present in biomedical images. Another aim is to provide a generic framework for image classification.

The following four biomedical imaging modalities are considered: terahertz (THz) imaging, dynamic contrast-enhanced MRIs (DCE-MRIs) including functional MRI (fMRI), retinal fundus imaging and optical coherence tomography (OCT). THz imaging is chosen as it is a very promising emergent diagnostic modality that complements MRI. Under certain circumstances, it can also be independently used to identify and assess disease proliferation. OCT is a non-invasive imaging technique relying on low-coherence interferometry to generate in vivo, cross-sectional imagery of ocular tissue, and it complements fundus photography. Furthermore, OCT data sets have a structure similar to that found in THz imaging and MRI. Commonalities in these data structures can be explored by developing a unified multichannel signal processing framework for biomedical image analysis. Integration of complementary data sets provides additional features which can assist in inferring disease proliferation.

This book also provides an account of recent advances in artificial intelligence (AI) algorithms that may be applied to the multichannel framework discussed. Feature extraction and classification methods taking into consideration recent advances in support vector machine (SVM) and extreme learning machine (ELM) classifiers are also explained, and these formulations are extended to higher dimensional spaces for multiclass signal classification. The discussion also provides some future directions for machine learning approaches using Clifford algebra classifiers and deep learning architectures with geometric neurons. These recent advances can potentially lead to particularly powerful artificial intelligence AI algorithms that may one day automate several diagnostic processes.

Because of the multidisciplinary exposure of the subject, this book should be useful to final-year undergraduate or graduate students and research practitioners in

Biomedical Engineering, Applied Physics and Computer Science departments, who have already some familiarity with the topics discussed and are interested in learning about the latest advances on the subject. The different topics covered should also provide new ideas for discipline hopping, improving employability and career progression.

In addition, Chaps. 3–6 this book provides a generic framework for biomedical signal processing and classification which should be useful to computer science practitioners and AI software developers entering the biomedical field. The proposed multichannel framework points towards the direction of developing an open software architecture for signal denoising and feature extraction upon which specialized routines – tailored to different biomedical applications – can be developed. This is also beneficial from a software standardization perspective.

One of the issues commonly encountered in biomedical image analysis is that scientists from different disciplines focus on the different aspects associated with an image. A molecular spectroscopist will be focusing on locations in an image where efficient energy exchange between the excitatory signal and the tissue under study has taken place. This process would include the identification of specific ro-vibrational lines (for gases) or bands (for liquids and solids) as biomarkers under different physiological conditions. In contrast, an engineer would be focusing on signal processing, whereas a computer scientist on identifying the boundaries between different types of tissues or identifying and suppressing artefacts arising from different illumination conditions. In contrast, clinicians would be mostly concerned with the identification of different types and the pathological state of tissue as well as the visualization of small regions in the body and the mapping of opaque objects using a particular imaging technique. All these scientists tend to operate at different levels of complexity across a range of hierarchy levels from molecules all the way to the cellular, tissue, organ or organism level. The diversity of processing algorithms and the fact that modelling at one level of hierarchy does not scale well to higher levels of complexity due to the multiparametric emergent properties of biological media, are major contributing factors that have impeded progress towards automating the diagnostic process. An effort has been made to account for these different perspectives.

This book is, therefore, structured as follows:

Chapter 1 provides a general introduction to THz spectroscopy and then focuses on THz-transient spectrometry. The different system configurations and types of signals recorded are explained. The MRI imaging modality is also introduced. The tensorial nature of the MRI signal is also explained. THz and MRI time series analysis are placed in a common signal processing framework on the basis of the data structures associated with single pixels or voxels. An introduction to retinal fundus imaging as well as optical coherence tomography is also provided. Similarities and differences between these four different measurement modalities are highlighted.

Chapter 2 provides an overview of clinical applications using the four imaging modalities discussed in Chap. 1. This includes biomedical applications of THz spectroscopy and MRI, contrast imaging on the basis of tissue water content, identification of biomarkers and the visualization of tissue oxygenation levels on the basis of the BOLD signal observed through fMRI. In addition, possibilities for combining THz spectroscopy and MRI with other sensing techniques using a multichannel framework are highlighted. Finally, recent advances in the application of fundus imaging to disease diagnosis and the application of OCT imaging for the visualization of increased vascularization in mammograms as well as the detection of abnormalities in infant brains are reported.

The following chapters take the view that the problem of developing automated classifier solutions for assessing disease progression should be seen as the tuning of three different modules that may be individually optimized for particular samples and data sets: the data acquisition imaging module, the data denoising pre-processing and feature extraction module and finally the classifier module. Tuning may be tailored separately for each module according to the features resolved by each measurement modality so as to optimize the classifier learning process.

Chapter 3 discusses different signal denoising methodologies applicable to both THz and MRI systems as well as fundus photography and OCT. Data windowing, apodization, parametric model fitting and multiresolution feature extraction methodologies with wavelets as well as adaptive wavelets for both THz and MRI data sets are also reviewed. The above discussions are effectively focusing on robust feature extraction and selection strategies, firstly from a single pixel perspective and then from an imaging perspective. Benefits from adopting a fractional order calculus approach to detect features in an image are explained. Recent advances in fundus image denoising are also highlighted. A multiresolution image fusion scheme that could be used to combine MRI with THz data sets is proposed. This chapter then discusses several feature selection strategies for both THz and MRI data sets. In the case of THz data sets features in time, frequency or wavelet domains associated with single pixels are considered. In the case of MRI data sets, the discussion focuses on features observed across entire images, taking into consideration textural information. Spatiotemporal correlations across different areas in an image, as identified through fMRI, are discussed. Advances in a graph-theoretical framework that can potentially elucidate such correlations are also mentioned. In addition, feature extraction and selection in retinal fundus imaging and OCT are reviewed.

Chapter 4 discusses recent advances in different classifier methodologies, with an emphasis on complex support vector machine and extreme learning machine approaches. An extension to multidimensional extreme learning machine classifiers is provided. Examples of binary as well as multiclass classification tasks using THz data sets are presented. The performance of other classifiers such as multimodal logistic regression, and naïve Bayesian, in performing classification of THz data sets is compared. In addition, some recent advances in clustering and segmentation techniques for THz data sets as well as for fundus images are discussed. Current methods for automatic retinal vessel classification are highlighted, as it is envisaged that the improved edge detection algorithms discussed in the previous chapters in conjunction with the proposed classification methodologies, can lead to better discrimination between arteries and veins. Finally, this chapter discusses some recent advances in automated image classification using performance criteria directly developed by clinicians.

Chapter 5 provides a more in-depth analysis of MRI data sets. A recently developed spatiotemporal enhancement methodology for DCE-MRIs that makes use of a tensorial multichannel framework is explained. Examples from breast tumour reconstruction are provided to showcase the proposed methodology. It is shown that tumour voxels registered in three-dimensional space can be reconstructed better after increasing contrast from background images using the proposed methodology. The algorithm can be used to perform both feature extraction and image registration. This chapter also discusses the general structure of supervised learning algorithms for functional MRI data sets. Advances in supervised multivariate learning from fMRI data sets that promise to further elucidate brain disorders are discussed. Finally, the general structure of topological graph kernels in functional connectivity networks is explained. The prospects for developing machine learning algorithms that would automatically provide spatiotemporal associations of brain activity across different regions using graph theory methodologies are discussed. A more critical view of what may be achieved taking into consideration limitations in the fMRI measurement modality is provided. Finally, some recent advances from the computer vision community of relevance are highlighted as possible future research directions.

Chapter 6 provides an outlook to future multichannel classifiers, incorporating multiple features in their input space. Such approaches are also suitable for classifying multidimensional tensorial data sets. The discussion focuses on Clifford algebra-based feature classification. A multichannel approach enables the fusion of information acquired from multiple images at different time stamps, so it can potentially elucidate disease progression. In addition, this chapter discusses recent advances in deep learning as related to MRI as well as THz imaging data sets. The use of geometric neurons which can combine information from complementary sensing modalities is highlighted as an important future research direction for feature extraction and classification in MRI. In addition, the proposed Clifford framework could also benefit the THz imaging community, providing improved classification results when these systems undergo clinical trials.

Chapter 7 provides some concluding remarks related to the recent advances in signal processing and classification across the four imaging modalities discussed throughout this book. It aims to highlight how progress in each of the above research areas can be shared to accelerate progress across different biomedical imaging modalities. Furthermore, this chapter summarizes some of the main aspects of the unified multichannel framework that was developed throughout this book. Finally, this chapter concludes by providing some future directions towards a generic framework for the automated quantitative assessment of disease proliferation. It is envisioned that in the near future, a combination of several biomedical sensing modalities will be integrated through sensor fusion and that artificial intelligence techniques will efficiently use the complementary information, to improve disease diagnosis.

The authors would like to gratefully acknowledge Dr. John W. Bowen from Reading University, Prof. Roberto K.H. Galvão from Instituto Tecnológico de Aeronáutica, São José dos Campos, Brazil, and Prof. Derek Abbott from the University of Adelaide for their valuable discussions over the years that have led to the development of our current understanding of the topics discussed in this book.

Melbourne, Australia — Xiao-Xia Yin
Reading, UK — Sillas Hadjiloucas
Melbourne, Australia — Yanchun Zhang
March 2017

Contents

Chapter 1
Introduction and Motivation for Conducting Medical Image Analysis

The demand for advanced image analysis techniques stems from the recent proliferation of new biomedical imaging modalities across the electromagnetic spectrum. The number of scans currently performed in most hospital environments has exploded placing unprecedented workloads on personnel associated with their interpretation. At the same time, we are also witnessing remarkable advances in artificial intelligence (AI). New algorithms are paving the way for the provision of automatic image interpretation which can lead to improved diagnosis and better understanding of disease progression. Furthermore, advances in biomedical equipment suitable for home use are also providing new opportunities for the further proliferation of AI systems and lead to advances in networked home care technologies which promise to make possible the remote diagnosis of the onset of disease much earlier than before, thus minimizing the need for consultation by experts. Such practice is also likely to provide almost expert opinion at reduced cost. Through these advances, one can foresee some inevitable developments that will affect how the provision of health care will be managed in the near future across the developed world.

From a signal processing and AI perspective, most of the imaging modalities display some underlining commonalities. In order to establish the generic underlying common problems encountered across the various imaging methods, this book focuses on just four representative modalities that operate at different parts of the electromagnetic spectrum: THz pulse imaging or TPI, MRI, fundus imaging and OCT. The aim of the first chapter is to introduce each measurement modality and explain how they complement each other. This will enable us to introduce in subsequent chapters a possible common framework that can lead to unified signal processing and image classification using machine learning. The common underlying theme in all four diagnostic methods considered is the imaging of tissue at various states of hydration and the possibility of providing diagnosis of the onset of disease or an assessment of disease proliferation on the basis of changes in the physicochemical environment of the cells, e.g. through changes in blood flow or through the use of biomarkers which can also lead to textural changes in the tissue. We first discuss

X. Yin et al., *Pattern Classification of Medical Images: Computer Aided Diagnosis*, Health Information Science, DOI 10.1007/978-3-319-57027-3_1

the technological aspects of THz spectroscopy, the different system configurations commonly used as well as the type of signals generated. An introduction to MRI and recent developments in contrast enhanced imaging is then provided. The need to develop a tensorial representation of the signal to account for anisotropy is also highlighted. This chapter also places THz imaging and MRI imaging in a common multi-dimensional signal processing framework. In addition, an introduction to retinal fundus imaging and OCT imaging is provided. Finally, similarities with the other two imaging modalities are highlighted. The similarity in these data structures naturally leads to a unified approach for data pre-processing and image classification extending pattern recognition to new application areas [1].

1.1 Introduction to Time-Resolved Terahertz Spectroscopy and Imaging

1.1.1 Time Domain and Frequency Domain THz Spectroscopy

Investigations at the terahertz (THz) part of the electromagnetic (EM) spectrum loosely defined between 100 GHz–10 THz are of much relevance to the biological sciences because THz radiation interacts strongly with polar molecules [2–4]. Biological tissue is generally composed of polar liquids so discrimination between tissue types can be made on the basis of water content. The technique is very sensitive in providing contrast between samples at various degrees of water saturation [5–7], and has applications in the evaluation of the severity of burns or partially necrotic skin samples [8] and the imaging of basal cell carcinomas [9–12] which can show an increase in interstitial water within the diseased tissue [5, 13].

Since THz photons have significantly lower energies (e.g. only 1.24 meV at 300 GHz) than X-rays, they have been considered by many as non-invasive. Although non-linear interactions between biological tissue and coherent THz radiation have been predicted by Fröhlich [14] and experimentally verified by the careful work of Grundler and the analysis of Kaiser [15] in the '90s, the current and widely held view is that any measurement technique that operates at THz frequencies should be evaluated using current guidelines on specific absorption rates. These are only associated with the thermal effects of the radiation with the tissue; so from a clinical perspective, such irradiation can be considered as non-invasive. Such a view is also further supported by noting that the Gibbs free energy conveyed in the THz light beam is insufficient to directly drive chemical reactions. For example, the molar energy at a frequency f of 100 GHz would be given from $E = Nhf$ where $N = 6.023 \times 10^{23}\,\mathrm{mol}^{-1}$, Avogadro's number), and $h = 6.626 \times 10^{-34}\,\mathrm{Js}$ (Planck's constant), resulting in a calculated value of only $E = 0.04\,\mathrm{kJ\,mol}^{-1}$ which is so low (approximately 100 times lower than the amount of molar energy required for ATP

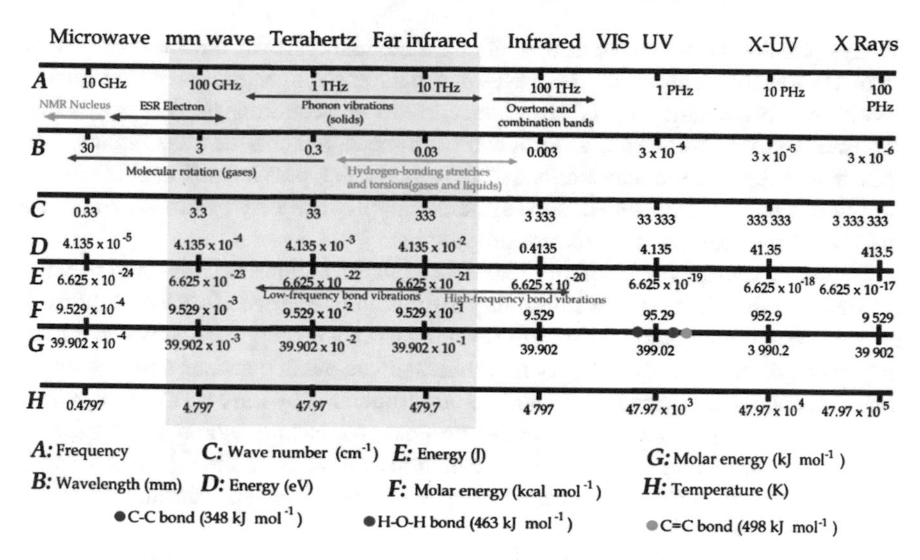

Fig. 1.1 Multidisciplinary interpretation of the electromagnetic spectrum

hydrolysis) that for most practical purposes; we may assume that the interference with biochemical processes would be minimal (Fig. 1.1).

Furthermore, in the THz part of the spectrum, many molecules have characteristic 'fingerprint' absorption spectra [16–18]. Substances in the condensed phase are held together by either ionic, covalent or electrostatic forces, and therefore the lowest frequency modes will be associated with intermolecular motion [19]. The interaction between THz radiation and biological molecules, cells, and tissues can be understood using assumptions of propagation of an angular spectrum of plane waves through the material [21]. Following standard postulates of dielectric theory, a medium may be characterized in terms of its permittivity ε (the ability of the medium to be polarized) and conductivity σ (the ability of ions to move through the medium). At higher frequencies, transitions between different molecular vibrational and rotational energy levels become increasingly dominant and are more readily understood using a quantum-mechanical framework [22]. THz pulse spectroscopy provides information on low-frequency intermolecular vibrational modes [23].

THz imaging can thus be remarkably informative regarding a sample's composition. The Fourier transform of the associated time domain waveform over a broad spectral range allows the calculation of the frequency dependent refractive index and absorption coefficients of the sample. Since wavelengths are longer in the THz part of the spectrum, there is sufficient phase stability in the experimental apparatus enabling the extraction of phase information by varying the time delay between the THz wave and the probe beam [16]. When some materials are sufficiently transparent to THz radiation, it is feasible to measure transmission responses and acquire spectral information. Reflectance imaging is also straightforward, and through the combination of transmittance and reflectance, a spectral absorbance may be inferred. This is not always possible at the infrared, optical and ultraviolet parts of the spectrum where errors, due to scattering of shorter waves due to the surface roughness of the samples, preclude direct calculations of absorbance. Reduced scattering of THz waves thus minimises errors in inferred absorbance from measurements of transmittance and reflectance. Alternative measurement topologies which provide differential absorption have also been developed; such systems can produce very informative contrast images for the evaluation of disease progression.

Further advantages of imaging using THz radiation include the improved penetration depth within the tissue and the ability to differentiate between organs on the basis of tissue water content. Since 70% of the human body is composed of water, a large proportion of the excitation energy is significantly attenuated and, as a consequence, the resultant spectra in many biomedical experiments may only be unambiguously resolved after the application of elaborate post-processing techniques. Excluding super-resolution techniques, imaging resolution is limited by the diffraction wavelength and is thus inferior to infrared or optical imaging but superior to microwave based imaging modalities.

Although much of the pioneering work in building interferometric spectroradiometers and other continuous wave measurement systems at the THz part of the spectrum took place at Queen Mary College over a period of almost 30 years under the guidance of D. H. Martin [20], it was only during the past two decades that THz science and technology has flourished as a universally accepted new sensing modality. Using continuous wave systems [24], there is a variety of instruments that may be assembled using quasi-optical active and passive components. The AB Millimetre vector network analyser, if available, is the preferred choice for continuous wave measurements with significant signal-to-noise per spectral bin all the way up to 1.2 THz. It is not, however, as user friendly for extracting scattering parameters as other commercially available solutions that operate at lower frequencies. An account of different topologies using null-balance methods can be found in [25] whereas polarimetric measurements for dichroic samples should ideally be performed using the topologies discussed in [26, 27] or Fabry-Perot structures, e.g. [28]. Alternative broadband experimental configurations may include Mach–Zehnder or Martin-Puplett configurations as discussed in [7, 20, 21]. When high power per spectral bin is needed, THz imaging may also be performed (at significant cost) with high-power THz sources under pulsed scanning mode and pulse-gated detection using large scale facilities (e.g. Jefferson lab, FELIX etc.). Currently, however, bio-medical investigations using these facilities are fewer than those performed in the physical sciences e.g. the semiconductor community.

Although there are several THz imaging systems that can be built using continuous wave sources by appropriately adapting the above configurations to perform raster-imaging of the sample [24], the focus of this book is on time domain spectroscopy (TDS) with ultrashort-pulse laser sources because of their recent proliferation. Such systems are more versatile for biomarker identification than their continuous wave counterparts because they are inherently very broadband without requiring liquid-helium cooled detectors (heterodyne based continuous wave systems are more narrow-band and lack such versatility because of the lack of such wide tunability of the sources). Furthermore THz pulse imaging (THz-TPI) has important applications in in vivo, in vitro and ex vivo biosensing [8, 16, 29, 33]; identifying 'fingerprint' resonances due to overtone and combination bands [5, 30].

At this point it is worth noting that there are several similarities between THz-TDS and the pulsed radar sensing modality. In THz-TDS, the time gated reflections are analysed directly in the time domain by observing their attenuation, phase delay and temporal spread after interacting with matter. Good temporal definition can provide localization of tissue interfaces on the basis of refractive index differences (the real part associated with impedance mismatch and the complex part with the attenuation due to the number of absorbers and their extinction coefficient). Studies in reflection geometry can occasionally also enable the indirect assessment of sample or layer thickness, as well as determining the position of embedded unknown objects, etc. [16].

An important advantage of time-domain systems over their continuous wave counterparts that are plagued by etalon effects is that of being able to perform pulse time gating. This is possible as long as the multiple reflections in the measurement system are sufficiently far apart so as not to be mixed with the molecular de-excitation signals of the sample. The typical time-resolved THz spectrometer used in most of the studies discussed so far, utilize a short coherence length infrared source (centered at around 800 nm) to generate a sub-100 femtosecond duration pulse train with repetition frequency of around 80 MHz. Each infrared pulse, is split into separate pump and probe beams. The pump beam is used to excite an optical rectification crystal, which acts as a T-ray emitter, and the T-rays produced (duration around 200 fs) are collimated and focused onto a sample by a pair of parabolic mirrors. The T-rays emerging from the sample are re-collimated by another pair of mirrors, before being combined with the probe beam in a T-ray detector crystal. As a result, the modification by the sample T-ray and the probe beams propagates through the THz detector crystal co-linearly. The pump beam, which is also transmitted through a chopper, travels through an optical delay stage that is modulated accordingly, so that the pump and probe beams arrive at the detector in a time-coincident manner. The electro-optic detector crystal produces an output that is proportional to the birefringence observed from the interaction of the THz pulse with the time-coincident infrared pulse replica within the crystal. This output is proportional to the T-ray response of the sample and this signal is measured with the use of a balanced optical photo-detection scheme. A lock-in amplifier (LIA) is also used to demodulate the signal, and this avoids $1/f$ (flicker) noise problems that are present in this detector-limited measurement scheme. Typically, THz-TPI is performed through a 2D raster scan after translating the sample in both the x and y direction, while keeping it at the focal plane of the parabolic mirrors. A typical setup [31, 34], is shown in Fig. 1.2.

Details of typical THz transient systems can be found elsewhere [33]. An interesting quasi-optical circuit topology for simultaneous measurements of both transmittance and reflectance that was reported by Ung et al. [35] is shown in Fig. 1.3. In that system, the frequency dependent reflectance $R(\omega)$ and transmittance $T(\omega)$ signatures are given from:

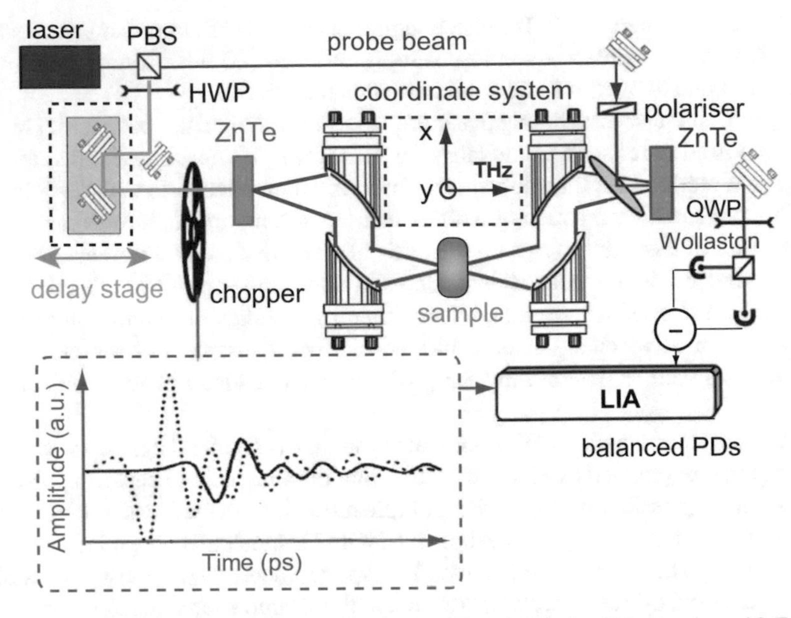

Fig. 1.2 A schematic experimental setup for electrooptic transmission THz imaging with ZnTe as EO generation and detection, illuminated by a femtosecond laser

$$R(\omega) = \frac{1-\widetilde{n}(\omega)}{1+\widetilde{n}(\omega)} + \frac{\frac{4\widetilde{n}(\omega)[\widetilde{n}(\omega)-1]}{(\widetilde{n}(\omega)+1)^3} \cdot \exp[-i2\widetilde{n}(\omega)\frac{\omega}{c}d]}{1-(\frac{\widetilde{n}(\omega)-1}{\widetilde{n}(\omega)+1})^2 \cdot \exp[-i2\widetilde{n}(\omega)\frac{\omega}{c}d]} \tag{1.1}$$

$$T(\omega) = \frac{4\widetilde{n}(\omega)}{[1+\widetilde{n}(\omega)]^2} \cdot \frac{\exp\{-i[\widetilde{n}(\omega)-1]\frac{\omega}{c}d\}}{1-(\frac{\widetilde{n}(\omega)-1}{\widetilde{n}(\omega)+1})^2 \cdot \exp[-i2\widetilde{n}(\omega)\frac{\omega}{c}d]} \tag{1.2}$$

where the normal incidence complex refractive index is $(\omega) = n(\omega) - ik(\omega)$ and the absorption coefficient is: $\alpha(\omega) = 4\pi k(\omega)/c$ where c is the speed of light, k is the wave number, d is the sample thickness and the tilde denotes a complex quantity. An alternative phase-sensitive topology is reported in the work by Pashkin et al. [36]. An interesting prospect for dispensing with the conventional x, y, z scanning stages for image formation at the focus of the paraboloids by adopting a metamaterials based scanning technique for image formation is discussed in [37, 38].

The resultant measurement at each pixel position of an image is an entire time-dependent waveform. Therefore, the result from TDS-TPI is a three-dimensional (3D) data set, which then can potentially be mapped to two-dimensional (2D) images [39], where structural and compositional discrimination based on a sample's optical properties may be conveniently performed using pattern recognition algorithms. In the following chapters, sample responses from multiple THz spectrometry experiments are used as examples to provide a generic pattern recognition framework.

The proposed approach extends the range of applications of pattern recognition to emergent sensing modalities [1, 40].

A further advantage of the associated phase stability in THz spectrometers (due to the associated longer wavelength) is that it enables direct measurement of both the real and imaginary (complex) components of the permittivity. A Debye relaxation model can be used to analyze the strong absorption of terahertz radiation in polar liquids at least up to 1 THz [5, 32]. This model can be directly related to the associated intermolecular dynamics. Spectroscopic studies can, therefore, potentially elucidate the way proteins influence the state of water and can lead to further understanding of the role of hydration shells in protein interactions [41, 42].

It is also worth noting that in all of the above experimental set-ups one needs to always consider that there may also be additional pseudocoherence errors because different parts of the beam across its aperture travel different paths through different regions of the sample (if it is of non-uniform thickness), interfering constructively or destructively with each other when they recombine. A recent account of advances in THz metrology discussing errors in both continuous wave as well as THz-transient systems can be found in [43]. Such errors are endemic to much of the THz literature although this is not extensively discussed. Management of these artefacts and their relevance to imaging applications is therefore an open issue requiring further consideration. For the case of reflectometric measurements using continuous wave sources, it is occasionally possible to de-embed the reflection signature from different layers as discussed in the work by Hadjiloucas et al. [44]. The technique has been applied to waveguide measurements but has yet to be applied to reflection measurements of biological tissue when the different strata contain different water content (Fig. 1.3).

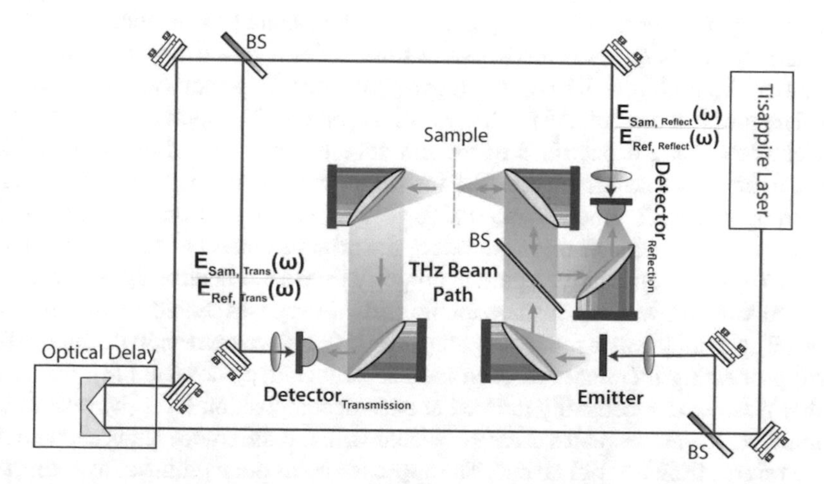

Fig. 1.3 Quasi-optical setup for simultaneous reflection and transmission THz-TDS measurements. The path of the 800 nm laser beam is depicted in *red*, while the THz beam path is shown in *green*, with all beams horizontally polarized. The sample is placed in the focus of the parabolic mirrors and, for a reference measurement in reflection geometry, a mirror is used adopted from [35]

From a technological point of view, THz imaging is thus an emergent complementary imaging modality of much interest within the biomedical community, potentially competing with positron emission tomography (PET) imaging which has picomolar sensitivity but poor spatial resolution and magnetic resonance imaging (MRI), which provides millimolar sensitivity with high spatial resolution. A diffraction limited imaging system operating at 2 THz would have a spatial resolution of 150 μm, which may be considered limiting for many biomedical applications for which this imaging modality offers niche applications (e.g. differential imaging of cancer cells in breast tissue of pregnant or lactating women). From a clinical perspective, tumours need to be identified at the earliest possible developmental stage and, unless suitable THz super-resolution techniques can be adopted (a difficult task since beams are diffractively spreading and the optics community has yet to extend existing algorithms from the infrared to the THz part of the spectrum), it is unlikely that current systems will be adopted by clinicians. Imaging systems integrating either PET or MRI modalities with THz pulse imaging to enable the generation of composite images is the most likely way forward for the integration of this technology in a clinical setting.

1.1.2 Recent Advances in Simultaneous Time-Frequency Dependent THz Spectroscopy

Time-frequency analysis methods have been developed to provide very parsimonious parametrizations of time series datasets and, in this sense, nicely complement other parametrization schemes performed in either time or frequency domains [45, 46]. The wavelet transform (WT) is a popular technique suited to the analysis of short-duration signals [47]. It decomposes the time series signal using two filter banks separating the high (detail) and low (approximation) frequency components of the signal assuming a pre-defined mother wavelet function. The approach provides very efficient de-noising capabilities in the presence of Gaussian white noise and has very parsimonious representation. An important feature of this transform is that it has orthogonal basis functions so that it enjoys perfect reconstruction symmetry, enabling its inverse transform to reproduce the original dataset without loss of information. This is a particularly important property from a biomedical signal processing perspective as software certification for biomedical purposes should require complete traceability of all the data processing steps. A further development in the biomedical signal processing literature has been the use of adaptive wavelets [48], where the mother wavelet is specifically tailored at each decomposition level (wavelet scale), to minimize the least squares error associated with the difference between the transformed signal from its original one. The approach holds great promise for optimizing the extraction of the spectroscopic information contained in each THz pulse transient as well as in THz TPI generally [49–52]. Figure 1.4 showcases the advantages of time-frequency analysis in terms of the reduction in classification errors. To generate this graph, the standard deviation of the noise was varied from 0.001 to 0.5. For

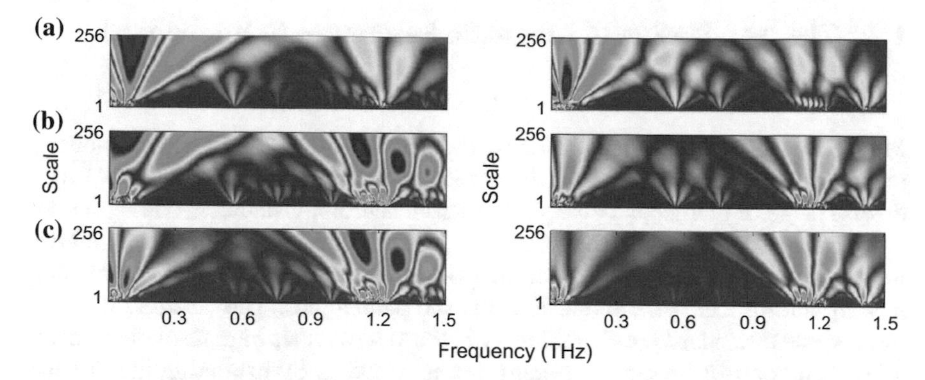

Fig. 1.4 Classification errors (%) as a function of noise level in the interferograms. Nonoptimized db4 wavelet (green), optimized wavelet (*red*) and Euclidean distance (*blue*) classifiers. The inset shows an inferogram of leather with (**a**) no artificially added noise and noise with standard deviation of (**b**) 0.1 and (**c**) 0.5. After [52]

each noise level, 250 noisy patterns were generated for each class (lycra and leather). As can be seen, the classification is much more robust to noise when carried out in the wavelet domain than in the original domain. Moreover, the robustness to noise is further increased by the optimization of the WT.

In addition to the above more elaborate routines, there have also been other examples of studies that incorporate WT pre-processing routines for signal-to-noise-ratio enhancement and classification of THz spectra [8, 53]. Such a pre-processing step enabled the successful discrimination of cancerous from normal tissue in wax-embedded histopathological melanoma sections as well as the classification of dentine and enamel regions in teeth [49]. It is now generally accepted that the performance of a classifier based on the output of a wavelet filter bank is improved over that of an Euclidean distance classifier in the original spectral domain [52]. Finally, an alternative very promising approach for the modelling of de-excitation dynamics, which has its origins to the theory of complex dielectrics, is through the use of fractional order calculus and the fitting of fractional order models. In this approach, the time series experimental datasets are modelled using very parsimonious pole-zero expressions associated with the dynamics of resistive, capacitive or inductive networks [54–56]. Although the fractional-order system identification literature is still in its infancy, it promises to provide much lower residual errors in the identified models, thus significantly advancing the science of chemometrics that is of significance to the further advancement of the discussed biomedical investigations. The approach can account for spectral shifts in amorphous materials as well as de-embed solvation dynamics.

Since dual modality THz/MRI tandem hybrid imaging systems have already been discussed in the literature [57], it is appropriate to look more closely at recent advances in MRI sensing before a combined signal/image processing framework is proposed.

1.2 The Application of Magnetic Resonance to Biomedical Imaging

Magnetic resonance imaging (MRI) was established as a new diagnostic modality in the early 1980s and rapidly gained wide acceptance as an imaging tool for a diverse range of biomedical disciplines such as neurology, oncology, obstetrics and gynaecology. In a clinical setting, it is now routinely used in cardiovascular, musculoskeletal, gastrointestinal and liver imaging as well as in neuroimaging, providing information on their physiological status and pathologies. This imaging modality has become a standard tool in radiology because it provides high resolution images with good contrast between different tissues. It works by exploiting the fact that the nucleus of a hydrogen atom behaves like a small magnet. MRIs employ powerful magnets which produce a strong magnetic field that forces protons from the nucleus of a hydrogen atom to align with that field. In a magnetic field, spins of protons can either align with or against the direction of the field. The magnetization is initially parallel to the magnetic field B_0. When a radio frequency (RF) current is then pulsed through the patient, the magnetic component of this electromagnetic wave generates a gradient magnetic field that exerts a force on the spinning top of a proton leading to a torque. The protons are stimulated and spin out of equilibrium. This causes the spinning top to precess around the gradient field. Excitation stops when the magnetization is tipped sufficiently into the transverse plane, forming a flip angle. When the radio frequency field is turned off, the precessing magnetization generates the energy released as the protons realign with the magnetic field. The time it takes for the protons to realign with the magnetic field, as well as the amount of energy released, changes depending on the environment and the chemical nature of the molecules. When a rotating field gradient is used, linear positioning information is collected along a number of different directions. Assuming the field strength to be 1 T, the protons are revolving 42.5 million times per second and it is at this frequency the molecular system under investigation is excited with a pulse (i.e. at the Larmor frequency). One of the principal determinants of the strength of the NMR signal from a given region is spin density, relating to the concentration of nuclei in the tissue precessing at the Larmor frequency. Using nuclear magnetic resonance (NMR), the hydrogen nuclei can be manipulated so that they generate a signal that can be mapped and turned into an image. A general schematic of the MRI excitation process in a clinical setting is illustrated in Fig. 1.5.

For a 90° flip angle, the produced NMR signal satisfies the following contrast equation:

$$\text{Signal} \propto \rho(1 - \mathrm{e}^{-\mathrm{TR}/\mathrm{T1}})\mathrm{e}^{-\mathrm{TE}/\mathrm{T2}} \tag{1.3}$$

where ρ denotes spin density, the $(1 - e^{-TR/T1})$ term indicates T1-weighting images, and $e^{-TE/T2}$ indicates T2-weighting images. Repetition Time (TR) refers to the time gap at which consecutive RF pulses are applied; while TE (Echo Time) refers to

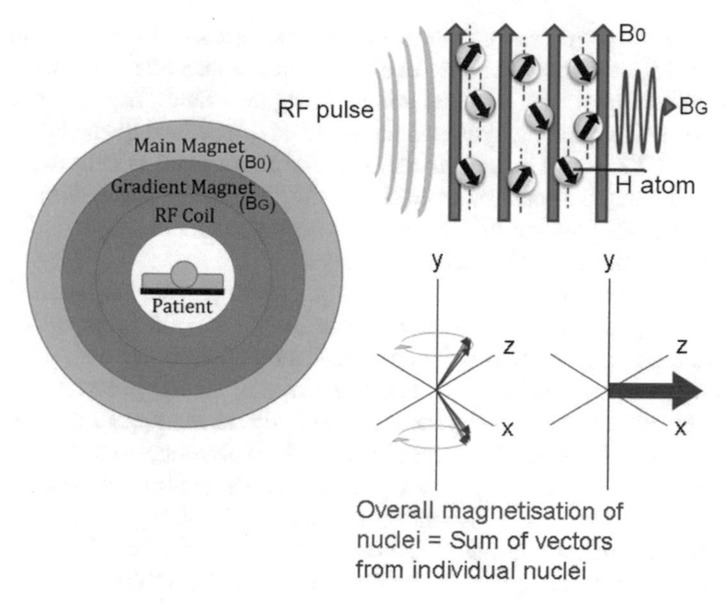

Fig. 1.5 Schematic of MRI in a clinical setting

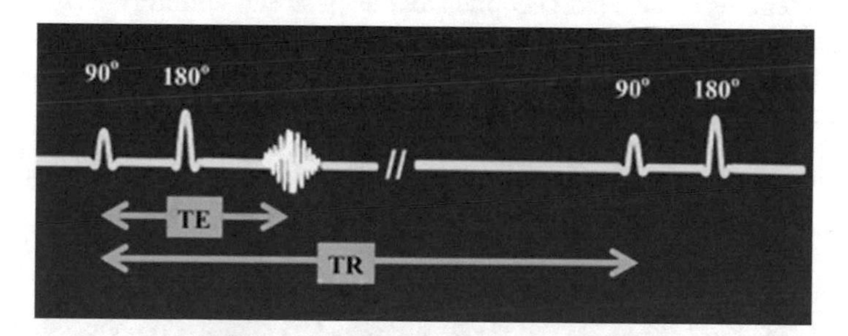

Fig. 1.6 Illustration of conventional (single echo) SE pulse sequence

the time delay between the applied RF pulse and its reception (echo). T1 weighted images (T1W) are produced by keeping TR and TE relatively short to minimize T2 relaxation effects, while T2 weighted images (T2W) are produced by keeping TR and TE relatively long to minimize T1 relaxation effects. The simplest form of the spin-echo (SE) pulse sequence consists of a 90°-pulse, a 180°-pulse, and then an echo. The time between the middle of the first RF pulse and the peak of the spin echo is called the echo time (TE). The sequence then repeats at time TR, the repetition time. Figure 1.6 illustrates a conventional (single echo) SE pulse sequence.

As illustrated in Fig. 1.5, a T1 weighted image relies on the longitudinal relaxation of a tissue's net magnetisation vector (NMV). Spins aligned to an external field (B_0) are aligned into the transverse plane by an RF pulse. They then slide back toward the original equilibrium direction based on B_0.

MRI de-embeds structural details of the various organs on the basis of the observation of hydrogen atom (proton) de-excitation rates as they arise following an excitation by an oscillatory radio signal within a magnetic field. The energy emission stemming from the spinning hydrogen molecules is determined by the two time constants, $T1$ and $T2$, and the contrast between different tissues is determined by the rate at which excited atoms return to the equilibrium state. The radio signals can be made to encode position information by varying the main magnetic field using gradient coils, enabling the formation of images.

Regions of fat present in the human tissue quickly realign its longitudinal magnetization with B_0, and it therefore appears bright on a T1 weighted image. Conversely, water has a much slower longitudinal magnetization realignment after an RF pulse, and therefore has less transverse magnetization after an RF pulse. Thus, regions composed of water produce a significantly lower signal and appear dark. Anatomical features can be identified fairly reliably by trained personnel to recognise regions with different water content. A T2W signal relies upon the transverse relaxation of the net magnetisation vector. T2 relaxation is seen only with gradient-echo (GRE) imaging because transverse relaxation caused by magnetic field inhomogeneities is eliminated by the 180° pulse at spin-echo imaging. T2 relaxation is one of the main determinants of image contrast with GRE sequences, and forms the basis for many magnetic resonance (MR) applications such as susceptibility-weighted (SW) imaging, perfusion MR imaging, and functional MR imaging [58–60]. For long TE imaging, tissues with short T2's (rapidly recovering) appear darkest. Compartments filled with water (e.g. CSF compartments) appear bright and tissues with high fat content (e.g. white matter) appear dark. This is sufficient for demonstrating various pathological conditions as most (but unfortunately not all) lesions are associated with an increase in water content. Figure 1.7 illustrates T1W and T2W images.

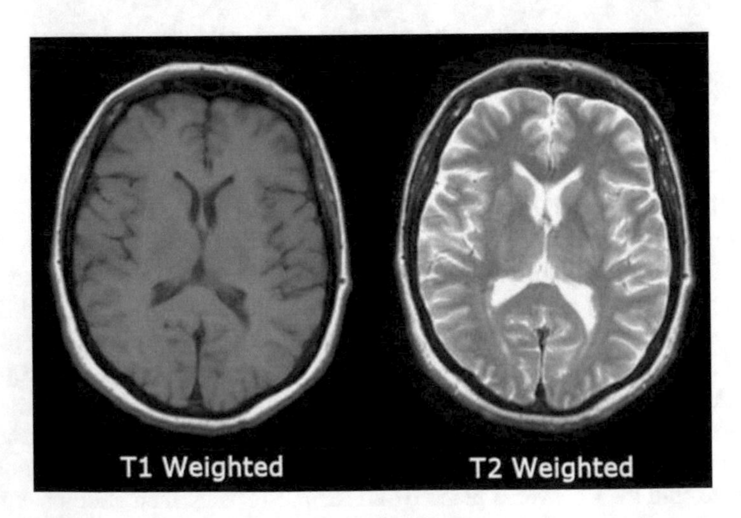

Fig. 1.7 Illustration of T1 weighted and T2 weighted images

An important advantage that MRI has over its computed axial tomography (CAT) counterpart is that it avoids the deleterious effects associated with X-ray irradiation. A recent advance in MRI methodology enabling the detection of tumour features with high sensitivity [61], has been the use of exogenous contrast agents, the well-known dynamic contrast enhanced MRI modality (DCE-MRI) [62]. The crucial advantage of DCE-MRIs over standard MRIs is that it provides registration of 3D spatial lesion information as well as temporal information regarding the progression of lesions. In addition, it provides additional information on vascularization by showing variations in contrast agent uptake rates, thus enabling a more accurate assessment of the extent of lesions and new opportunities for their better characterisation [63–65]. From a classification perspective, DCE-MRI produces a sequence of three-dimensional (3D) patterns recorded at different time instances. These datasets are therefore four-dimensional, with three spatial dimensions and a quantization in the time domain defined by the image interval lapse time. The detection of anomalies in spatiotemporal datasets is an emergent interdisciplinary topic that requires the development of completely new software tools [66]. Furthermore, as discussed in [67–70], analysing spatiotemporal patterns is critical for the correct identification of tumour anomalies in DCE-MRIs, establishing whether they are malignant or benign.

An important advance in MRI technology is its ability in detecting tumour anomalies with high sensitivity [61], has been the use of exogenous contrast agents, the well-known dynamic contrast enhanced MRI modality (DCE-MRI). The crucial advantage of DCE-MRIs over standard MRIs is that it provides registration of 3D spatial lesion information as well as temporal information regarding the progression of lesions. In addition, it provides additional information on vascularization by showing variations in contrast agent uptake rates, thus enabling a more accurate assessment of the extent of lesions and new opportunities for their better characterisation [63–65].

An important advance of relevance to the neuroimaging community, which was introduced in the 1990s and greatly improved temporal resolution (on the order of seconds), has been that of blood oxygen level dependent (BOLD) functional magnetic resonance imaging (fMRI). In this modality, the BOLD fMRI signal has no stable, absolute interpretation and tends to slowly drift up and down over time. Other recent developments in clinical MRI that need to be considered are that of high field fMRI e.g. using 4 T magnets (which have the advantage of improving T1 times) and the emergence of low-field techniques (milli-Tesla systems) which are combined with cryogenically cooled phased array detectors. In the case of low field techniques, these developments are likely to lead to the proliferation of more versatile imaging systems which will be less claustrophobic to patients and provide improved compatibility for patients with implants. Such systems are likely to have different requirements for de-noising and classification, placing them in a unified algorithmic context at such an early stage of development is useful.

Much of the work on MRI focuses on the measurement of an effective diffusion tensor of water in tissues [71], following nuclear induction [72–75]. MRI provides unique characterization of the biological tissue (in terms of tissue composition, the physical properties of its tissue constituents, and microstructure and its architectural organization) as well as clinically relevant information that is not available from other imaging modalities. Brain gray matter is sufficiently homogeneous so a scalar representation of the apparent diffusion coefficient (ADC) is used. The need for a tensorial representation arises most often when considering diffusion in skeletal and cardiac muscle [76–78], and in white matter where the measured diffusivity is known to depend upon the orientation of the tissue [79–81].

Processing of the MR signal entails relating the measured echo attenuation in each voxel with the applied magnetic field gradient sequence [82, 83]. In its simplest form, the measurement provides a scalar b-factor value which is calculated for each diffusion-weighted image (DWI). The b-factor summarizes the attenuating effect on the MR signal of all diffusion and imaging gradients in only one direction [75]. It effectively measures the projection of all molecular displacements along one direction at a time. For non-homogeneous samples, a symmetric b-matrix is used [84]; this again is calculated for each DWI. The b-matrix captures the attenuating effect of all gradient waveforms as applied in all three directions(x, y and z) [84, 85]. The effective diffusion tensor, $\mathbf{D}$, is similarly estimated from a series of DWIs.

A commonly used expression relating the effective diffusion tensor to the measured echo is:

$$\begin{aligned}\ln\left(\frac{A(\mathbf{b})}{A(\mathbf{b}=\mathbf{0})}\right) &= -\sum_{i=1}^{3}\sum_{i=1}^{3} b_{ij}D_{ij} \\ &= -(b_{xx}D_{xx} + 2b_{xy}D_{xy} + 2b_{xz}D_{xz} + b_{yy}D_{yy} \\ &\quad +2b_{yz}D_{yz} + b_{zz}D_{zz}) = -\mathrm{Trace}(\mathbf{bD})\end{aligned} \tag{1.4}$$

where A($\mathbf{b}$) and A($\mathbf{b}=\mathbf{0}$) are the echo magnitudes of the diffusion weighted and non-diffusion weighted signals respectively, and b_{ij} is a component of the symmetric b-matrix, $\mathbf{b}$. When the medium is isotropic, $\mathbf{b} = b_{xx} + b_{yy} + b_{zz} = \mathrm{Trace}(\mathbf{b})$.

The first moment of the diffusion tensor field, or the orientationally averaged value of the diffusion tensor field can be calculated at each point within an imaging volume:

$$\begin{aligned}< D > &= Trace(\mathbf{D})/3 = (D_{xx} + D_{yy} + D_{zz})/3 \\ &= (\lambda_1 + \lambda_2 + \lambda_3) =< \lambda >\end{aligned} \tag{1.5}$$

where λ_1, λ_2, λ_3 are the three eigenvalues and $< \lambda >$ labels their mean. An estimate of $< D >$ is obtained by taking the arithmetic average of ADCs acquired in all possible directions.

In contrast, in a trace-weighted image, the geometric mean of N DWIs $A(\mathbf{b}^i)$ is used to produce a trace weighted intensity: TWI $= \sqrt[N]{\sum_{i=1}^{N} A(\mathbf{b}^i)}$.

If the DWI signal attenuation is given by:

$$A(\mathbf{b}^i) = A(\mathbf{0}) \times e^{-(b^i_{xx}D_{xx}+2b^i_{xy}D_{xy}+2b^i_{xz}D_{xz}+b^i_{yy}D_{yy}+2b^i_{yz}D_{yz}+b^i_{zz}D_{zz})} \tag{1.6}$$

then the conditions for producing a Trace-weighted DWI are:

$$\sum_{i=1}^{N} b^i_{xx} = \sum_{i=1}^{N} b^i_{yy} = \sum_{i=1}^{N} b^i_{zz} = N\beta > 0 \tag{1.7}$$

i.e. that the total diffusion weighting along the $x, \; y, \; z$ directions is the same, and

$$\sum_{i=1}^{N} b^i_{xy} = \sum_{i=1}^{N} b^i_{yz} = \sum_{i=1}^{N} b^i_{xz} = 0 \tag{1.8}$$

i.e. that the sum of each of the off-diagonal elements of the b-marix is zero. In this way,

$$\mathrm{TWI} = A(\mathbf{0})e^{-\beta \mathrm{Trace}(\mathbf{D})} \tag{1.9}$$

which results in an image whose intensity is 'weighted' by Trace($\mathbf{D}$).

When selecting a model for the dataset, one needs to consider that gray matter, white matter and cerebrospinal fluid (CSF) could all occupy the same macroscopic voxel. As a result, a three compartment model can be built:

$$\frac{A}{A_0} = f_1 e^{-\mathrm{Trace}(\mathbf{bD}_{\mathrm{wm}})} + f_2 e^{-\mathrm{Trace}(\mathbf{bD}_{\mathrm{gm}})} + f_3 e^{-\mathrm{Trace}(\mathbf{bD}_{\mathrm{csf}})}$$

where $\mathbf{D}_{wm}$ represents the diffusion tensor for white matter, and $\mathbf{D}_{gm}$ and $\mathbf{D}_{csf}$ represent the apparent diffusion coefficients for gray matter and for CSF, respectively, which are assumed to be isotropic. This is a model requiring 11 parameters, therefore ARX and subspace signal processing schemes become appropriate. Addition of intracellular and extracellular compartments to the above model increases rapidly the number of parameters that need to be estimated. This gives rise to parametrization issues which can overwhelm a classifier.

For N non-interacting compartments, with the same T1 and T2, each described by its own diffusion tensor, a simplification in the processing can be made by taking a Taylor series expansions of the signal about Trace($\mathbf{bD}_{\mathrm{i}}$) $= 0$:

$$\frac{A}{A_0} = \sum_{i=1}^{N} f_i e^{-\mathrm{Trace}(\mathbf{bD}_\mathrm{i})} \approx \sum_{i=1}^{N} f_i \left[1 - \mathrm{Trace}(\mathbf{bD}_\mathrm{i}) + \frac{1}{2}(\mathrm{Trace}(\mathbf{bD}_\mathrm{i}))^2 \ldots \right] \tag{1.10}$$

or

$$\frac{A}{A_0} \approx \sum_{i=1}^{N} f_i - \mathrm{Trace}\left(b \sum_{i=1}^{N} f_i \mathbf{D}_i \right) + \cdots = 1 - \mathrm{Trace}(\mathbf{bD}_\mathrm{eff}) + \cdots \tag{1.11}$$

$$\frac{A}{A_0} \approx e^{-\mathrm{Trace}(\mathbf{bD}_\mathrm{eff})} \tag{1.12}$$

where $\mathbf{D}_\mathrm{eff} = \sum_{i=1}^{N} f_i \mathbf{D}_i$.

Looking at the problem from a systems identification perspective, if the parameters of the above model need to account for non-linear interactions resulting from the exchange of spins in each compartment, a Wiener of Hammerstein model needs to be identified. This formulation would account for a multi-compartment/multi-component model, where differences in relaxation parameters can lead to different rates of echo attenuation in each compartment, making it more difficult to explain the cause of signal loss within a voxel. In practice, there are irregular boundaries between macromolecular and microscopic-scale compartments that need to be taken into account. In addition, the different macromolecular structures comprising these boundaries may affect the displacement distribution of water molecules differently, necessitating the formulation of even more complex models or potentially nonlinear models with fractional order dynamics. Assuming the system dynamics are described in state space, the problem may be formulated as a multiple-input multiple output problem with a deficient rank in the observability matrix that would require additional information for it to be uniquely solved. Furthermore, one can potentially address the deficient matrix problem by using the complementary information from THz-TPI measurements.

Diffusion weighted intensities as a function of the *b* factor also tend to vary when there is an exchange of blood between compartments [91]. A multi-exponential fractional order calculus methodology can provide a good model of long range interactions as this can be associated with the change in the relaxation rates of the spin system. Furthermore, models for the movement of water within and between compartments have been proposed. These vary in terms of complexity and number of components considered so their application for the interpretation of clinical datasets is at its infancy. The best way to address this is to place the problem explicitly within a biophysical context and assign reflection coefficients for the membranes present in different parts of the tissue. Then, a model should be derived after assuming a diffusion process due to potential chemical changes.

Since often there are also thermal gradients in a tissue there are differences in blood flow and thermal conductivity, and temperature cannot be assumed to be uniform throughout a tissue sample. Temperature gradients can be associated with changes in the measured diffusivity (to the extent of about 1.5% per $1\,^{\circ}C$) [91–94], and changes in the DWI from adjacent voxels limit the precision of the technique. This is, again, another area where THz imaging in tandem can potentially be used to minimize these artefacts by providing an independent measure of flow.

Finally, it is worth noting that a source of artefacts in MRI stems from eddy currents associated with large, rapidly switched magnetic field gradients produced by the gradient coils during the diffusion sequence. As a consequence, the field gradient at the sample differs from the prescribed field gradient, resulting in a difference between the actual and prescribed b-matrix. Furthermore, a slowly decaying field during readout of the image causes geometrical distortion of the diffusion-weighted images. These issues may be addressed by adopting pule shaping methodologies.

Progress in machine learning offers new opportunities for automated tumour screening. In addition, it can also potentially provide associations and correlations through the time series analysis of datasets, thus elucidating disease progression [95–100]. Image processing techniques can be used to extract quantitative information on lesion morphology, volume and kinetics, as well as to distinguish viable from nonviable tissue [63, 98]. Techniques for processing large volumes of medical image datasets with high dimensionality are not, however, sufficiently mature. Experts often distinguish tissue states on the basis of tumour information from radiological reports by characterizing lesions either as malignant or as benign [63, 101–104]. Current tumour detection methodologies based on analysing a series of two-dimensional texture features is not only time consuming, but can also be problematic as experts are often unable to take into consideration more complex morphological features of tumour anomalies across the entire tissue volume [70, 98, 105].

1.3 Placing THz Imaging and MRI Time-Series in a Common Signal Processing Framework

In addition to molecular fingerprinting, another motivation for using THz pulse imaging in conjunction with MRI stems from the possibility of separately performing fiber tractography, following fiber-tract trajectories within the brain and other fibrous tissues [86–88]. This has important applications to neuroscience as it enables the tracking of neuronal fiber pathways [90]. An important question that still needs to be addressed in THz transient spectroscopy is whether the extinction coefficient of water at THz frequencies, as well as the de-excitation dynamics observed in the time domain sequences associated with a single voxel, are different when the water is free or bound. The energy state of water (water potential) provides additional information regarding the surrounding tissue, because different tissue has different osmotic and matric potential. It is also very common for diseased tissue to be accompanied by a dramatic change in cellular water potential as stressed cells over-produce certain amino-acids e.g. proline. Correlating potential osmotic measurements with water absorbance at the THz part of the spectrum, should, therefore provide information complementary to that associated with the diffusion tensor of the MRI modality.

Of relevance to both THz pulse imaging as well as DCE-MRI systems, is the need for multi-channel acquisition [89]. In the case of DCE-MRI this is necessary to account and correct for patient movement during the scan (often by fusing information from heterogeneous sensing modalities) [106]. Correlations with breathing, enables pixel de-blurring at the post-processing stage, minimizing artefacts [107]. Similarly, in THz pulse imaging, hyperspectral imaging may be used to improve the signal-to-noise ratio (SNR) at each pixel or voxel in an image. This is possible because a single femtosecond pulse from the spectrometer is associated with a very broad spectrum, so differentiation between tissues can be performed after integrating the differences in the complex insertion loss function over a large number of frequencies (making use of Fellgett's multiplex advantage).

Both MRI as well as THz pulse imaging systems have shortcomings in that they require comparatively long integration time for the acquisition of an image. Thus, in order to speed-up measurement time, different approaches are considered: either accepting a higher noise level per pixel or voxel or limiting the resolution (number of pixels or voxels) or reducing the number of tomographic projections. A common shortcoming with such practices is to introduce undesirable image artefacts due to an inadequate Nyquist sampling rate in the spatial domain [108, 385]. A pre-processing step that can reduce the dimensionality of the hyperspectral or multi-channel datasets by compressing them to more parsimonious representations can potentially minimise the dimensionality of the input dataset presented to a classifier. This can help improve its classification accuracy and generalization ability. An additional advantage from compression is the potential signal-to-noise ratio improvement.

Algorithms for material extraction parameters on the basis of the expressions provided above are discussed in the work by Duvillaret et al. [109, 110] as well as the work by Mittleman's group [111] and Koch's group [112–114]. Suppression of etalon effects (interference caused by multiple reflections from dielectric layers) in THz reflection spectroscopy is possible by fitting a Lorentzian dispersion model as discussed by Kniffin and Zurk [115]. The treatment of errors in THz spectroscopy is discussed extensively in the recent book edited by Naftaly [43]. Such considerations have also significant ramifications in image reconstruction and registration as there is a danger that classifiers will be trained on features resulting from systematic errors.

At this point it is worth noting that, in all these approaches, in experiments with samples of complex composition, one has to evoke an effective medium theory if absorption bands are too close together or if the modelling process assumes a frequency-dependent multi-exponential composite transmittance response of the type $T(\omega) = e^{-\sum_{i=1}^{N} \varepsilon_i \int_0^d c_i(d)\mathrm{d}d}(\omega)$ to account for the presence of multiple (N) absorbers.

This is often the case when the modelling process assigns a different concentration c_i (with subscript i denoting the number of absorbers), and molar extinction coefficient ε_i for each of the chemical species present. Such modelling is usually performed on the basis of the Beer-Bouguer-Lambert Law assuming the medium is homogeneous within the considered interaction volume (over a path length dd of uniform composition). The fitting of these multi-exponential expressions requires the assumption of a linear interaction of the components in the mixture (which is not always the case), as well as a large number of calibration samples so that a sufficiently large number of linearly independent equations can be obtained (over-parametrization). From a mathematical perspective, this problem is similar to that encountered in MRI where a number of lifetimes can be observed either because of instability of a signal at longer timescales (e.g. in BOLD fMRI) as discussed by Aguirre et al. [116], or as a result of changes in neuro-vascular coupling, or in complex mixtures using multiple spin labels (e.g. in Arterial Spin Labelling ASL perfusion fMRI which is analogous to ^{15}O PET imaging and the labelled protons act as a diffusible tracer, as implemented in either continuous CASL or pulsed PASL mode), or when spatiotemporal correlations affecting T1/T2 ratios need to be weighted and extracted. In addition, in a neuroimaging context, the variance in T1/T2 ratios across different populations (groups of subjects) can also be placed in a more informative context using a multi-exponential fit algorithm. Finally, similar problems can be encountered in multi-pulse-field-gradient experiments [117].

Every measurement at each pixel position of a TDS-TPI image is an entire time-dependent waveform, i.e. a three-dimensional (3D) data set, which then can potentially be mapped to two-dimensional (2D) images [39], where structural and compositional discrimination can be performed on the basis of a sample's frequency dependent complex refractive index using pattern recognition algorithms. In cases where the user has to process multi-channel or tensorial datasets, the needed exponential data fitting can be performed using multilinear algebra routines. A particularly elegant formulation can be found in the work by Papy et al. (2005) [118].

1.4 Introduction to Retinal Fundus Imaging

Fundus photography is the acquisition of images (nowadays digitally) of the back of the eye, to resolve features of the retina, optic disc, and macula [119, 226, 345]. The technique can be used clinically to diagnose and monitor the progression of a disease through the measurement of vessel width, colour, and reflectivity [227].

In fundus retinal photography, the camera records color images of the condition of the interior surface of the eye. Repeated photography at regular intervals provides an assessment of relative changes of specific features over time (Fig. 1.8).

In both cases, the camera system comprises a low power microscope with an attached camera designed to photograph the interior surface of the eye, including the retina, retinal vasculature, optic disc, macula, and posterior pole (i.e. the fundus). An example of such system is illustrated in Fig. 1.9.

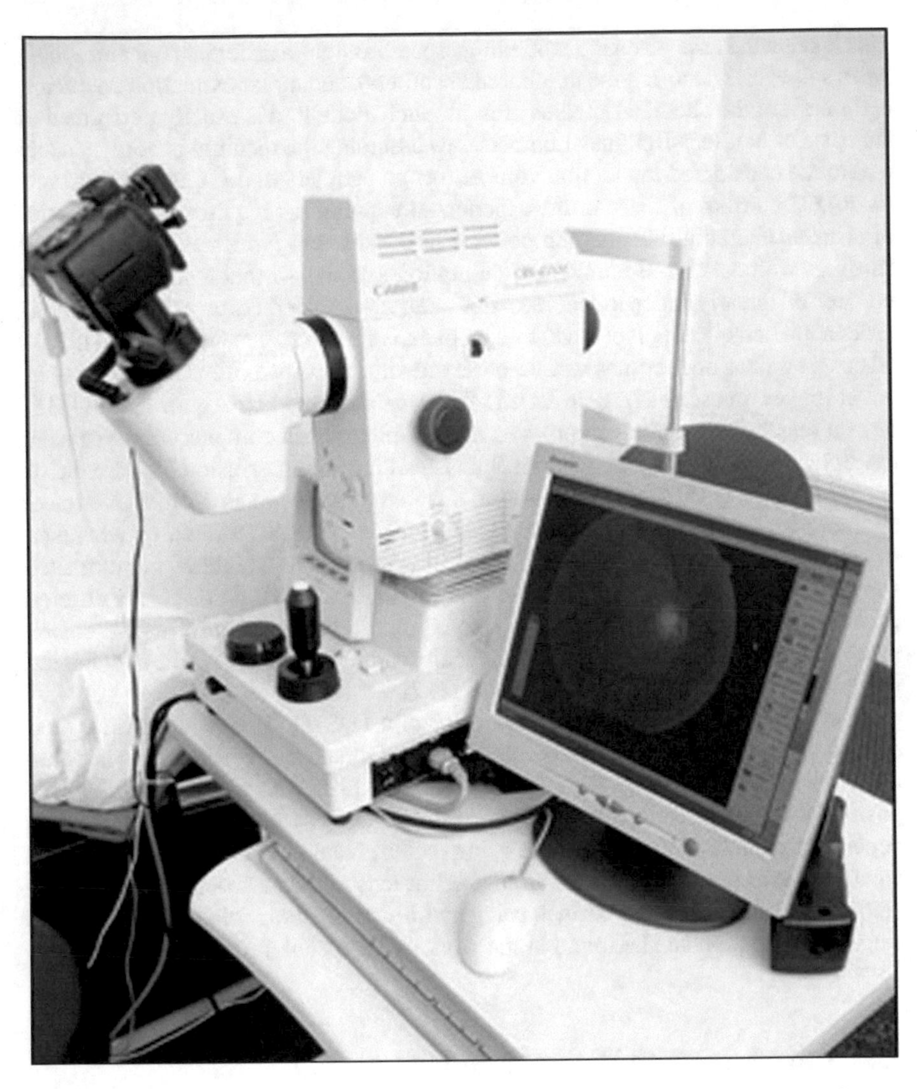

Fig. 1.8 Typical fundus photography set-up comprising high resolution imaging system that can resolve features at the back of the eye (retina); informative features include the appearance and size of the optic nerve or macula and the presence of freckle (choroidal nevus)

Fundus photography can also be performed with the use of colored filters, or with specialized dyes including fluorescein and indocyanine green. The optical design of a fundus camera is based on the indirect ophthalmoscope. Fundus cameras are characterized by the angle of view—the optical angle of acceptance of the lens. An angle of 30°, is considered the normal angle of view, this creates an image with a magnification factor of 2.5. Wide angle fundus cameras capture images between 45

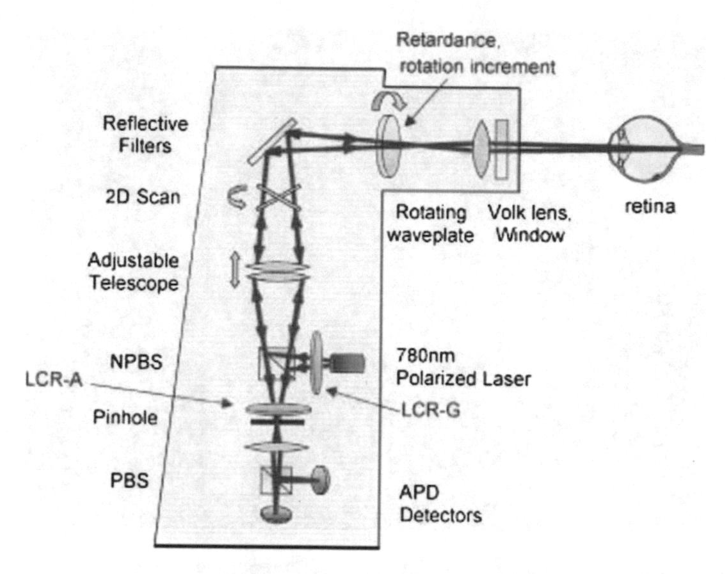

Fig. 1.9 GDx-MM (MM for Mueller Matrix) optical and polarization path. NPBS: non-polarizing beam splitter; PBS: polarizing beam splitter; APD: avalanche photodiode; LCR: liquid crystal retarder. Modifications from the GDx path are emphasized in *red* and include the following: insertion of LCR-G in generator path; insertion of LCR-A in analyzer path; and changing the retardance and rotational increment of the rotating wave plate. After [228]

and 140° and provide proportionately lower retinal magnification. A narrow angle fundus camera has an angle of view of 20° or less.

An evolution to the above design is the Mueller matrix polarimeter [228]. Such system has recently been used to image the retinas of normal subjects; a system of this type is illustrated in Fig. 1.9. Light from a linearly polarized 780 nm laser was passed through a system of variable retarders and scanned across the retina. In this configuration, light returned from the eye passes through a second system of retarders and a polarizing beam splitter to reach two confocal detection channels. The accuracy and repeatability of polarization parameter measurements are typically within $\pm$ 5%. At the signal processing stage, optimization of the polarimetric data reduction matrix can be achieved using a condition number metric.

The GDx, is an incomplete polarimeter, which can be used to probe the increase of scattered light concomitant with retinal disease [228–231]. It is a scanning laser polarimetry (SLP) with a linearly polarized 780 nm laser source, a rotating half wave plate, and a polarizing beam splitter which directs the co- and cross- polarized return light to two detection channels. A two-dimensional retinal scan is usually performed at 20 different wave plate orientations. The signals from the co- and cross-polarized detectors are processed to produce a linear retardance map of the scanned region. A constant birefringence factor is then used to convert the retardance map to a thickness map of the retinal nerve fiber layer. The resolution at the retina is about 15 μm, and the scan covers a visual field of 15°. Scanning is normally performed using a slow

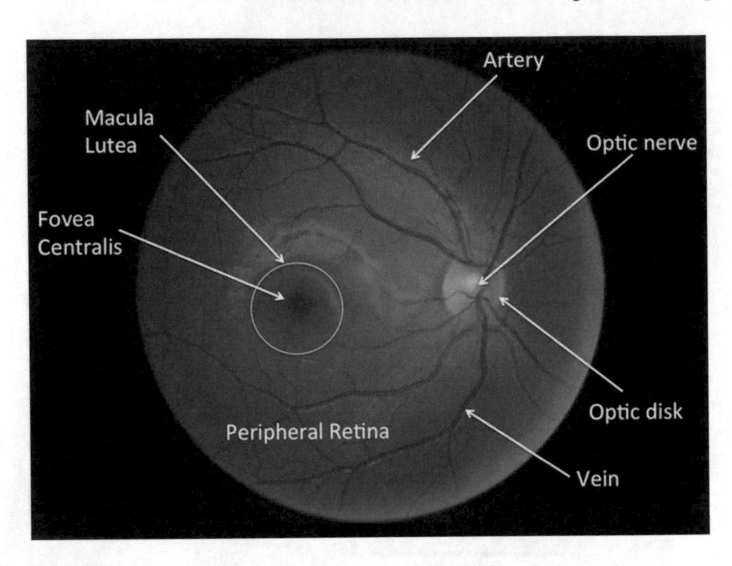

Fig. 1.10 A normal retinal image registered using retinal fundus photography

scan galvanometer driven at 26 Hz coupled to a fast resonant scanner oscillating at 4 kHz.

The retina is a layered tissue lining the interior of the eye that enables the conversion of incoming light into a neural signal that is suitable for further processing by the visual cortex of the brain. Because the retina is used in all visual tasks, all ocular structures have to be optically transparent for image formation. This makes the retinal tissue accessible for imaging noninvasively, as illustrated in Fig. 1.10. Because the retina's function makes it a highly metabolically active tissue constantly needing significant volumes of blood supply, the retina allows direct noninvasive assessment of circulation [119].

1.5 Introduction to Optical Coherence Tomography (OCT)

Since its introduction in 1959, fluorescein angiography has been the preferred method for performing retinal imaging. After 1991, however, a new modality, that of Optical Coherence Tomography (OCT) was introduced [232]. OCT is a novel imaging technology that produces high resolution cross-sectional images of the internal microstructure of living tissue [238, 239]. Its roots lie in the early work on white-light interferometry that led to the development of optical coherence-domain reflectometry (OCDR), a one-dimensional (1-D) optical ranging technique [240]. Since its introduction, OCT has played a pivotal role in improving retinal diagnostic imaging. An important recent advance that is likely to significantly benefit the range of application of OCT for vascular imaging is the use of cowpea mosaic virus (CPMV) nanoparticles

[120]. The bioavailable cowpea mosaic virus (CPMV) can be fluorescently labelled to high densities with no measurable quenching, resulting in exceptionally bright particles with in vivo dispersion properties that allow high-resolution intravital imaging of vascular endothelium for periods of at least 72 h. There is significant potential for example to perform intravital visualization of human fibrosarcoma-mediated tumor angiogenesis using fluorescent CPMV as it provides a means to identify arterial and venous vessels and to monitor the neovascularization of the tumor microenvironment. OCT uses 3D imaging technology to achieve highly detailed internal imaging of the human eye with an optimal resolution of just a few micrometres. It generates cross sectional images by analyzing the time delay and magnitude change of low coherence light as it is backscattered by ocular tissues. An infrared scanning beam is split into a sample arm (directed toward the subject) and a reference arm (directed toward a mirror). As the sample signal returns to the instrument it is correlated with the signal at its reference arm. Minute imbalances between the two arms of the instrument are registered at the photodetector plane; these are highly sensitive to the distance of the sample from the instrument port. The resulting change in signal amplitude provides tissue differentiation by analysis of the reflective properties of each layer in the tissue. As the scanning beam moves across the tissue studied, the sequential longitudinal signals, or A-scans, can be reassembled into a transverse scan yielding cross-sectional images, or B-scans, of the subject. The scans can then be analyzed in a variety of ways providing both empirical measurements (e.g. RNFL or retinal thickness/volume) and qualitative morphological information. A generic block diagram of different OCT system configurations is illustrated in Fig. 1.11. An example of an OCT fundus image showing the multiple de-embedded tissue layers is illustrated in Fig. 1.12.

OCT uses 3D imaging technology to achieve highly detailed internal imaging of the human eye with an optimal resolution of just a few micrometres. It generates cross sectional images by analyzing the time delay and magnitude change of low coherence light as it is backscattered by ocular tissues. An infrared scanning beam is split into a sample arm (directed toward the subject) and a reference arm (directed toward a mirror). As the sample signal returns to the instrument it is correlated with the signal at its reference arm. Minute imbalances between the two arms of the instrument are registered at the photodetector plane; these are highly sensitive to the distance of the sample from the instrument port. The resulting change in signal amplitude provides tissue differentiation by analysis of the reflective properties of each layer in the tissue. As the scanning beam moves across the tissue studied, the sequential longitudinal signals, or A-scans, can be reassembled into a transverse scan yielding cross-sectional images, or B-scans, of the subject. The scans can then be analyzed in a variety of ways providing both empirical measurements (e.g. RNFL or retinal thickness/volume) and qualitative morphological information. A generic block diagram of an OCT system is illustrated in Fig. 1.11. OCT imaging provides similar information to an ultrasound or MRI. The use of OCT enables optometrists to determine, track and manage the health of human eyes, as illustrated in Fig. 1.12.

Over the past few years, OCT technology has continually evolved and expanded within ophthalmology. Furthermore, its uses have been adopted in other medical

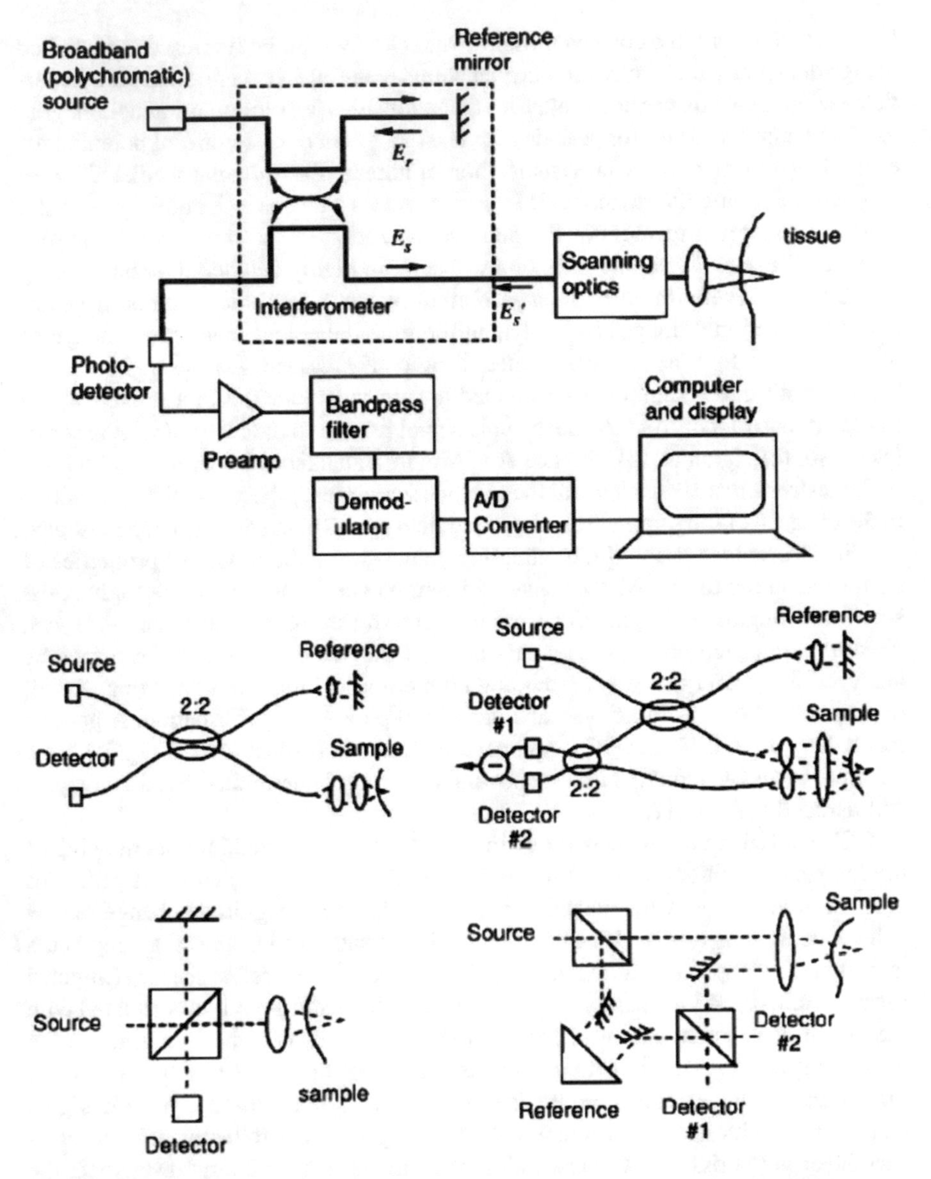

Fig. 1.11 *Top*: Generic block diagram of an OCT system based on white light interferometry, at the center (*left*) fiber optic interferometric implementation, and on the right balanced configuration based on 2 × 2 fiber optic couplers, at the bottom free-space Michelson (*on the left*) and Mach-Zehnder topologies (*on the right*). After [238]

environments [242, 243]. In the skin and other highly scattering tissues, OCT can image small blood vessels and other structures as deep as 1–2 mm beneath the surface. A variance of the technique, called ultrahigh resolution (UHR) OCT was introduced

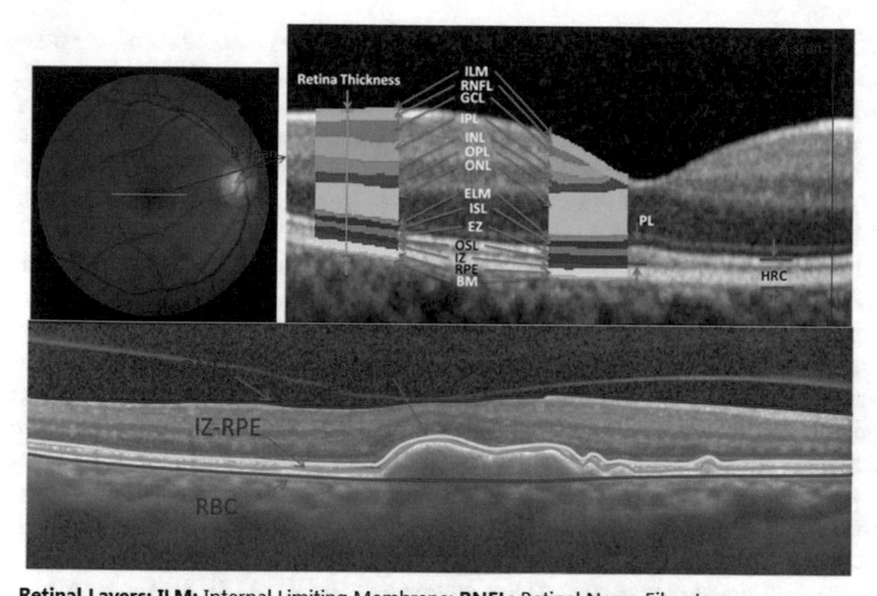

Retinal Layers: ILM: Internal Limiting Membrane; **RNFL:** Retinal Nerve Fiber Layer;
GCL: Ganglion Cell Layer; **IPL**: Inner Plexiform Layer; **INL**: Inner Nuclear Layer;
OPL: Outer Plexiform Layer; **ONL**: Outer Nuclear Layer; **ISL**: Inner Segment Layer;
ELM: External Limiting Membrane; **PL**: Photoreceptor Layer; **RPE**: Retinal pigment epithelium.
IZ: Interdigitation Zone, a layer which is not always distinguishable even in the normal eyes.
PL is comprised with three segments and they are ISL + EZ + OSL; **HRC**: Hyper Reflective Complex.
EZ: Ellipsoid Zone; **OSL**: Outer Segment Layer; **RBC**: The complex of the RPE/BM/choriocapillaris;

Fig. 1.12 A color fundus image showing the retinal surface (*top left*) and a macula center SD-OCT B-scan image (*top right*), a portion of the cross section across *green line* (*top left* image), defining the layers in the SD-OCT B-scan image. Proposed segmented boundaries are delineated in an SD-OCT image (*bottom*). After [241]

in 2004 [244]. This significantly improves image quality and enables better visualization of individual retinal layers. Anterior segment OCT scanners have become widely available since 2005 and the introduction of Spectral (Fourier) Domain OCT (SD-OCT, FD-OCT) technology now provides greater tissue resolving power, significantly higher scan density, and faster data acquisition than that achieved with the original Time Domain OCT systems [245]. Swept source OCT (SSOCT) is a popular alternative technique.

Optical coherence tomography angiography (OCTA) is currently the most successful functional extension of OCT, due to the fact that it can be implemented in any OCT platform and it meets an immediate clinical diagnostic needs [246, 247]. The main aim of OCTA is to sense dynamic structural changes between successive tomograms [248]. The simplest approach is to calculate the average of pairwise differences of a set of linearly or logarithmically scaled intensity tomograms taken at the same position [250, 251]. This can be conveniently implemented using functional extensions of OCT such as Doppler OCT (DOCT) or Time Domain OCT (TD-OCT)

[252, 253] as both are extensively used nowadays to assess blood flow. Using these techniques, the flow signature may also be used to contrast vascular structure. With the advent of high-speed Fourier domain OCT (FDOCT), the full potential of DOCT to perform non-invasive volumetric angiography was realised [254]. The phase information of the FDOCT signal obtained after the Fourier transform of spectral data can also be used to this effect [255, 256]. Alternative techniques include heterodyning of the signal so as to directly extract phase information [257].

In many respects, OCT imaging with pulsed sources has the same structural characteristics (displaying attenuation, delay, frequency dependent dispersion) as that of an ultrasound scan, a THz scan or an MRI scan in the sense that different layers in the image are systematically de-embedded from their individual signatures, provided there is sufficient contrast between the layers and the scanning system has transversally oversampled the individual layers of the imaged tissue. As this is an interferometric technique, the associated expressions of the intensity that impinges on the photodetector are very similar to those found in systems designed to perform reflection THz spectroscopy (continuous wave or pulsed configurations) [239]. Finally, a recent non-invasive structural and microvascular contrast imaging modality is a phase difference swept source OCT angiography (pOCTA) [258]. The advantage of pOCTA is its independency of backscattering intensity changes, yielding potentially better vascular contrast for highly scattering tissue [130]. At the forefront of these OCT developments are the clinical studies of UHR-OCT and pOCTA currently underway at the New England Eye Center (NEEC) in collaboration with Drexler's group at the Medical University of Vienna.

Chapter 2
Overview of Clinical Applications Using THz Pulse Imaging, MRI, OCT and Fundus Imaging

After establishing the technological aspects of the four different imaging modalities in the previous chapter, this chapter focuses on their biomedical applications. First, THz pulse imaging is discussed within the context of assessing tissue vascularization, tissue water content, and the possibility of developing molecular fingerprinting. A similar discussion of recent applications of MRI to bio-imaging is also provided. The complementarity of the two imaging methods is also highlighted. Finally, the use of fundus photography and OCT to perform disease diagnosis are also discussed.

2.1 Recent Advances in the Application of THz Pulse Spectroscopy to Biomedical Imaging

As discussed earlier, THz-TDS is a time-domain technique, where time gated reflections are analysed directly in the time domain by observing their attenuation, phase delay and temporal spread after interacting with matter. Their temporally good definition can provide localization of tissue interfaces on the basis of their different refractive index. Different tissues have a different frequency dependent refractive index. The real part of the refractive index is associated with the impedance mismatch of the excitation THz wave, whereas the complex part is associated with the absorbance. Studies in reflection geometry enable the indirect assessment of sample or layer thickness, and can be used to determine the position of embedded unknown objects, etc. [16, 24]. In addition to their relatively non-invasive interaction with biological tissue T-rays have significant potential in advancing both in vivo and in vitro biosensing applications [8, 16, 29]. Furthermore, a significant number of biomolecules have several characteristic 'fingerprint' resonances due to discrete molecular vibrational, torsional and librational modes, both in liquids and solids [4, 5, 30].

X. Yin et al., *Pattern Classification of Medical Images: Computer Aided Diagnosis*, Health Information Science, DOI 10.1007/978-3-319-57027-3_2

2.1.1 THz Radiation Absorption and Detection in Tissue

THz radiation interacts strongly with polar molecules, a prime example being water [2]. Polar water molecules are active in the infrared region and have various vibrational modes [3]. In the mid- to far-infrared, the vibrations involve combinations of the symmetric stretch ($\nu 1$), asymmetric stretch ($\nu 3$), and bending ($\nu 2$) of the covalent bonds. The vibrations of water molecules may be thought of as restricted rotations, resulting in a rocking motion, as shown in Fig. 2.1a. In liquid water, since hydrogen bonds are much weaker than the covalent bonds (intra-molecular), their bond lengths are much longer (1.97 Å versus 0.96 Å), as shown in Fig. 2.1b. Steric effects from dipole moments in water clusters vary according to hydrogen proximity and, as a consequence, shifts in ro-vibrational modes at THz frequencies are encountered. Furthermore, these shifts are expected to be loosely correlated with different water potential values, which indirectly affects molecule's ability to interact with its surrounding molecules. This has further important ramification on the way proteins influence the state of water. An analysis of steric forces can lead to further understanding of the function of hydration shells in proteins [17, 41, 42].

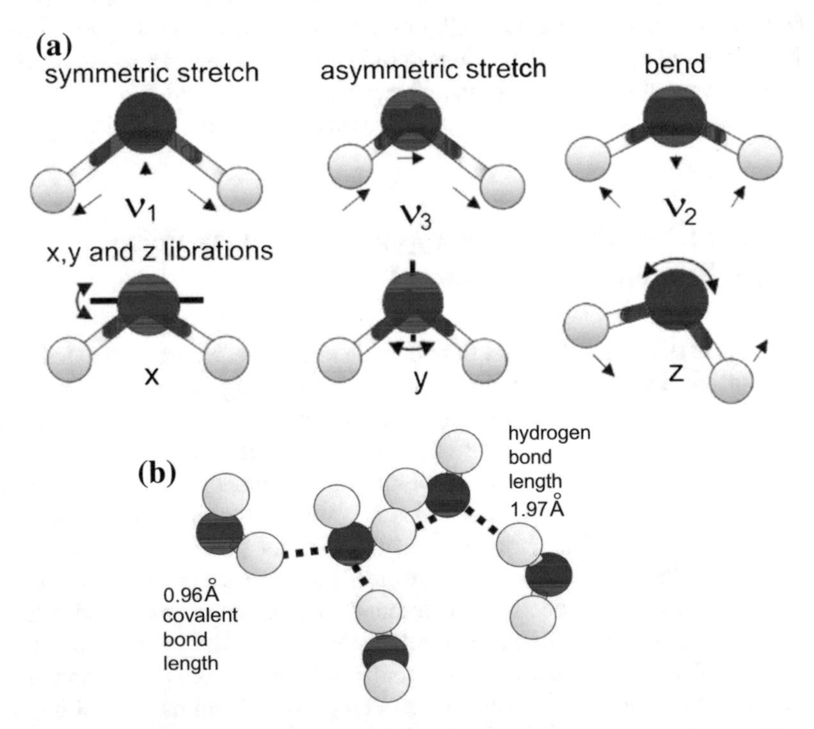

Fig. 2.1 **a** The main vibrational modes in water. **b** A schematic diagram illustrating the differences between intra- and inter-molecular bonding in water. After [3]

As discussed earlier, THz-TDS provides a direct measure of the real and imaginary components of tissue permittivity. A Debye relaxation model can be used to analyze the strong absorption of THz radiation in polar liquids at least up to 1 THz [5, 32]. This model can be directly related to the associated intermolecular dynamics.

Biological tissue is generally composed of polar liquids. Due to the exceptionally high absorption losses of polar liquids at THz frequencies and the low source power in TPI systems, it is difficult for the THz radiation to propagate through biological tissue along a substantial distance. However, the same high absorption coefficient that limits penetration in tissue also provides extreme contrast between samples at various degrees of water saturation [5]. This property has proven advantageous in the examination of the properties of water uptake and distribution in plants [6, 7], as well as in the evaluation of the severity of burns through the study of necrotic skin samples [8]. In addition, [9, 10] describe the application of TPI techniques for imaging of basal cell carcinomas (BCC) *ex vivo* and *in vivo*. Note that BCCs typically show an increase in absorption of THz radiation compared to normal tissue. This may be attributed to either an increase in interstitial water within the diseased tissue [13] or a change in the vibrational modes of water molecules through interactions with other functional groups. Systematic studies in tissue identification are reviewed in [5].

2.1.2 Identification of Compounds with Complex Composition

T-ray spectroscopic studies also provide complementary information on low-frequency bond vibrations, hydrogen bond stretching and torsions in liquids and gases with the lowest frequency modes associated with intermolecular motion [19, 22, 23], as illustrated in Fig. 1.1. The vibrational spectral characteristics of bio-molecules, which lie in this range (wavenumbers between 3.3 and 333 cm^{-1}) make T-ray imaging systems a promising sensing modality for clinical diagnosis. Another advantage of performing spectroscopic investigations at this part of the spectrum is that many molecules have characteristic 'fingerprint' absorption spectra [16, 18], thus making T-ray imaging systems a promising sensing modality for clinical diagnosis. The identification of pure compounds using molecular signatures with THz-TDS systems, however, is still not straightforward because of the inherently broad spectral signatures in liquids and solids. Nevertheless, there is a growing number of multiple confirmed observations of particular resonant signatures that may be attributed to the presence of compounds in pure form [142]. Of particular relevance here is the growing interest in studying the conformational structure, binding states, and vibrational or torsional modes of proteins and oligonucleotides [131, 132] through the analysis of spectral features [133]. Different reflection or absorption signatures may also be attributed to a change of density or polarizability, and these can be further associated with a dehydration state, or a denaturing process which give rise to a new amorphous absorption band or a temperature related absorption band shift [24, 33].

Pulsed THz wave technology has been applied extensively in biosensing [4]. Many pioneering investigations in biomolecule characterization were performed by the Aachen group [136] and Jepsen's group [134]. These were followed by a rapid growth of investigations by other researchers worldwide [135, 137, 138]. An interesting example is that of an affinity biosensor monitoring of the binding between biotin and avidin molecules on supported membranes composed of biotin layers on a quartz surfaces treated with octadecanol, as proposed by Menikh et al. [139]. In that work, an amplified detection of biotin-avidin binding was very clearly observed through the dithering of the samples in a THz beam. This was attributed to the conjugation of agarose particles and avidin molecules and a change in contrast due to a change of the refractive index resulting from the chemical binding process [30, 140]. Avidin has a very strong affinity for biotin and is capable of being bound to any biotin-containing molecules. The importance of the work is that it showcases THz pulse sensing as a generic detection technique that can potentially be used to detect DNA hybridization and antigen-antibody interactions [30]. THz transient spectrometry has also been used to successfully distinguish between two artificial RNA single strands, composed of polyadenylic acid (poly-A) and polycytidylic acid (poly-C), from their different THz spectral transmission responses [17, 141].

The identification of pure compounds using molecular signatures with THz-TDS systems is still not straightforward because of the inherently broad spectral signatures in liquids and solids. Nevertheless, there is a growing number of multiple confirmed observations of particular resonant signatures that may be attributed to the presence of many compounds in pure form [142]. Of particular relevance here is the growing interest in studying the conformational structure, binding states, and vibrational or torsional modes of proteins and oligonucleotides [131, 132] through the analysis of spectral features [133]. Different reflection or absorption signatures may also be attributed to a change in density or polarizability, or may indicate a dehydration state, or a denaturing process leading to a new amorphous absorption band or a temperature related absorption band shift. A compilation of readily identifiable spectral signatures of complex biomolecules in an atlas has already been considered at Durham University, and significant progress has been made to include a significant variety of different tissue types. Yet there is a wider recognition by the THz community that this approach although very useful it is unlikely to have the universal applicability that can be found in other databases such as HITRAN, because of the variability in the location of the spectral bands observed. Such problems are further compounded by noting the variation in spectra of similar substances when these are recorded at different labs. Different sample preparation techniques and a lack of protocol standardization have been a problem within the THz community. Sample standardization which is normally found in the crystallographic community could be significantly beneficial in that respect.

In addition to the above, there are also other relevant studies based on frequency specific fingerprinting of biomolecules that have been discussed in the literature. Nishizawa et al. [144] illustrated the use of a widely tunable coherent THz scanning system for THz transmission spectroscopy to study samples consisting of nucleobases and nucleotides in crystalline form to further gain an insight of the composition of

RNA and DNA molecules. The THz spectra of those samples were measured in the 0.4–5.8 THz range. These studies showed that the molecules have quite different characteristic spectral patterns in this frequency region, furthermore, the absorption signature patterns observed were sufficiently clear and reproducible for identifying and discriminating between these molecules.

Using pulsed THz spectroscopy [31, 131], it has also been possible to study the low frequency collective vibrational modes of bio-molecules, i.e. DNA, Bovine Serum Albumin and Collagen in the range 0.1–2.0 THz. It is generally accepted that for most samples, broadband absorption increases with frequency and a large number of the low frequency collective modes for these systems is also deemed as IR active. Herrmann et al. [143] also carried out measurements of THz spectra of Poly(dA-dT)-Poly(dT-dA) DNA and Poly(dG)-Poly(dC) DNA and used new signal processing routines to infer the THz complex refractive index. The resultant spectral features showed that those samples were indeed distinguishable in the range 0.1–2.4 THz. Several research groups in Germany and Australia, have also studied the photo-isomerization of retinal chromophores [145, 146] focusing on the conjugated polyene chain of the biologically important chromophore retinal and its low-frequency torsional vibration modes. In that work, the absorption and dispersion spectra of different retinal isomers (all-trans; 13-cis; and 9-cis retinal) in the far-infrared region between 10 and 100 cm^{-1} were measured by THz-TDS at 298 and 10 K. At low temperatures, it was observed that the broad absorption bands resolve into narrow peaks that directly correlated to torsional modes of the molecule. The study also confirmed that vibrational modes within the molecule can be approximately localized through a comparison of the absorption spectra of different retinal isomers.

An alternative important research direction vigorously pursued by Teraview Ltd., Cambridge, U.K., aims to put an end to patent infringements within the pharmaceutical industry by detecting the presence of drug polymorphs [23, 147, 148]. Such studies, for example, have successfully used TPI to examine the variation in the crystalline structure of Ranitidine Hydrochloride polymorphs. Significant differences in the spectra of two different polymorphs were clearly observed at around 1.10 THz enabling their correct identification. A recent account on advances in the identification of the crystalline structure of drugs using TPI is provided in [149]. Furthermore, the observation of the crystallization of compounds has also been possible [150].

2.1.3 Recent Advances in the Application of DCE-MRI Imaging Techniques to Biomedical Imaging

MRI has proven to be of clinical importance to the classification, grading, and diagnosis of tumours. Clinical management of many tumour types is now reliant on MRI. Clinical information for both surgical planning and clinical management is derived from tumour morphology and the relationship of lesions to neighbouring structures that are revealed using MRI. Magnetic resonance provides images for clear identification of some cases of pathological change, as well as delineation of organ location and the identification of anatomical features.

An evolution of this imaging modality since the 1980s has been an alternative high-performance imaging modality which is called dynamic contrast enhanced DCE-MRI. This is now widely used in the diagnosis of cancer and is becoming a promising tool for monitoring tumour response to treatment [151]. DCE-MRI patterns can be affected by a wide range of physiological factors; these include vessel density, blood flow, endothelial permeability and the size of the extravascular extracellular space in which contrast is distributed [151, 152]. The crucial difference from traditional medical imaging (i.e. X-rays) is that the DCE-MRI modality provides 3D spatial information about lesions as well as temporal information about lesion physiology (showing variations in contrast agent uptake rates), allowing for more accurate assessment of lesion extent and improved lesion characterisation [68, 89].

Typically, DCE-MRI images are acquired with the use of a conventional gradient echo (GRE) pulse sequences that repeatedly image a volume of interest after injecting a contrast agent, such as gadolinium diethylenetriamine pentaacetic acid (Gd-DTPA) into the patient's blood stream. The DCE imaging employs a full *k*-space sampling strategy, (where the *k*-space relates to the associated wavenumber, a terminology originally introduced by the semiconductor industry to denote momentum space but in MRI is associated with spatial frequency). Three dimensional (3D) volume acquisition of slice profiles is normally performed. These are generally rectangular and always contiguous slices. By registering slices in a contiguous manner, the signal is recorded and integrated uniformly from all tissue coordinates in each slice, thus avoiding cross-talk.

One of the biggest advantages of the gradient-echo pulse sequence is that it can be performed quickly enough to enable 3D FT (3DFT) data acquisitions. In 3DFT imaging, a volume or slab of tissue is excited, rather than merely a thin slice of tissue. This means the 3D MRI data acquisition consists of three different phase encoding directions: the transaxial plane, the sagittal plane, and the coronal plane. Images are obtained sequentially every few seconds over a period of up to 5 to 10 min. There is always a trade-off between spatial (sRes) and temporal (tRes) resolution. Usually, most radiologists clinical protocols show a preference for scans at high sRes allocating only 1–2 min for tRes data acquisition [153].

A typical DCE-MRI dataset consists of one baseline 3D MR image which is used as a reference before contrast agent injection [31, 62]. Additional scans are performed to acquire post-contrast images at the second, third, and subsequent slices (usually 6 or 7). Each time slice has a typical time interval of 60 s.

Following the terminology introduced independently by Ljunggren [154] and Twieg [155] we shall refer to the, *k*-space to denote the spatial (either 2-D or 3-D) frequency domain of the imaging system. Within the context of temporal image processing the *k*-matrix, is composed of digitized MR signals stored during the data acquisition process before any reconstruction computations. The complex data entries are associated with the pulse sequence of the accurately timed radio frequency and gradient pulses.

In clinical practice e.g. during a DCE-MRI mammogram, reducing the signal acquisition time is desirable, and this is normally achieved by undersampling the k-space. Undersampling may be achieved by adopting a random partial k-space updating [156] protocol. The HASTE sequence, which samples half the k-space [157], is now routinely used in clinical MRI.

Aliasing from sampling the k-space below the Nyquist rate, however, introduces imaging artifacts [385]. Since there is always a need for better tRes while preserving adequate SNR and sRes, several groups [158–160] have shown that it is possible to accelerate DCE-MRI (without employing parallel imaging) by a factor of ten using compressed sensing (CS) based for image reconstruction as proposed in [108]. The approach allows the filling of missing k-space data using a constrained optimization technique to interpolate the values between under-sampled adjacent data points in the spatial domain.

Recent work by Yin et al. [65] based on the broad principles of compressed sensing represents an important advancement in the above mentioned CS modality. The technique makes use of the fact that, when under-sampling the k-space, it is possible to use variable density sampling schemes in a Cartesian coordinate system to widely distribute the resulting artifacts and reduce their visual impact. Such an approach was further explored using a model-based method for the restoration of MRIs with sparsity representation in a transformed domain, e.g. spatial finite-differences (FD), or after using the discrete cosine transform (DCT). The reduced-order model, in which a full-system-response is projected onto a subspace of lower dimensionality, has been used to accelerate image reconstruction by reducing the size of the linear system associated with the measurement space. The singular value threshold technique [161] (SVT) was used in the denoising scheme to reduce and select the model order of the inverse FT image, and to restore multi-slice breast MRIs that have been compressively sampled in k-space. Restored MRIs with SVT de-noising show reduced sampling errors compared to direct MRI restoration methods via spatial FD, or DCT. The difference image related to IT, shown in Fig. 2.2b, contains a relatively large number of noisy (error) pixels that are located around the boundary of the imaged section. Reconstruction with the identity transform (IT) also shows some blurring at the image edges. In contrast, the reconstructed image using SVT denoising illustrated in Fig. 2.2a, shows a reduced number of error pixels compared to the reconstructed image in Fig. 2.2b.

2.1.4 Recent Advances in the Application of fMRI Imaging to Biomedical Imaging

Functional Magnetic Resonance Imging (fMRI) is a non-invasive imaging technique that does not require the injection of contrast agent [59]. Functional MRI has relatively high spatial and reasonable temporal resolution, and can be acquired in the same session as structural MRI. It effectively captures the changes in the Blood Oxygenation Level Dependent (BOLD) contrast, allowing the evaluation of brain

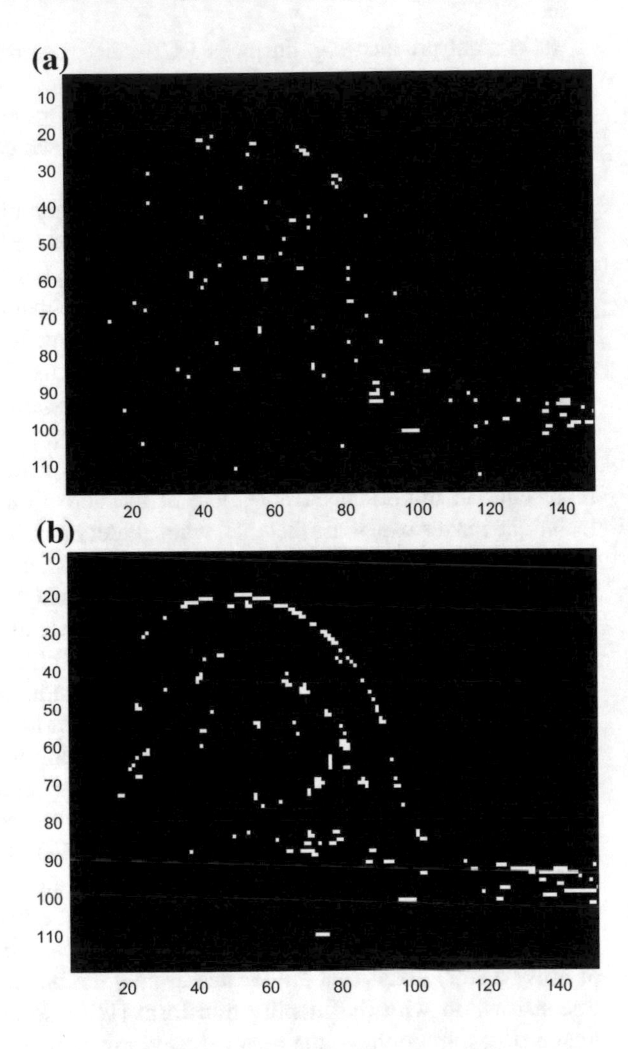

Fig. 2.2 **a** Illustration of the difference image segment between the measured MRI and reconstructed image using SVT for denoising. **b** The difference image segment between the measured MRI and transformed image from sampled *k*-space

activity due to external stimuli. The low signal-to noise ratio (SNR) of fMRI data makes detection of the activations-related signal changes difficult; hence most of the data is collected from periodic stimulation after alternating with the rest condition. The temporal dynamics of the activation response, which is delayed and is relatively slow compared to actual brain activity, is another problem that must be dealt with during analysis. Most of the present methods rely on exclusive modelling of the hemodynamic response function to detect this delayed activation. The most extensively used fMIR data analysis techniques are variants of the general linear models based on the t-test, the F-test, on correlation coefficients (between observed responses and stimulus function) or multiple linear regression. A general drawback in all these techniques is that they require accurate knowledge of the actual stimulus function.

At this point it is also worth noting that, in experimental NMR studies, the transverse magnetization decays at rates much faster than what would be theoretically predicted by natural atomic or molecular mechanisms; this accelerated rate is commonly denoted as T2* ('T2-star'). These T2* relaxations relate to the decay of transverse magnetization caused by a combination of spin-spin relaxation and magnetic field inhomogeneity. For this reason, the MR sequences obtained using gradient echoes and relatively long TE values are also called T2*-weighted. They are often used to accentuate local magnetic homogeneity effects to aid in the detection of hemorrhages or calcification. T2*-sensitive sequences also form the basis for functional MRI (fMRI) using the BOLD technique. From the above description it may be concluded that T2* is always less than or equal to T2.

Figure 2.3 illustrates the general principle of fMRI. Oxygen is delivered to neurons by haemoglobin in capillary red blood cells. When neuronal activity increases there is an increased demand for oxygen and the local response is an increase in blood flow to those regions of increased neural activity. Haemoglobin is diamagnetic when oxygenated but paramagnetic when deoxygenated. This difference in magnetic properties leads to small differences in the MR lifetime signal in the blood in that region according to its level of oxygenation. Since blood oxygenation varies according to the levels of neural activity, these differences can be used to spatially localise and temporally resolve brain activity. Brain fMRI BOLD imaging is one of the most promising emergent measurement modalities with several applications in neuroscience, neurosurgery, rehabilitation and psychology. An overview of recent advances of functional imaging in oncology can be found in the comprehensive book edited by Luna et al., (2014) [163]

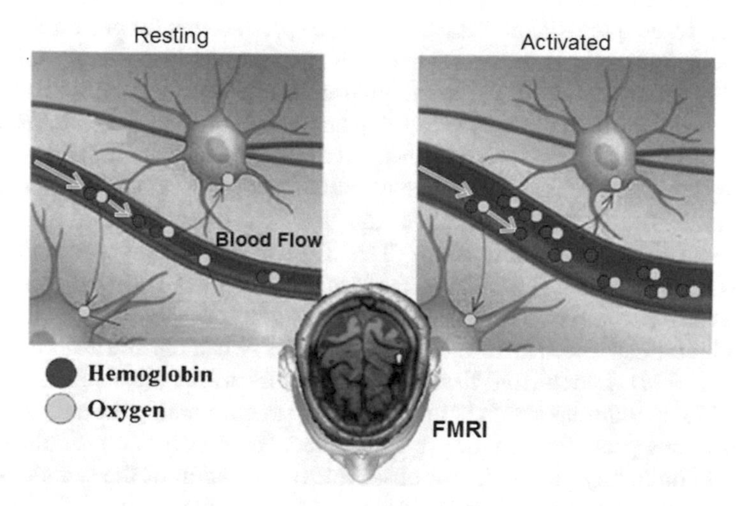

Fig. 2.3 Simplified illustration of different levels of oxygenation in blood on the basis of a resting or activation state of a nearby neuron as observed through fMRI. After [162]

2.1.5 Advantages and Shortfalls of T-Rays and DCE-MRI & FMRI

As TPI and MRI time series are becoming more widely available in conventional clinical practice, it is envisaged that data acquisition and analysis will be performed in tandem to benefit from the complementarity of each signal, thus capitalizing on the inherent differences in signal generation and tissue contrast mechanism. One of the primary advantages of THz imaging over MRI, is the availability of various spectroscopic signatures within a frequency band which may be attributed to changes of THz biomarker concentration.

Although, a number of papers discuss spectroscopic investigations of biomolecules such as DNA [4, 17, 131, 143, 144], unfortunately the responses of many biological tissues are unknown in this band. A further related problem is the current lack of development of reliable computer aided diagnostic algorithms for interpreting the multispectral images obtained by T-ray imaging [164]. A number of authors have partly addressed this question by fitting the measured data to linear models and using the filter coefficients as a means of classifying different tissue types [11]. One of the most important potential applications for THz technology along this line of research is the detection and identification of specific biological and chemical agents [165]. Although it is widely recognized that T-rays can be used to image tumour microvasculature, most reports focus on the feasibility of using TPI to image breast tumours [166, 167] and skin cancer [168]. In both these cases, the contrast observed is mainly due to the absorption of THz waves by the water that is present in biological tissue and the actual state of hydration of the tissue under study. A recent review carried out by Yu et al. [169], extensively discusses such investigations and relates them to the future potential of THz imaging and spectroscopy for performing cancer diagnosis. A further important development in THz tumour image analysis has been reported by Huang et al. [170], where gold nanorods were used in vitro as novel contrast agents for both molecular imaging and photothermal cancer therapy. With the aid of a laboratory microscope, those investigations showed that, as a result of the strongly scattered red light from gold nanorods in the dark field, malignant cells can be clearly visualized and identified from non-malignant cells.

As THz time domain spectroscopy (THz-TDS) and imaging are being extended to address new biomedical problems, the identification of specific proteins is likely to be the focal point in those investigations. Such research direction can draw upon previous investigations on histo-morphology studies of healthy and diseased excised tissue [171, 172]. Lyophilized tissue samples from various organs have also been imaged [173] and this approach has the advantage of eliminating the effects of water absorption thus providing a more reproducible THz signature by eliminating the variability commonly present in various levels of hydration of the sample. A good application example for such investigations would be the study of the collective vibrational modes of protein deposits found in amyloidosis. In humans, the accumulation of protein deposits in tissue occurs as part of the natural ageing process. An unnaturally rapid accumulation of deposits, however, can occur in diseases such as

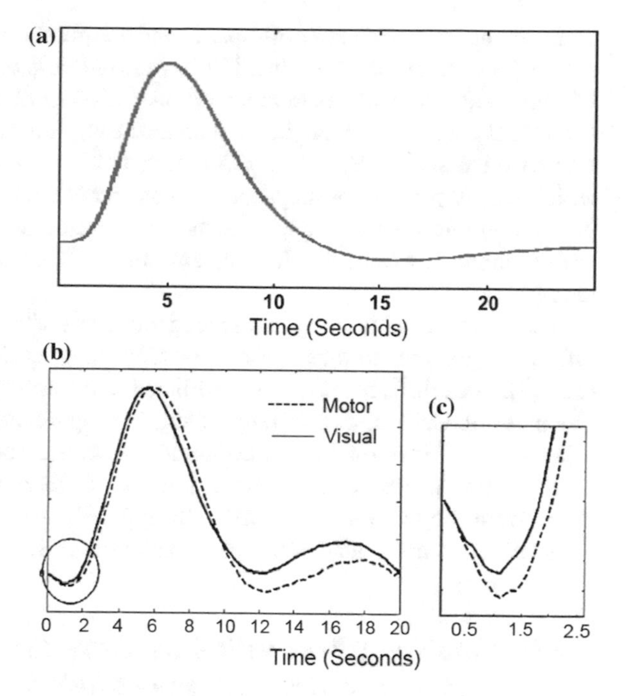

Fig. 2.4 **a** The standard canonical model for the HRF used in fMRI data analysis illustrates the main features of the response. **b** Examples of empirical HRFs measured over the visual and motor cortices in response to a visual-motor task. **c** The initial 2 s of the empirical HRFs give strong indication of an initial decrease in signal immediately following activation. After [175]

Alzheimer's Disease (AD), resulting in the functional decline of the tissue, leading to dementia. This is a particularly promising research direction for THz spectroscopy investigations as the early detection of AD can lead to a much better management of the disease.

Furthermore, as mentioned earlier, fMRI is often used to identify brain areas activated by a stimulus. The observed change in the fMR signal, however, is the result of an indirect effect related to the changes in both blood flow rates as well as level of oxygenation following changes in neural activity. The underlying evoked hemodynamic response to a neural event is typically referred to as the hemodynamic response function (HRF). Figure 2.4 shows the typical shape of such a curve after modelling the HRF; this is sometimes also called the canonical HRF. The increased metabolic demands due to neuronal activity lead to an increase in the inflow of oxygenated blood to active regions of the brain. Since more oxygen is supplied than actually consumed, this leads to a decrease in the concentration of deoxy-hemoglobin which, in turn, leads to a small, but measurable, signal increase because deoxyhemoglobin is paramagnetic.

When considering the complementarity between BOLD-fMRI and THz-TDI in the above example, it is worth noting that the BOLD-fMRI modality is correlated to both levels of hemoglobin oxygenation as well as flow rate, and an independent measurement of water content spatially resolved using THz-TDI can enable a better differentiation between the two signals. This becomes particularly useful, for example, when standard diffusion tensor models are deemed inaccurate.

From the perspective of both spatial and temporal resolution, the two techniques are complementary to each other [175]. In fMRI, it is impossible to simultaneously increase both, as increases in temporal resolution limit the number of k-space measurements that can be made in the allocated sampling window and thereby directly influence the spatial resolution of the image. Unlike conventional enhanced MRI, which simply provides a snapshot of enhancement at one point in time, DCE-MRI permits a more complete depiction of the wash-in and wash-out contrast kinetics within tumors. Signal intensity data are often normalized to concentration prior to analysis [174].

THz measurements with femtosecond transients of tumours produces significantly different signatures to those produced when imaging normal adipose (fatty) tissue [11, 12]. Such differences may be attributed to the absorption coefficient and refractive index of each tissue. Similarly, changes in signal intensity taken from DCE-MR images are different for healthy and tumour tissues according to the different degree of absorption of the contrast agent. A further difference between the two datasets stems from the fact that DCE-MRIs are typically acquired at several time frames. This process is associated with a restricted temporal resolution.

2.1.6 Combining MRI with Alternative THz Spectrometric Systems and Other Imaging Modalities

2.1.6.1 Alternative THz Spectrometric Imaging Modalities for Biomedical Applications

Over the years, several alternative THz systems to the ones described in Sect. 1.1 have also been proposed [176–181], and these may also form the basis of THz spectrometric systems which can eventually be combined with MRI or fluorescence imaging modalities. Of particular note in such systems are the spectrometers based on the asynchronous optical sampling (ASOPS) scheme [182–185]. The technique uses two pumped femtosecond Ti:sapphire ring oscillators which produce femtosecond pulses with a repetition rate f and $f + \Delta f$ as set by the optical path length of each resonator (around 1 GHz when free running). Using beam splitters, a small portion of the signal (ratio 90:10) is directed to fast photodiodes which produce electrical trigger signals which are further amplified by low-noise high bandwidth microwave amplifiers (e.g. model ZFL 1000LN from Mini-circuits) operated in a trans-impedance configuration (converting a photo-current into a voltage). Although the photodetectors are not preserving the shape of the pulse, this is of no consequence to the stabilization scheme as the goal is to just generate a triggering event for the synchronization process. The difference in repetition rate ($\Delta f \approx 10\,\text{kHz}$) is obtained using a microwave mixer and the signal is subsequently sent to a frequency-to voltage converter which serves as an input to a proportional integral derivative (PID) controller that drives the piezoelectric transducer that controls the path length in the slave resonator cavity. Figure 2.5 illustrates the asynchronous optical sampling scheme.

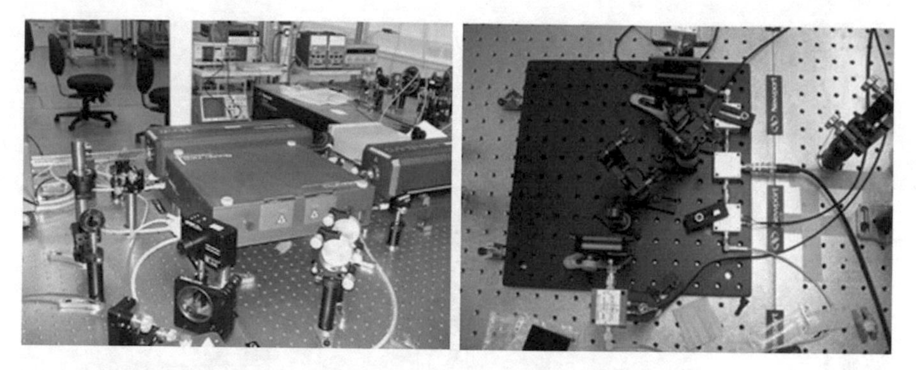

Fig. 2.5 ASOPS spectrometer and external frequency difference stabilization scheme that controls the repetition rate of the slave ring laser resonator to be always offset by a small amount e.g. 10 kHz to that of the master laser resonator

The close-loop system has a large linear gain in the forward path (composed of the cascaded PID signal, high voltage amplifier signal, the transducer voltage to displacement conversion, and the conversion of resonator path length to frequency comb repetition rate) and unity gain in the feedback path. With reference to Fig. 2.6, using transfer function notation and using $A \gg 1$:

$$V_{\text{out}} = \frac{A}{1+AB} V_{\text{REF}} \approx \frac{A}{AB} V_{\text{REF}} = \frac{V_{\text{REF}}}{B} \tag{2.1}$$

so that the characteristics of the system are governed by the stable characteristics of the feedback path B. The difference in the repetition rate between the two resonators is set by V_{REF}. More recently, an alternative version of that system (TL-1000-ASOPS) incorporating substantially improved locking between the two femtosecond resonator lasers as well as carrier envelope phase stabilization options, have been made available by Laser Quantum Ltd to complement their HASSP-THz system. The bandwidth of this spectrometer is up to 6 THz when operated with their proprietary Tera-SED planar large-area GaAs based photo-conductive emitters.

An important advantage of eliminating the translation stage from the spectrometer is that the spot size of the optical beam propagating through the reference path of the interferometer is no longer of variable size (due to diffractive spreading of the infrared beam) for different path lengths imposed by the translation stage, as is in the case for a conventional THz transient spectrometer. This is a very important advantage in ASOPS as a dilution of the gate pulse in an Auston receiver changes its multimoded antenna pattern in both amplitude and phase delay. This type of error has not been systematically addressed by the THz community although careful work [186] has shown that changing the spot size dramatically alters the recorded time-domain signature and hence the corresponding Fourier transformed spectrum. Such errors are endemic to most THz transient spectrometers and can be exacerbated

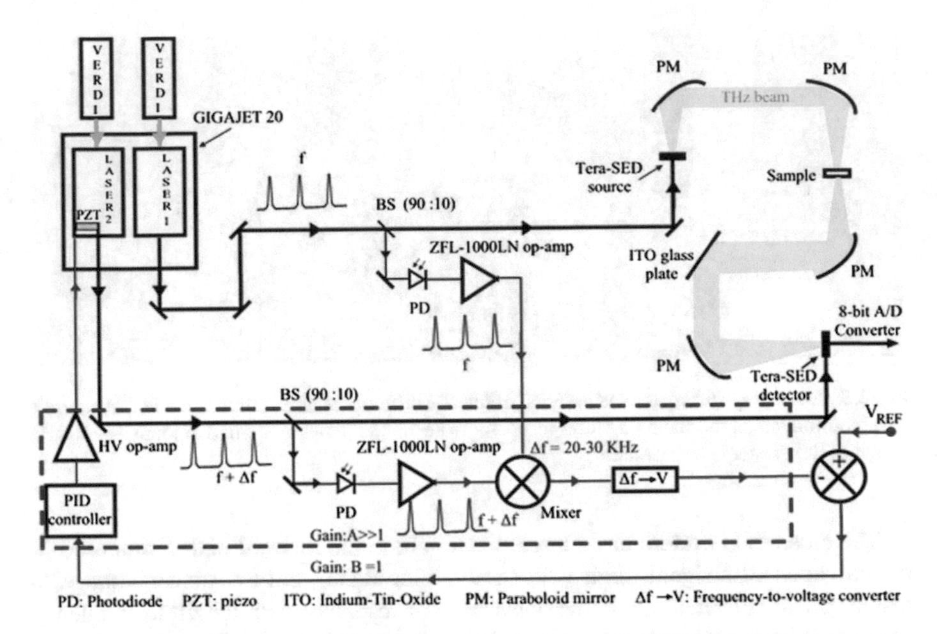

Fig. 2.6 Explanation of the feedback locking scheme found in ASOPS THz transient spectrometers currently marketed by Laser Quantum Ltd. Adopted from [185]

when ratioing the background and sample spectra. This is particularly important when interpreting spectra from imaged biological tissue.

An interesting alternative to the above scheme for the 9–12 μm part of the spectrum that may also be combined with other imaging modalities is that proposed by Keilmann's group (2004) [201, 202]. In this technique, the mid-infrared radiation from two electromagnetic waves (femtosecond duration pulses) is focused onto 0.5 and 1 mm GaSe crystals respectively, and through second order non-linearity 2 pulses whose overlapping bandwidth is centered at different frequencies is obtained. The two outputs of slightly different frequency are then superimposed to interfere on a power detector as shown in the figure below. A ZnSe combiner is used to direct the two beams to the detector and the down-converted signal is captured by a fast HgCdTe detector. The detector output signal contains a modulation ("beat") at the difference frequency Δ, which is conveniently selected to lie at the RF part of the spectrum (the technique is also known as multi-heterodyne spectroscopy), i.e. $f_r' = f_r - \Delta$. Interference modulation is produced by each heterodyne element. All modulations together may be viewed as a time-domain interferogram, that when Fourier transformed in the frequency domain, results in a harmonic radio frequency comb spectrum that is an exact replica of the dual beam's spectrum. A particularly attractive feature of the technique is that it can provide video-rate chemical imaging. Figure 2.7 illustrates the general principles of frequency comb spectrometry.

Such systems may also be further modified to perform imaging at subwavelength scale using near-field microscopy by observing the elastic light scattering from a tip

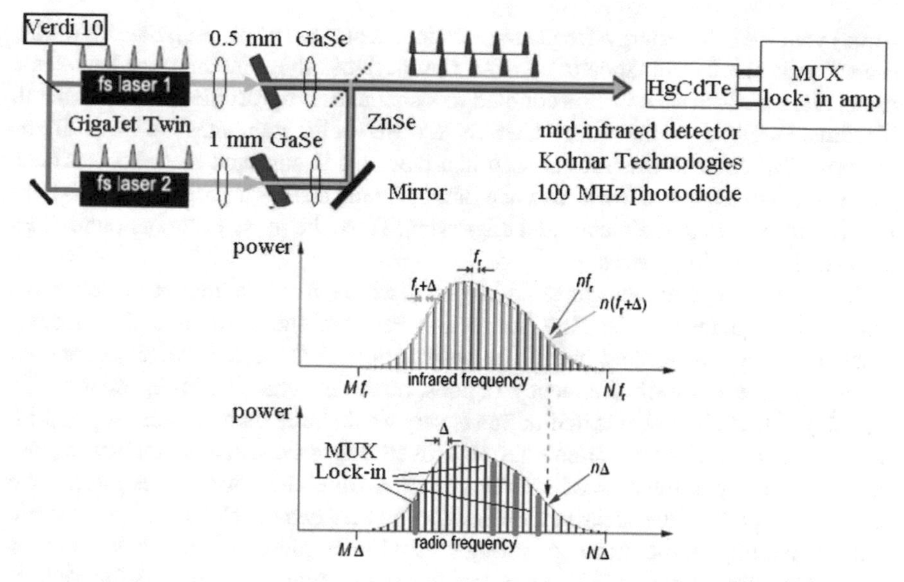

Fig. 2.7 Frequency comb spectrometry where a beat frequency signal at the RF part of the spectrum is generated after heterodyning the femtosecond pulses of two lasers (these are offset by a few Hertz). Multiplexed (MUX) lock-in amplifiers are subsequently used to select specific signatures for further chemometric analysis. After [202]

[188–191, 201]. The s-SNOM technique which provides vibrational contrast especially in the mid-infrared fingerprint spectral region, uses a light focused beam to illuminate the tip region of an atomic force microscope (AFM). By recording the scattered light in the backward direction, an optical image is simultaneously generated. The tip oscillates at the cantillever's mechanical resonance frequency (trapping mode) with the important consequence that the near-field optical image becomes modulated at the cantillever's resonance harmonics allowing electronic filtering against otherwise overwhelming scattering coming from the shaft and cantilever.

2.1.6.2 Combining MRI with THz and Other Imaging Modalities

The case for adopting a dual MRI-THz modality has been made clear in the seminal works by Oh et al. [192] as well as Park et al. [57], where the authors applied the technique to detect the onset of ovarian cancer. The diagnostic performance of such imaging has been significantly enhanced by the use of nanoparticle probes (NPPs). Multimodal probes enable the combination of various imaging techniques. THz waves for example, can efficiently interact with surface plasmons (SPs) associated with the injected nanoparticles. Such interactions are of a polaritonic nature. Polaritons are the product of combining an exciton (a bound state of an electron and an electron-hole which are attracted to each other by the electrostatic Coulomb force) with Planck's energy-frequency relation. A surface plasmon polariton (SPP), therefore, is an electromagnetic wave that propagates along the interface between a metal and a dielectric; it is thus coupled to a charge density oscillation in the metal. The imaginary part of the wave's transverse wave vector attenuates the wave amplitude perpendicular to the interface, so that the wave is confined near the interface. The wave also extends a finite distance into the metal so that it propagates with both loss (ohmic losses in the metal) and dispersion. Thus, the most strongly bound SPPs are also the most lossy ones.

In the visible and near-infrared regions, where many common metals have relatively large resistivities, the interaction between the wave and the electron plasma is very strong, and hence the propagation distance is relatively short. At the microwave and radio-frequency regions, however, where metallic resistivity is typically extremely low, this interaction is very weak. Such plane waves propagating parallel to the interface are often referred to as surface waves, and do not have a plasmonic character. In the case of THz frequencies, which lie between the microwave and infrared parts of the spectrum, the interaction between the electromagnetic mode and the electrons in the metal are stronger than in the microwave range, but weaker than in the infrared region. This gives rise to several unique possibilities for medical imaging. For example, if a metal surface of an injected nanoparticle is curved, a significant fraction of the propagating THz wave will follow the curving metal. This is in contrast to the case in the microwave region, where almost none of the electromagnetic energy of a surface wave follows the curved surface. Furthermore, THz SPPs can have propagation distances of hundreds or thousands of wavelengths, whereas SPPs at higher frequencies typically have propagation lengths of only a few tens of wavelengths. If near-infrared (NIR) excitation of NPPs targeted to cancer cells is used, SPs around the nanoparticles will be generated, increasing the temperature of the water inside the cells, inducing a change in the THz signal. The combination of THz waves and NPPs, and the use of differential detection techniques, can thus result in more accurate imaging of cancerous tumours with high sensitivity. The excitation of localized nanoparticles with waves of different electromagnetic frequencies, can, therefore, provide complementary information which can assist clinicians in more accurately establishing the boundaries of different type of tissue. Furthermore, they may provide an assessment of molecular and cellular activities.

A typical example of such a multifunction probe is that of $Feridex^{®}$ (Gurbet Group, Paris, France), superparamagnetic iron oxide nanoparticles (SPIOs). When these are used, they can enhance the magnetic resonance image contrast by reducing the RF relaxation time of the water protons. $Feridex^{®}$ SPIOs consist of a metallic nanoshell with a core size of 10–15 nm which is coated with dextran (to improve MRI by helping the nanoshell travel in the body). These particles, however, can also be utilized as a contrast agent for THz imaging, following induction of SPs by an NIR laser. Figure 2.8 illustrates the response of a SPIO to a THz pulse and an RF pulse.

This type of system follows other recent trends in combining multiple imaging modalities for the early detection of cancer; for example MRI with fluorescence imaging as discussed by Lee et al. [193] or positron emission tomography with near-

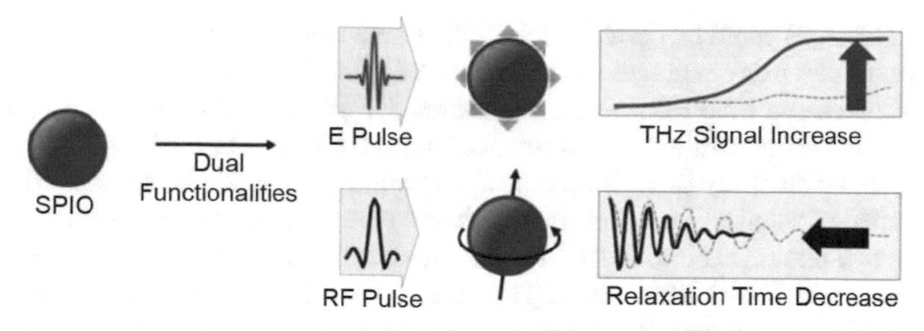

Fig. 2.8 Response of a SPIO to a THz pulse and an RF pulse. The SPIO has two functionalities, firstly it reduces the relaxation time of water protons in response to RF pulses in a strong magnetic field and raises the THz signal amplitude through SPs induced on the SPIO surface when exposed to an electric field. The magnetic feature is used for MRI and the electrical feature is used for THz imaging. After [57]

infrared fluorescence to characterize tumour vasculature as discussed in the work by Cai et al. [194], which combines positron emission tomography with fluorescent semiconductor nanocrystals (quantum dots) [195]. The use of quantum dots has significant advantages over their conventional organic fluorophore counterparts in that they have reduced photo-bleaching and a broad excitation spectrum with a narrow emission spectrum (with a sharp well-defined symmetric emission peak as opposed to a red tail) [196–199]. The resulting fluorescence is thus 10–20 times brighter so the associated images have better signal to noise ratio. A further advantage is that they have a large Stokes shift (difference between peak absorption and peak emission wavelengths) which reduces auto-fluorescence thus increasing sensitivity and clarity of the resulting images [200]. Because such nanocrystals can also be tailor-made to various sizes and shapes (which enables them to emit at different frequencies) their active uptake to different compartments in a cell can be identified and visualized simultaneously using wavelength multiplexing techniques [203–205]. Their inorganic composition also makes them more robust toward metabolic degradation which contributes to their longevity in vivo [206]. The multi-colour emission property of quantum dots allows the use of many probes to track several targets in vivo simultaneously [207, 208]. Furthermore, the yield obtained from quantum dots is almost 90% at room temperature [209]. Finally, they can also be easily functionalized [210]. An alternative is also to use lanthanide ion metal coordination complexes as luminescent molecular probes e.g. Yb(III), Er(III) and Nd(III) Eu(III) and Tb(III) complexes [211].

Following a critical review of MRI's ability to detect ovarian tumours [212], the need for imaging modalities with improved sensitivity has been established. The use of multifunction magnetic nanoparticles not only improves contrast in imaging [193], but also provides new opportunities for localized drug delivery [213, 214]. Furthermore, it opens-up the possibility of gaining further understanding of the biophysical environment and metabolic properties of the targeted cells [215]. The general idea of further combining multiple imaging modalities which can provide complementary information to existing imaging techniques is a rapidly evolving research topic that merits future exploration. For example, one could envisage that 2-photon microscopy

[217, 218, 222] could be combined with THz transient spectrometry since the femtosecond laser, used to create the seed pulses for the 2-photon system, can also be used at the same time to generate the pulses for the Auston switch or non-linear crystal for THz generation. Fluorescence lifetime imaging is a particularly useful experimental modality to the biomedical community as the de-excitation lifetime of the excited molecules is proportional to their concentration. Near-infrared radiation used in two-photon excitation suffers from significantly less absorption in biological specimens than UV or blue-green light, making the technique more appropriate for imaging thick specimens. The gradual loss in intensity (or 'attenuation') of excitation light from scattering is also reduced, as scattering decreases with decreasing excitation frequency. The technique can be label free and can rely on the natural fluorescence of compounds within the cell, so no additional dyes or quantum dots need to be added for the measurements. This can have important advantages since the physicochemical environment of the cells is not altered during the measurement process. Furthermore, because the technique relies on the use of short duration pulses for the excitation, there is less photo-bleaching of and photo-damage to the cells. The associated pulses may also be used for simultaneous chemical photoactivation or the activation of optogenetic switches. A further advantage of 2-photon microscopy over confocal microscopy is that it achieves confocality by using the emission pinhole aperture to reject out-of-focus light. However, inside thick specimens, scattering of the fluorescent photons is inevitable, resulting in significant loss of photons at the confocal pinhole. Two-photon microscopy limits the excitation volume, requiring no pinhole aperture, thus minimizing signal loss.

Alternative imaging modalities include variances of the well-known electron spin resonance (ESR) technique. The theoretical basis of ESR spectroscopy is similar to that of nuclear magnetic resonance (NMR), except that an electron spin, rather than a nuclear spin, is the focus [219]. Unpaired electrons in biological systems are in much lower abundance than nuclei, so ESR is a technique that focuses on local sites while NMR is more global. When biomolecules exhibit paramagnetism as a result of unpaired electron spins, transitions can be induced between spin states by applying a magnetic field and then supplying electromagnetic energy, usually in the microwave range of frequencies.

The interaction of an external magnetic field with an electron spin depends upon the magnetic moment associated with the spin, and the nature of an isolated electron spin is such that two and only two orientations are possible. The application of the magnetic field thus provides a magnetic potential energy which splits the spin states by an amount proportional to the magnetic field (Zeeman effect), and then radio frequency radiation of the appropriate frequency can cause a transition from one spin state to the other. The resulting ESR absorption spectra (also known as electron paramagnetic resonance (EPR) spectra) can be particularly useful to the study of radicals. This is because radicals typically produce an unpaired spin on the molecule from which an electron is removed. ESR is particularly suitable for studying basic molecular mechanisms in membranes and proteins by using nitroxide spin labels. In particular, nitroxide spin label studies with high-field/high-frequency ESR and two-dimensional Fourier transform ESR enable one to accurately determine distances in biomolecules, unravel the details of the complex dynamics in proteins, characterize the dynamic structure of membrane domains, and discriminate between bulk lipids and boundary lipids that coat transmembrane peptides or proteins [220]. The semi-conductor community has already combined an ASOPS THz transient spectrometer with a high magnetic field pulser for the characterization of materials [221]. It is therefore, appropriate to consider in the near future the adaptation of such a set-up to perform spectrometry of biomolecules.

Finally, it is worth mentioning the new opportunities to study biomolecules using dynamic nuclear polarization (DNP) techniques which increase the sensitivity of NMR spectroscopy by using high frequency microwaves to transfer the polarization of the electrons to the nuclear spins. The enhancement in NMR sensitivity can amount to a factor of well above 100, enabling faster data acquisition and greatly improved NMR measurements. With the increasing magnetic fields (up to 23 T) used in NMR research, the required frequency for DNP falls into the THz band (140–600 GHz) [223, 224].

2.1.7 Recent Advances in the Application of the Fundus Camera to Disease Diagnosis

As stated earlier, a fundus camera or retinal camera is a specialized low power microscope with an attached camera designed to photograph the interior surface of the eye, including the retina, retinal vasculature, optic disc, macula, and posterior pole (i.e. the fundus). The fundus enables direct observation of microcirculation non-invasively [225].

Many important eye as well as systemic diseases manifest themselves in the retina [119, 226, 227]. Changes in microcirculation can damage the retina. Assessment of vascular characteristics plays an important role in various medical diagnoses, such as diabetes [267, 268] hypertension [269] and arteriosclerosis [270]. Since the retina is normally not illuminated internally, external illumination projected into the eye, as well as the light reflected by the retina, must traverse the pupillary plane. Thus, the limited size of the pupil and the small opening in the iris (usually between 2 and 8 mm in diameter), has always been the primary technical challenge in fundus imaging [119]. Fundus imaging is further complicated by the fact that the illumination and imaging beams cannot overlap because this results in corneal and lenticular reflections, which tend to diminish image contrast. Consequently, separate paths are used in the pupillary plane resulting in optical apertures of the order of only a few millimeters. Because the resulting imaging setup is technically challenging, fundus imaging historically involved relatively expensive equipment and highly trained practitioners. Over the last ten years or so however, there has been a major effort to make fundus imaging more accessible, resulting in a reduced dependence on personnel expertise. This has also contributed to the wider proliferation of the technique.

One of the main applications for the fundus camera is in diagnosing microcirculation problems when the flow of blood in the smallest blood vessels in the network become blocked [225]. These changes in microcirculation can damage the retina. The

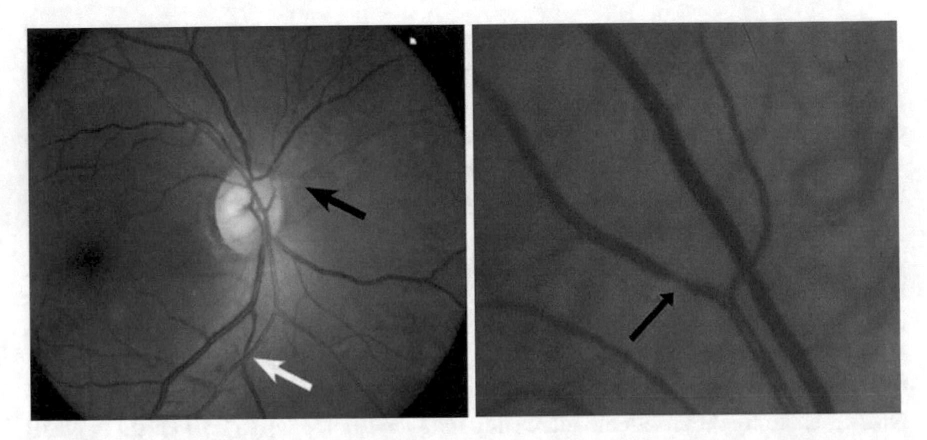

Fig. 2.9 (*Left panel*) Mild hypertensive retinopathy: generalized and focal arteriolar narrowing (*black arrow*) with arteriovenous nicking (*white arrow*). After [272]. (*Right panel*) An example of focal arteriolar narrowing. After [273]

abnormalities seen on a retinal image can be divided into two groups, those related to vascular changes and those related to extravascular changes. Both abnormalities can be used to predict the onset of hypertensive retinopathy, diabetic retinopathy, or a minute stroke. In addition there are features that are well correlated with anemia. Retinal arteries subjected to chronic hypertension show areas of focal or generalized narrowing. The light reflex is also narrowed. The arterial wall also thickens and becomes less transparent. As illustrated in the left panel of Fig. 2.9, mild hypertensive retinopathy shows generalized and focal arteriolar narrowing (black arrow) with arteriovenous nicking (white arrow). The right panel of Fig. 2.9 shows a retinal image with significant focal arteriolar narrowing.

A hallmark of diabetic retinopathy has been the identification of microaneurysms. Such a case is illustrated in the left panel of Fig. 2.10. The condition is characterized by tiny, round, red spots commonly seen in and around the macular area. These spots correspond to minute dilations of very small retinal vessels; the vascular connections are too small to be seen with an ophthalmoscope. In the right panel of Fig. 2.10, a case of non-proliferative diabetic retinopathy is illustrated. In the superior temporal quadrant, one can observe a large retinal hemorrhage between the two cotton-wool patches, this is accompanied by some beading of the retinal vein just above them, and by the presence of tiny tortuous retinal vessels above the superior temporal artery.

Stroke affects many elderly people, and sadly is a leading cause of death and disability. A simple and non-invasive method that predicts risk of stroke and stroke mortality which has been investigated developed by The Centre for Vision Research at Sydney University's Westmead Millennium Institute involves the use of fundus photography of the retina. An image that simultaneously shows the onset of a micro-aneurysm, the narrowing of retinal vesicles and athero-venous nicking which is typical of a patient who might have a stroke in the near future is illustrated in Fig. 2.11.

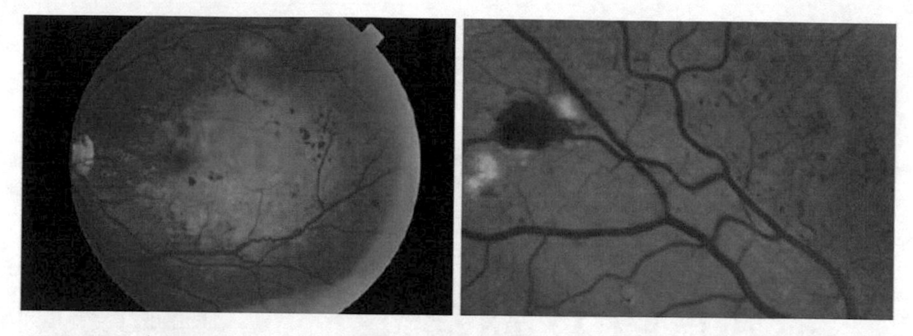

Fig. 2.10 The *left panel* shows tiny, round, *red* spots commonly seen in and around the macular area, which are the hallmark of diabetic retinopathy. The image on the *right panel* depicts nonproliferative retinopathy related to severe diabetic retinopathy. After [272]

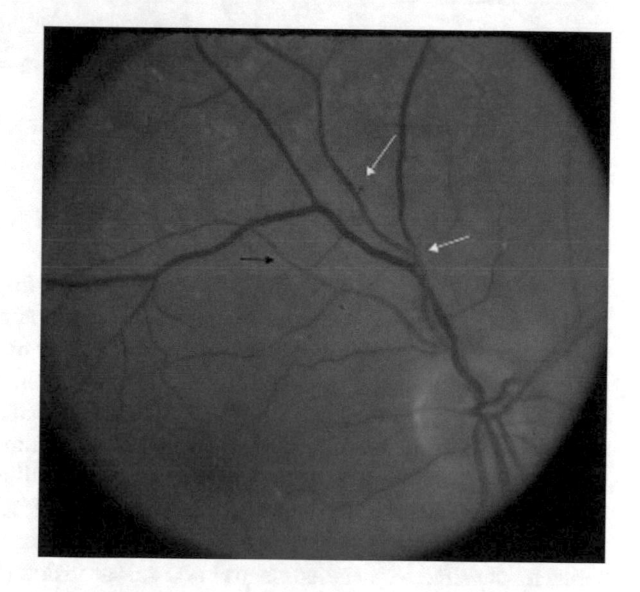

Fig. 2.11 A retina showing patient predisposition to stroke—The arrows indicate (clockwise from the *top arrow* in the picture). *White arrow* 1—A micro-aneurysm/haemorrhage; *Black arrow*—Narrowing of retinal vesicle; *White arrow* 2—Athero-venous nicking

2.1.8 Recent Advances in the Application of OCT Techniques to Disease Diagnosis

Optical coherence tomography (OCT) [232] has been used in a wide range of biomedical applications. [233, 234] OCT noninvasively acquires high-resolution, cross-sectional images of the retina [235]. A time-domain OCT system, such as the Stratus OCT device (Carl Zeiss Meditec, Dublin, CA), is capable of acquiring OCT reflectivity data at a rate of 400 axial scans per second. In addition, spectral-domain OCT (SD-OCT) systems, such as the Cirrus HD-OCT (Carl Zeiss Meditec) for example, have recently gained U.S. Food and Drug Administration approval. SD-OCT technology improves on time-domain systems, allowing performance of up to 27,000 axial

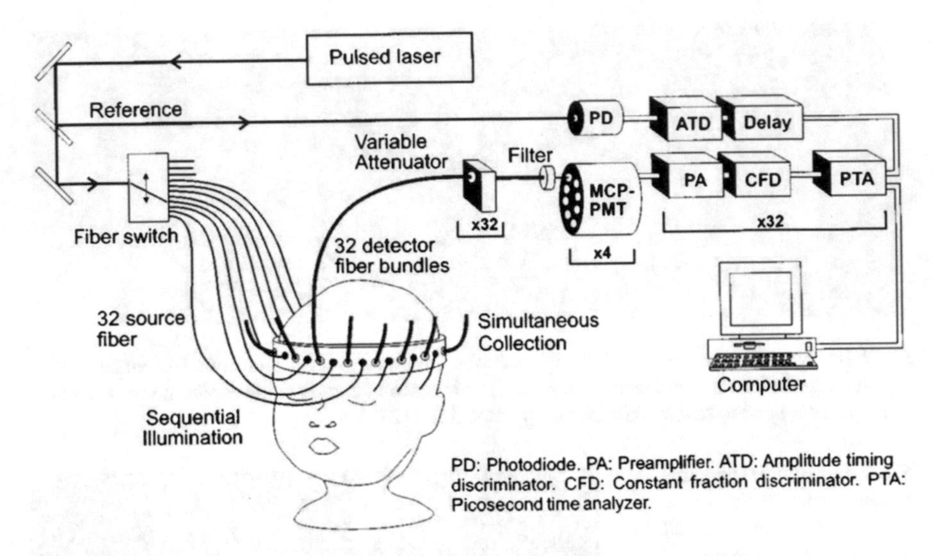

Fig. 2.12 A 32-channel time resolved OCT imaging system. After [266]

scans per second [237, 245]. The increased axial scan rate results in approximately 50 times faster data acquisition rates in practice.

OCT scanning can detect a number of eye diseases at their initial stages (sometimes years before symptoms become obvious), making treatment much more effective and reducing the chances of irreversible damage. For example, it can help provide early detection or rule out diseases such as glaucoma, macular degeneration and diabetic maculopathy. Macular hole disease is associated with a hole in the retina that can result in deterioration of vision. Prior to treatment, the loss of vision can vary depending on the size of the hole. This is further illustrated in Fig. 2.12. A case of age-related macular degeneration is illustrated in Fig. 2.14. Deterioration of the macula can interfere with a patient's central vision because it affects the part of the retina responsible for detailed central and colour vision.(Fig. 2.13)

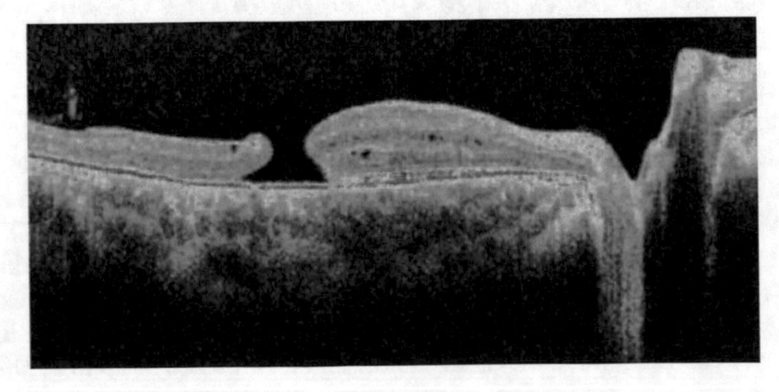

Fig. 2.13 Illustration of typical macular hole case, the hole in the retina that can result in deterioration of vision

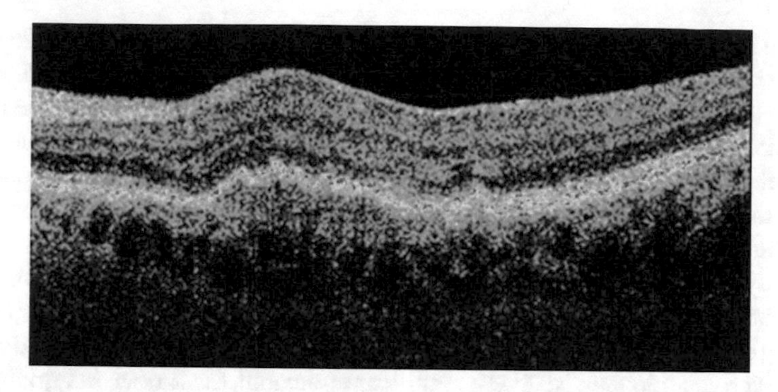

Fig. 2.14 Illustration of a case of macular degeneration. The condition is associated with a partial or complete loss of a patient's central vision

2.1.9 Alternative Multichannel and MEMS Based OCT Imaging Modalities

Beyond the applications of OCT described in the previous sections, there are also alternative multi-channel implementations which are particularly useful to biomedical imaging e.g. for the visualization of increased vascularization in mammograms as well as the detection of abnormalities in infant brains [259]. Using Ti:sapphire lasers or alternative fibre lasers (e.g. ytterbium-doped femtosecond fiber lasers as well as large-mode-area fibre based systems) [260, 261] which can achieve high-power using chirped-pulse amplification techniques [262, 263] to generate femtosecond or few picosecond pulses, the signal-to-noise ratio of such imaging techniques has been steadily improving over the past 20 years. These multi-channel techniques use transmitted light between pairs of points to perform reconstruction of an arbitrary three-dimensional distribution of internal scatterers and absorbers. As this type of imaging suffers from significant scattering, the Radon transform [264] which is used in MRI, may not be used and alternative algorithms for the extraction of the effective refractive index and scattering coefficients have been developed [265, 266]. An excellent example of such imaging system is the one developed at University College London known as the multichannel optoelectronic near-infrared system for time-resolved image reconstruction (MONSTIR). This system has now evolved to provide multispectral imaging at 4 wavelengths between 650 and 900 nm [122] and has significant potential for generating functional images of newborn brain [123].

This multi-spectral approach to diffuse optical imaging leads to the generation of independent images of changes in concentration of oxyhemoglobin and deoxyhemoglobin so current efforts focus on the development of data-driven approaches for optimum wavelength selection [124]. Another interesting aspect of current work in this area is the application of spatio-temporal regularisation techniques [125] which can provide real-time three-dimensional dynamic reconstruction of the optical properties of a hemispherical infant head phantom, taking into consideration the moving absorption as well as scattering targets. These signal processing techniques are of much relevance to the THz transient tomography community, if adapted accordingly so that the THz scattering component associated with the shortest wavelengths of the broadband signal is significantly suppressed.

Finally, it is worth noting that alternative implementations of OCT using micro-electromechanical systems for endoscopic applications [126, 127] are also rapidly evolving and have important biomedical applications e.g. in bladder cancer diagnosis [127]. Such techniques also show significant potential for further integration with alternative complementary imaging techniques such as photoacoustic microscopy and ultrasound imaging [128, 129]. The development of new image processing algorithms that can perform de-noising, image segmentation as well as classification that can lead to improved spatio-temporal correlations for improved functional imaging across different tissues is a unifying theme that will be discussed in the following chapters.

Chapter 3
Recent Advances in Medical Data Preprocessing and Feature Extraction Techniques

This chapter discusses different feature extraction and selection strategies for the four imaging modalities considered. Windowing and model fitting parametric approaches are first considered. Then, recent advances in multi-resolution algorithms and wavelet analysis are presented. The algorithms discussed can provide de-noising as well as a generic multi-resolution sensor fusion framework. The focus is on robust feature extraction and selection strategies, firstly from a single pixel perspective and then from an imaging perspective. The benefits from adopting a fractional order calculus approach to detect features in an image are explained. Recent advances in fundus image denoising are also highlighted. A multiresolution image fusion scheme that could be used to combine MRI with THz datasets is proposed. This chapter then discusses several feature selection strategies for both THz as well as for MRI datasets. In the case of THz datasets, features in time, frequency or wavelet domains associated to single pixels are considered. In the case of MRI datasets, the discussion focuses on features observed across entire images, taking into consideration textural information. Spatio-temporal correlations across different areas in an image, as identified through fMRI are also discussed. Advances in a graph-theoretical framework that can potentially elucidate such correlations are also mentioned. In addition, feature extraction and selection in retinal fundus imaging and OCT are reviewed.

X. Yin et al., *Pattern Classification of Medical Images: Computer Aided Diagnosis*, Health Information Science, DOI 10.1007/978-3-319-57027-3_3

3.1 Overview of Medical Image Data Preprocessing Strategies

3.1.1 Data Windowing and Model Fitting Parametric Approaches

In the case of THz TPI datasets, data pre-processing aims to isolate the real T-ray responses from the effects of amplitude and phase noise associated with the pulse-to-pulse THz emitter instability and laser beam pointing stability, which is temperature dependent, and related to translation stage movement uniformity and detector shot noise, thus reducing artefacts that could compromise the classifier performance. Co-averaging multiple measurements improves signal-to-noise-ratio per pixel but at the expense of significantly increased measurement time and image acquisition rate. Since there is only a square root advantage in signal-to-noise ratio as a function of time by co-averaging, post-processing for de-noising is essential in the THz community. Furthermore, long integration times are unsuitable in applications where the THz response is time-dependent, for example, in sample drying. Signal processing can partly alleviate some of these issues. Window apodization, for example, reduces frequency domain Gibbs ripple due to the data discontinuities at the edge of the recorded time domain interferograms. Optimization of the apodization function is now possible even for dispersive samples using algorithms accounting for the asymmetry of the propagating femtosecond THz pulses [274]. The proposed approach also has important applications in a completely different context, potentially improving time resolution in perfusion MRI datasets.

Well established techniques for filtering include Wiener filtering [276], principal component analysis [277], artificial neural networks [278], and Maximum-Entropy techniques [226, 279]. These are applicable to both THz-TPI and MRI datasets, as well as retinal fundus images. A recent advance in the modelling of de-excitation dynamics which has its origins to the theory of complex dielectrics is the use of fractional order calculus and the fitting of fractional order models. In this approach, the time series experimental datasets are modelled using very parsimonious pole-zero expressions. Such filters can be implemented in real time using resistive, capacitive or inductive networks [54–56]. Although the fractional-order system identification literature is still in its infancy, it promises to provide much lower residual errors in the identified models of a given process, thus significantly advancing the science of Chemometrics as applicable to both THz TPI as well as DCE-MRI and functional MRI datasets. The essence of such parametrization is that a fractional order model of the form:

$$G(s) = \frac{b_0 + b_1 s^{\beta_1} + b_2 s^{\beta_2} + \cdots + b_m s^{\beta_m}}{1 + a_1 s^{\alpha_1} + a_2 s^{\alpha_2} + \cdots + a_n s^{\alpha_n}} \tag{3.1}$$

where $b_0,\ b_1, \ldots b_m, a_1,\ a_2, \ldots a_n$ are coefficients to be identified and $\beta_1,\ \beta_2, \ldots \beta_m$, $\alpha_1, \alpha_2, \ldots \alpha_n$ are positive real valued exponents, can account for collective interactions from multiple species and intermolecular forces (such as charge screening at a distance) providing a very parsimonious model of the interactions. In this context the approach can account for spectral shifts in amorphous materials as well as de-embed solvation dynamics. As discussed in [280], the application of fractional order calculus for MRI datasets is still in its infancy but already there have been cases where a Debye relaxation in combination with a Kohlrausch-Williams-Watts function [281] and a Rigaut type asymptotic fractal expression [282] have been used to represent such datasets. These studies are leading to Bloch-Torrey type diffusion expressions [283–285], which can be placed in a system identification framework along the lines of the generic polynomial expression above.

A well-established methodology for extracting fractional order dynamics is through the use of the CRONE toolbox for Matlab [286–289].

3.1.2 Multi-resolution Wavelet Analysis for Noise Removal

Wavelet denoising [47, 309–312] complements other parametrization schemes performed in either time or frequency domains [45, 46]. In THz TPI, multiresolution techniques such as wavelet transforms are particularly effective to further de-noise mean-centered apodized interferograms. Furthermore, they enable direct time-frequency information to be extracted while at the same time ensuring very parsimonious parametrizations of these time series datasets. A typical de-noising procedure consists of decomposing the original signal using the Discrete Wavelet Packet Transform (DWPT) or the Discrete Wavelet Transform (DWT) [304–306], thresholding the detail coefficients, and reconstructing the signal by applying the appropriate inverse transform (IDWT or IDWPT respectively). For the de-noising of femtosecond THz transients, a three-level decomposition is usually sufficient [307], and unnecessary computational load associated with more decomposition levels can be avoided.

A wavelet filter bank decomposes a time series signal by separating the high (detail) and low (approximation) frequency components of the signal assuming a pre-defined mother wavelet function. The approach has very efficient de-noising capabilities in the presence of Gaussian white noise and provides very parsimonious representation of the THz TPI signal. An important feature of this transform is that it is orthogonal so that it enjoys perfect reconstruction symmetry. This enables its inverse transform to reproduce the original dataset without loss of information. The approach provides a way forward for easier biomedical software certification as it provides complete traceability of all the data processing steps. More specifically, in a wavelet filter bank, the low-pass filtering result undergoes successive filtering iterations with the number of iterations N_{it} chosen by the analyst as shown in Fig. 3.1.

The final result of the decomposition of data vector $\mathbf{x}$ is a vector resulting from the concatenation of row vectors $\mathbf{c}(N_{it})$ (termed approximation coefficient at the largest scale level) and $\mathbf{d}(s)$ (termed detail coefficients at the sth scale level, $s = 1, \ldots, N_{it}$) in the following manner:

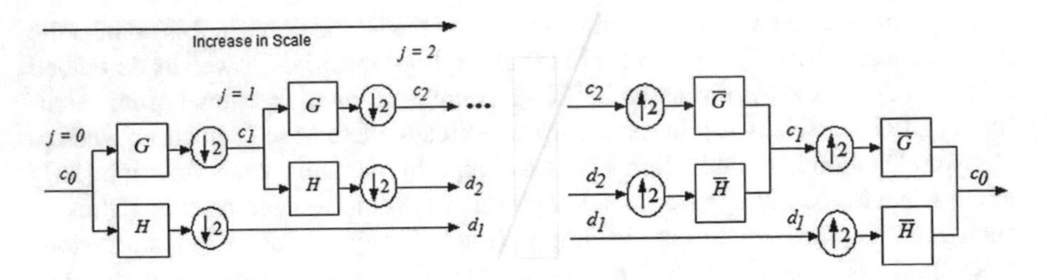

Fig. 3.1 Two-channel filter bank implementation of the wavelet transform applied to data vector **x**. Blocks **H** and **G** represent a low pass and a high-pass filter respectively and the ↓ 2, ↑ 2 symbols denote the dyadic down-sampling and up-sampling operators respectively. The decomposition can be carried out to more resolution levels by successively splitting the low-pass channel Bars indicating reconstructed channels (after either hard or soft thresholding). The large arrow indicates adaptive filtering

$$t = [\mathbf{c}(N_{it})|\mathbf{d}(N_{it})|\mathbf{d}(N_{it} - 1)| \cdots |\mathbf{d}(1)] \tag{3.2}$$

with coefficients in larger scales (e.g. $\mathbf{d}(N_{it})$,$\mathbf{d}(N_{it}$ - 1),$\mathbf{d}(N_{it}$- 2),. . .) associated with broad features in the data vector, and coefficients in smaller scales (e.g. **d**(1),**d**(2),**d**(3),. . .) associated with narrower features such as sharp peaks. The filter bank transform can be regarded as a change in variables according to the following operation,

$$t_j = \sum_{n=0}^{J-1} x_n v_j(n), \qquad j = 0, 1, \ldots, J - 1 \tag{3.3}$$

where t_j is a transformed variable and $v_j(n) \in \mathscr{R}$ is a transform weight. The transform can be written in matrix form as:

$$\mathbf{t}_{1\times j} = \mathbf{x}_{1\times J}\mathbf{V}_{J\times J} \tag{3.4}$$

where $\mathbf{x} = [x_0\ x_1, \ldots, x_{J-1}]$ is the row vector of original variables, **t** is the row vector of new (transformed) variables and V is the matrix of weights. Choosing **V** to be unitary (that is, $\mathbf{V}^T\mathbf{V}$ = **I**), the transform is said to be orthogonal. For $\{h_0, h_1, \ldots, h_{2N-1}\}$ and $\{g_0, g_1, \ldots, g_{2N-1}\}$ impulse responses of the low-pass and high-pass filters respectively, a circular convolution consisting of flipping the filtering sequence and moving it alongside the data vector. This is used for generating the approximation coefficients from the data vector **x**. The approximation **c** and detail **d** coefficients are stacked in vector **t** = [**c**|**d**], so the wavelet transform can be expressed in matrix form as follows:

$$\mathbf{V} = \left[\begin{array}{ccccc|ccccc} 0 & 0 & \cdots & h_{2N-4} & h_{2N-2} & 0 & 0 & \cdots & g_{2N-4} & g_{2N-2} \\ h_{2N-1} & 0 & \cdots & h_{2N-5} & h_{2N-3} & g_{2N-1} & 0 & \cdots & g_{2N-5} & g_{2N-3} \\ h_{2N-2} & 0 & \cdots & h_{2N-6} & h_{2N-4} & g_{2N-2} & 0 & \cdots & g_{2N-6} & g_{2N-4} \\ h_{2N-3} & h_{2N-1} & \cdots & h_{2N-7} & h_{2N-5} & g_{2N-3} & g_{2N-1} & \cdots & g_{2N-7} & g_{2N-5} \\ \vdots & \vdots & \vdots & \vdots & \vdots & \vdots & \vdots & \vdots & \vdots & \vdots \\ h_0 & h_2 & \cdots & 0 & 0 & g_0 & g_2 & \cdots & 0 & 0 \\ 0 & h_1 & \cdots & 0 & 0 & 0 & g_1 & \cdots & 0 & 0 \\ 0 & h_0 & \cdots & 0 & 0 & 0 & g_0 & \cdots & 0 & 0 \\ \vdots & \vdots & \vdots & \vdots & \vdots & \vdots & \vdots & \vdots & \vdots & \vdots \\ 0 & 0 & \cdots & h_{2N-2} & 0 & 0 & 0 & \cdots & g_{2N-2} & 0 \\ 0 & 0 & \cdots & h_{2N-3} & h_{2N-1} & 0 & 0 & \cdots & g_{2N-3} & g_{2N-1} \end{array}\right] \quad (3.5)$$

where the following conditions for orthogonality need to be satisfied:

$$\sum_{n=0}^{2N-1-2l} (h_n h_{n+2l}) = \begin{cases} 1, & l = 0 \\ 0, & 0 < l < N \end{cases} \quad (3.6)$$

$$g_n = (-1)^{n+1} h_{2N-1-n}, \quad n = 0, 1, \ldots, 2N-1 \quad (3.7)$$

The above expressions have universal applicability to both THz transient time domain sequences as well as MRI and OCT signals.

An important development in the wavelet signal processing literature has been the use of adaptive wavelets [48, 313, 314] where the mother wavelet is specifically tailored at each decomposition level (wavelet scale) accordingly, to minimize the least squares error associated with the difference between the transformed signal from its original one. The general structure of the algorithm is shown in Fig. 3.2.

This approach provides a remarkably efficient way for extracting information contained in each THz pulse transient associated with each pixel in an image [12, 17, 18, 33, 49–52, 59, 60, 226, 350, 447]. The transform can also be applied to datasets acquired using continuous wave systems. Figure 3.3 showcases the advantage of optimal wavelet de-noising in a classification context. To generate this graph, the standard deviation of the noise was varied from 0.001 to 0.5. For each noise level, 250 noisy patterns were generated for each class (lycra and leather datasets acquired using a continuous wave Fourier transform spectometer). As can be seen, the classification is much more robust to noise when carried out in the wavelet domain than in the original domain. Moreover, the robustness to noise is further increased by the optimization of the wavelet transform (green line) as opposed to the application of standard db4 wavelets. The work clearly supports the notion that the performance of a classifier based on the output of a wavelet filter bank is better than that of an Euclidean distance classifier in the original spectral domain [52].

Other interesting parametrizations of relevance are the ones discussed in [315], those in [316] and more recently in the work by Galvão's group [317, 318]. These

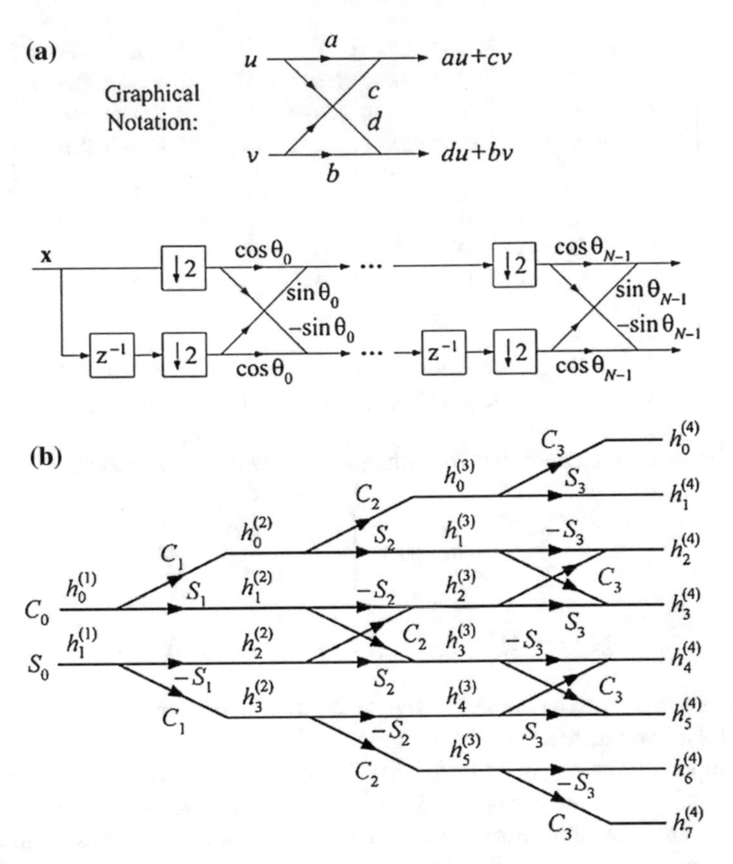

Fig. 3.2 **a** Procedure for parameterizing wavelet filter banks by N angles. **b** Recursive generation of low-pass filter weights $\{h_n^{k+1}\}$ in terms of $\{h_n^k\}$ by adding one additional angular parameter at a time. S_k and D_k represent the sine and cosine of angular parameter θ_k respectively. By using this procedure, any set of N angles $\{\theta_0, \theta_1, \ldots, \theta_{N-1}\}$ leads to a sequence of low-pass filter weights that satisfies the orthogonality condition

algorithms, with minimal modification (appropriate tuning of the mother wavelet) can also be used for de-noising in fundus photography studies.

Other examples of wavelet transform pre-processing routines for signal-to-noise-ratio enhancement and classification of THz spectra can be found in [8, 53]. Such pre-processing steps have enabled the successful discrimination of cancerous from normal tissue in wax-embedded histopathological melanoma sections as well as the classification of dentine and enamel regions in teeth [49]. It is, nowadays, generally accepted that the performance of a classifier based on the output of a wavelet filter bank, is better than that of an Euclidean distance classifier in the original spectral domain [52].

An alternative promising pixel de-noising method involves the use of wavelet power spectrum estimation techniques (WPSET), as discussed by Kim et al. [255]. This approach may remove spectral artefacts without distorting spectral features.

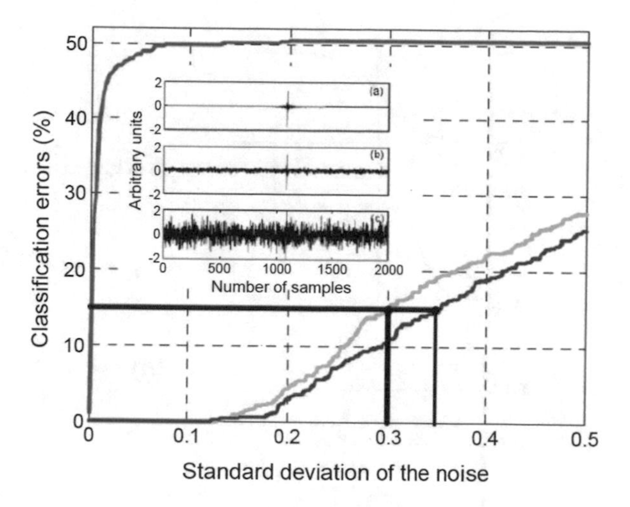

Fig. 3.3 Illustration of the classification errors (%) as a function of noise level in the interferograms. Nonoptimized db4 wavelet (*green*), optimized wavelet (*red*) and Euclidean distance (*blue*) classifiers. The inset shows a leather interferogram with (**a**) no artificially added noise and noise with standard deviation of (**b**) 0.1 and (**c**) 0.5. After [52]

This is a nonparametric approach based on a wavelet representation of the logarithm of the power spectrum [320]. The authors applied the WPSET to the transmission spectrum of water vapor and verified the effectiveness of the approach. Alternative signal pre-processing methods for de-noising include base line correction [321], smoothing [322], first and second derivative [322, 323], multiplicative scatter or (signal) correction [324], and standard normal variate analysis [325]. All these methods have their own merit under different experimental conditions, and further confirm the universal applicability of wavelets for de-noising THz TPI datasets. [326].

3.1.3 *Current Standards and Recent Developments in Multiresolution Feature Representation in Imaging*

Extending the discussion from time domain sequences to an imaging perspective, the discrete cosine transform (DCT) using Wang factorization, Lee's power of two block lengths DCT scheme [290], Arai's scheme [291], Loffler's algorithm or Feig-Winograd factorization [292] are particularly useful. The attractiveness of the DCT algorithm stems from the fact that it is asymptotically equivalent to the Karhunen-Love transform which possesses optimal de-correlation as well as optimal energy compaction properties. Two-dimensional wavelet transforms are also well established in multimedia coding standards (H.265 and JPEG2000) [293] are of interest to all the imaging modalities discussed so far, as well as retinal fundus photography. Because of the possible preservation of information in the signals in the wavelet transform when a perfect reconstruction orthogonal transform is used, these multi-resolution approaches have unique advantages and can be part of any signal pre-processing routine where classification is the end goal. Further examples of the application of these algorithms are discussed in more detail in the following sections.

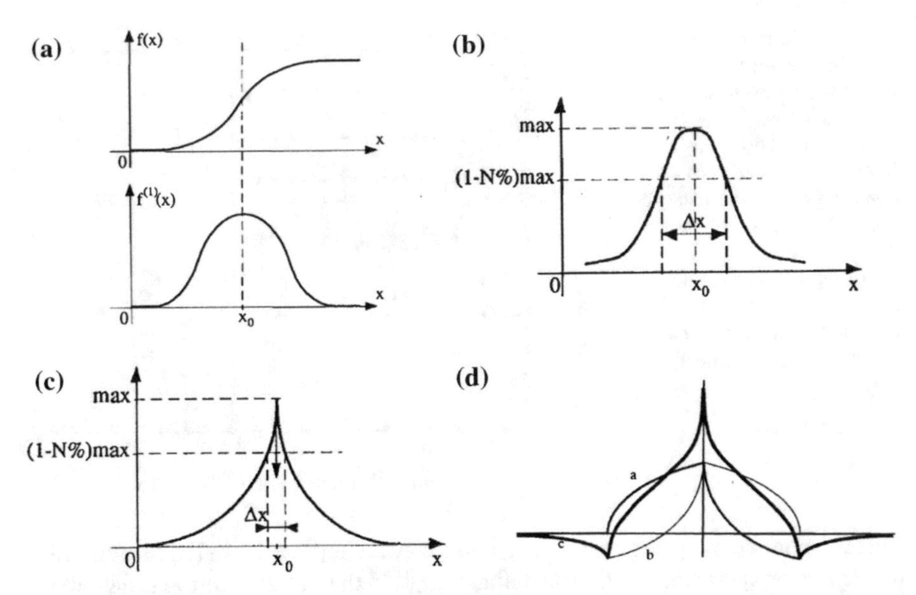

Fig. 3.4 **a** The maximum of the derivative $f^{(1)}(x)$ determines the abscissa x_0 of the inflexion point of transition $f(x)$. **b** The ratio $1/\Delta x$ defines detection selectivity, **c** Selectivity improvement by creating a cusp, **d** Construction of the response of the CRONE detector for $1 < n < 2$: (i) $f^{(n)}(x)$ calculated with increasing x; (ii) opposite $f^{(n)}(x)$ calculated with decreasing x; (iii) detector response. Adopted after [299]

It is also worth noting that fractional order signal processing can significantly benefit current segmentation practices across all the four imaging modalities discussed throughout this book. An image can be interpreted as a function of two variables which are defined within a bounded area. The function's value always lies within a bounded interval, and through a discretization step, the image is normally spatially sampled so that quantification of its luminous intensity is performed. The extraction of contours consists of detecting all inflexion points of luminance transitions. In most of the current image processing literature, edge detection is performed using integer-order differentiation operators. Normally these operators are first order on the basis of the gradient in the image or second order on the basis of the Laplacian (finding an inflexion point where the slope is maximal). The application of a differentiation operation, however, ensures amplification of high frequencies which can be unwanted if the image is noisy. In [294–299], the authors demonstrated that an edge detector based on fractional differentiation can improve the existing criterion for thin features detection, or can improve detection selectivity in the case of parabolic luminance transitions and the criterion of immunity to noise, which can be interpreted in terms of a general robustness to noise. A comparison of integral order and fractional order transitions generated using the CRONE detector along a single dimension are shown in Fig. 3.4 above, the authors also discussed the case of using two vectorial operators with two independent components (horizontal and vertical) to account for the 2-dimensioinal case.

From the above discussion, it may be concluded that such fractional order image processing modalities are an important emergent research area which is likely to be adopted by the biomedical imaging community. The proposed approach should be seen within a more general framework for constructing fractional generalized orthogonal bases [301, 302] which are likely to be soon also adopted for image processing. An object-oriented approach to the CRONE toolbox has already been proposed [288], and this could provide better integration of the signal processing algorithms discussed with the classification approaches proposed in the subsequent chapters of this book.

3.1.4 Recent Advances in MRI Wavelet Denoising

The rationale for a wavelet-based statistical analysis of fMRI data can be found in the work by Dinov et al. [327] and Weaver [328]. An important consideration in this type of filtering is that the noise in magnitude MR images is signal-dependent (Rician), whereas most de-noising algorithms assume additive Gaussian (white) noise [329].

In [330], a bilateral filter was introduced at the low pass filter bank corresponding to the highest scale of MRI images to suppress Rician noise in an image, a task more difficult than the removal of Gaussian noise. Because filtering was introduced at the approximation coefficients of the filter bank, this had the effect of preserving the edge features in the image. Subsequent soft thresholding and Neigh Shrink thresholding on a power basis were adopted for the reconstruction of the signal. The structured similarity index, the root mean square error or the Bhattacharrya coefficient, which is normally used for finding the statistical similarity between two data samples can be used for validation purposes of the proposed decomposition and reconstruction. The work in [330] followed the pioneering investigations by Nowak [331] who first proposed the removal of Rician noise using wavelets. An alternative to the above mentioned wavelet thresholding approaches is also proposed in [332]. The idea behind the proposed algorithm is to perform a preliminary coefficient classification to empirically estimate the statistical distributions of the coefficients that represent useful image features. The approach however, although shown to be particularly effective, still requires further evaluation.

Rather than power based signal decomposition, an alternative is to preserve the real and complex aspects of a signal by performing filtering separately [333]. There is significant merit in this approach when considering that the output of a dual channel filter bank can be coupled directly to the input stage of a complex support vector machine classifier (as will be discussed in the following chapters). A similar approach where the complex part of the signal was treated separately was adopted in [334] for diffusion-weighted imaging.

An important difference between standard MRI images and fMRI ones (e.g. BOLD) is that the noise distribution in BOLD images has recently been shown to follow a Gaussian model, which simplifies denoising [335, 336]; this is not necessarily the case for all types of fMRI, however. In the particular case of BOLD fMRI datasets, the spatial coherence features associated with individual time series are related to specific voxels within the image [337]. Spatial coherence is very closely related to the "smoothness", encountered across an image, but also includes components of spatial correlation that cannot be captured by a continuously differentiable auto-covariance function (e.g., measurements of full-width at half-maximum smoothness). Spatial coherence is in effect a measure of the degree to which power at a particular temporal frequency shares phase across space. In BOLD fMRI, spatial coherence has been found to vary systematically across temporal frequency. Lower temporal frequencies tend to share phase to a greater extent across space than high frequencies [337]. Algorithms developed for spatial smoothing of BOLD datasets often augment temporal noise in the low frequency range, and can deleteriously impact experimental fidelity [338]. Because perfusion fMRI data do not possess temporal autocorrelation in time, there is less of an influence of temporal frequency upon spatial coherence [339]. A multi-resolution de-noising framework is therefore most appropriate to BOLD datasets. Perfusion fMRI data will also usually benefit from spatial smoothing during pre-processing [340], although the standard caveats regarding the optimal detection of the activation function at different scales still remains an open problem [341].

3.1.5 Recent Advances in Fundus Image Denoising

Because of the difficulty in taking pictures of the eye fundus, as stated earlier, captured images often have inadequate contrast, lighting variations across the image, localized noise and anatomic variability affecting both the retinal background texture and the blood vessel structures [226, 342]. Yin et al. [226] observed that textured features in retinal photography can show either fine-grained or coarse-grained noise. Speckle noise can be reduced at a post-processing stage by applying a connectivity constraint on the extracted curvature based enhanced image. This constraint is varied over the image according to each noise region's predominant blood vessel size. Figure 3.5 provides an illustration of texture-based partitioning that can be applied in a fundus photograph.

Thin vessel detection in a noisy retinal image presents the biggest challenge from a software post-processing perspective. Aggressive noise suppression is associated with the loss of true blood vessel features so must be exercised cautiously as it can lead to registration of false positive classification readings. The denoising process involves transformation of noisy images into some domain where noise components are more easily recognized. To remove noise, a thresholding procedure is implemented and the transformation is reversed to reconstruct a noise-free image. The most commonly used denoising method in fundus photography is based on the use of a complex valued log-Gabor wavelet filter where amplitude information is decomposed while preserving important phase information across the image [343]. The process begins by calculating amplitude and local phase at each point of a retinal image and then applying the previously mentioned log-Gabor wavelet filter

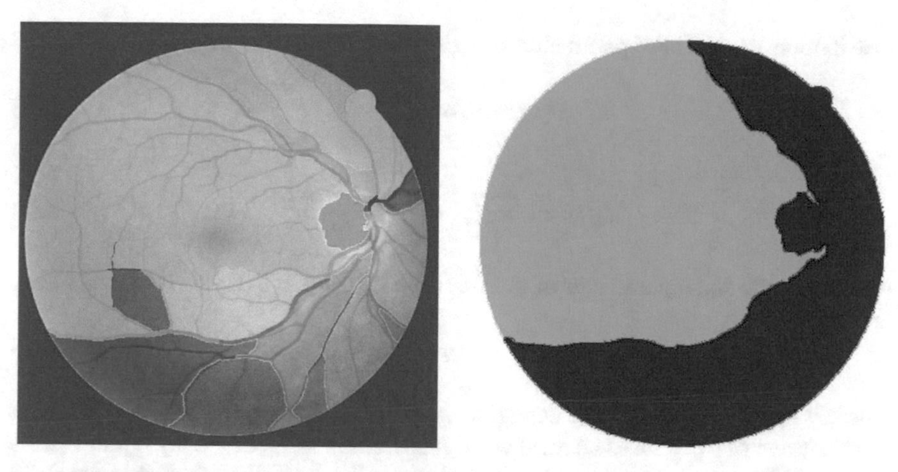

Fig. 3.5 Illustration of the texture-based partitioning of a fundus photograph. On the *left panel*, colour-coded mapping of the vessel texture is illustrated with the original image selected from the DRIVE database. The *right panel* illustrates colour-coded mapping of the two partitions on the basis of vessel texture: one region is dominated by small blood vessels (labeled in *blue*) and the other region is dominated by large blood vessels (labeled in *red*). After [226]

[344] which has a Gaussian transfer function on a logarithmic frequency scale. The amplitude information of the wavelet filtered image shows that most of the energy is concentrated in the centre of the image. However, the local phase information is distributed throughout the image across all frequencies. Amplitude or phase information alone is not capable of reconstructing the image efficiently. Hence, it is advisable to adopt a phase preservation technique while shrinking the amplitude information at different scaling factors and at different orientations. For an image $\mathbf{I}(x, y)$, the image response for even symmetric (M_n^e) and odd symmetric (M_n^o) wavelets at scale n is given by Eq. 3.8. The amplitude $A_n(x, y)$ and phase $\phi_n(x, y)$ at a wavelet scale n are calculated as Eqs. 3.9 and 3.10 respectively.

$$[Re_n(x, y), Im_n(x, y)] = [I(x, y) \times M_n^e, I(x, y) \times M_n^o] \tag{3.8}$$

where $Re_n(x, y)$ and $Im_n(x, y)$ are the real and imaginary parts of the complex valued frequency component.

$$A_n(x, y) = \sqrt{Re_n(x, y)^2 + Im_n(x, y)^2} \tag{3.9}$$

$$\phi_n(x, y) = \mathrm{atan2}(\mathrm{Im_n(x, y)/Re_n(x, y)}) \tag{3.10}$$

During the denoising procedure, a noise threshold at each wavelet scale is determined and the amplitude of the filtered vector is attenuated leaving the phase unchanged. An image can be reconstructed by summing the remaining even-symmetric filter responses over all scales and orientations. The above procedure ensures preservation of phase across different wavelet scales. The estimation of noise threshold is determined on the basis of the mean μ_R and variance σ_R^2 of the Rayleigh distribution $R(x)$. These parameters are given by:

$$R(x) = x/\sigma^2 e^{-(x)^2/2\sigma^2} \tag{3.11}$$

$$\mu_R = \sigma\sqrt{\pi/2}, \ \ \sigma_R^2 = \frac{4-\pi}{2}\sigma^2 \tag{3.12}$$

where σ is the scale parameter of the Rayleigh distribution. The noise threshold τ_1 is calculated as

$$\tau_1 = \mu_R + c\sigma_R \tag{3.13}$$

where, c specifies the standard deviation values of noise to reject. It is assumed that a lower value of c produces an ideal wave shape. If the value of c is high, thin vessels are treated as noise and removed. In practical applications, therefore, the value of c is tuned close to 1.

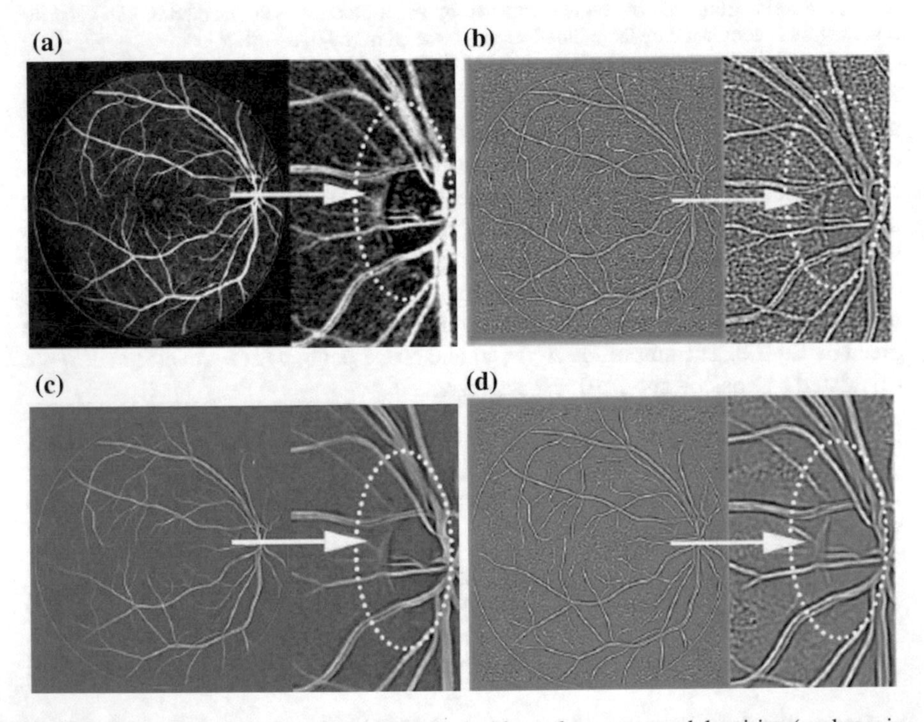

Fig. 3.6 Illustration of resultant images obtained without phase preserved denoising (as shown in **a** and **b**) and with (as shown in **c** and **d**) phase preserved denoising. **a** The image before using line detection. **b** The resultant image after using local normalization. **c** The denoised image with scale factor of 2 and 15 degrees of orientation before using line detection. **d** The denoised image with scaling factor of 8 and 15 degrees of orientation. After [345]

Figure 3.6 compares the resultant retinal fundus images with or without the use of phase preserving denoising. Figure 3.6a, b are the results before using line detection and after local normalization, both are processed in the absence of phase preserving denoising. Similarly, Fig. 3.6c, d are the results before using line detection and after using the local normalization operation but with phase preserving denoising. It is clearly seen that the denoising technique is able to remove a significant amount of noise without losing vessel features.

3.1.6 *The Need for a Multiresolution Image Fusion Approach*

Another area where wavelet transforms have proven to be useful is in cases where images are acquired using parallel MRIs as the technique introduces spatially varying noise levels [346]. In this case, wavelet based de-noising can be used to extract the edges from the original image and then generate a noise map from the wavelet coefficients at finer scales. The noise map is zeroed at locations where edges have been detected and directional analysis is used to calculate noise in regions of low-contrast edges that may not have been detected. An advantage of the proposed methodology is that it is fully automated and can be applied on final reconstructed images without requiring sensitivity profiles or noise matrices of the receiver coils.

A further application of wavelet transforms is in combining information present in multiple images of the same scene. It is also worth noting that the application of wavelet transforms represents an evolution of the standard pyramid transform which is extensively used by the sensor fusion community. The result of image fusion using wavelet transforms is, therefore, a new image which is more suitable for human and machine perception or further image-processing tasks such as segmentation, feature extraction and object recognition [347]. This becomes particularly important in multi-channel tensorial datasets as will be discussed in the following chapters, and is of much relevance to the future integration of both THz-TPI and MRI datasets as shown in Fig. 3.7.

Finally, as discussed in the excellent paper by Lustig et al. [108], wavelet transforms have applications in sparse MRI and compressed sensing. These algorithms are of much relevance to the THz imaging community.

From the discussion so far, it may be concluded that pre-processing techniques focusing on dimensionality reduction in the feature space as well as the fusion of information are at the core of a successful pattern recognition system. Inclusion of more features improves classifier performance but may compromise the generalization ability of the classifier. This is the well-known curse of dimensionality [348], which becomes quite prominent if the number of features is large. An overview of informative features suitable for selection is provided in the next section.

3.2 Overview of Feature Selection Strategies

In both THz TPI as well as MRI, after the de-noising pre-processing step, input data vectors must be grouped together into sets of feature vectors [1]. The choice of parameters for grouping is fundamental to the subsequent performance of the classifier. As a requirement for a classification system is to automatically make generalizations on its input space, often on the basis of its training set [349], the feature selection process is crucial to the subsequent efficiency of the classifier. A very large input space can overwhelm the classifier and a non-representative feature can lead to classification errors or have the training after a number of epochs converge to local minima. Furthermore, the chosen features should be well selected so as to ensure they are representative of the samples. There is a wide range of parameters one can select, and these can display non-transformed structural characteristics: moments, power, amplitude information, energy, etc., as well as transformed structural characteristics: phase and amplitude spectra, coefficients from wavelet decomposition etc.

3.2.1 Feature Selection Strategies in THz TPI Datasets

In the case of THz TPI based feature extraction, every measurement at each pixel position of an image is an entire time-dependent waveform, for example, a four-dimensional data set (x, y, z co-ordinates associated with a peak signal in amplitude or phase delay or maximum group velocity dispersion, the area under a portion of the time-domain waveform, the value corresponding to the logarithm of the absorbance or a differential absorbance value with reference to another wavelength). A good example of using selected features in the spectrum can be found in the work by Yin et al. [17, 18], which was applied to identify six different powder samples: sand, talcum, salt, powdered sugar, wheat flour, and baking soda in a multiclass classification context. An advantage of this approach is the small dimensionality of the feature vectors.

Alternatively, it can also be beneficial to consider a higher-dimensional dataset, taking into consideration real and complex coefficients of a Fourier transformation, principal components (PCs) from PCA, wavelet coefficients from time-frequency

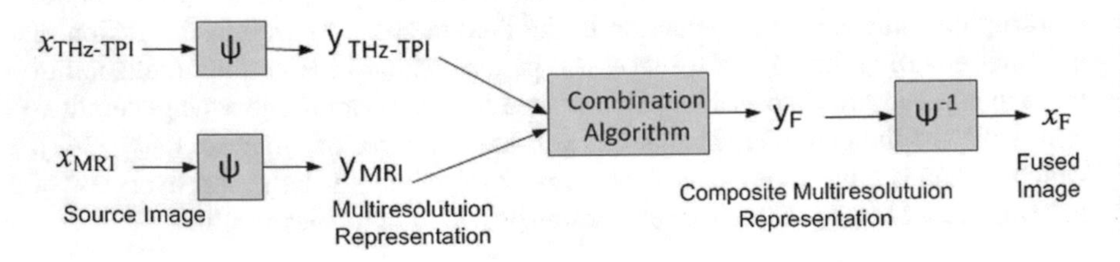

Fig. 3.7 Multiresolution image fusion scheme combining MRI and THz-TPI datasets

analysis, Auto Regressive (AR), Auto Regressive Moving Average (ARMA), coefficients, or a mixture of wavelets with AR and ARMA coefficients [11]. The selection of features in the PCA domain are discussed in [45, 166]. The usual problem with such an approach is the need to have a reliable set of calibration samples.

To achieve effective feature extraction, the fast WT may be adopted. The features presented to the classifier, in this case, become the extracted wavelet coefficients [17]. The use of AR and ARMA models on the WTs of measured T-ray pulse data has been previously discussed elsewhere [11]. In that work, the features of a processed THz signal are eventually classified by an Mahalanobis distance classifier. The effectiveness of this method was demonstrated by performing cancer cell discrimination from normal tissue (a binary classifier); the same classifier was also used in the multi-class classification task of recognising different kinds of powders.

Furthermore, coefficients derived using subspace identification methods from state space analysis of the corresponding time series (e.g. from Multivariable Output Error State sPace (MOESP) or Canonical Variable (CVA) Algorithms), or fractional order identification expressions which may be in the form of Cole, Harviliak -Negami, Fröhlich-mixture or Debye screening expressions, or parameters associated with fractional deconvolution information can also be used. Other characteristics in the signal that can be associated with additional features with discriminative power are as follows: [350] mean, standard deviation, skewness, kurtosis, 1st quartile (Q1), 3rd quartile (Q3), inter-quartile range (IQR), median, maximum and minimum as calculated from entire cross-correlation sequences between samples or samples and a reference. As will be discussed in the following section, it is beneficial to augment the classifier input space by treating real and complex parts of the signal separately so that the classification is performed on the basis of a sample's frequency dependent complex refractive index (or complex insertion loss) or to further augment it by providing additional channels to further accommodate structural and textural information. This can often be necessary due to either a channel spectrum or because of pseudo-coherence issues in the sample which can lead to an overestimation of the complex insertion loss due to a variation in the thickness or composition of the sample across the aperture. Problems in sample uniformity across the aperture arise more often is spectroscopy at the THz part of the spectrum because THz imaging systems have a diffraction limited minimal aperture that is larger than that of other conventional optical or infrared spectrometers. The resulting features n can be viewed as a vector in a n dimensional space, known as a *pattern space*.

Linear transforms are useful both for noise extraction and for representing the information in the data using fewer coefficients. Noise extraction can be performed by assuming that the system is detector noise limited rather than source noise limited. In this case, the noise spreads equally among all transform coefficients, while useful information will generally be concentrated in fewer coefficients. Examples of commonly used linear transformations for the processing of spectroscopic data include the FT, windowed FTs, WTs, and principal-component analysis (PCA). A comprehensive evaluation of various linear transforms that may be used for the denoising of spectra from continuous wave THz spectrometers can be found in [45]. The main conclusions of the work are summarized in Table 3.1.

Table 3.1 Advantages and drawbacks of linear transforms

Transform	Advantages	Disadvantages
PCA:Y=U Δ V^T	Maximum information compression	Each PC is related to the whole spectrum. No a priori assumption on a particular model associated with the dataset structure so no artefacts "Problematic" regions in the spectrum cannot be excluded after the computation of the PCs Since the analysis functions are obtained from the statistics of the data, many calibration samples may be required to obtain reliable PCs
Fourier	The analysis functions are fixed.	Spatial information is lost. Problematic regions in the spectrum cannot be excluded after the transform. Compacting a waveform using Fourier coefficients is not as efficient when samples have complex spectra and filtering too many Fourier coefficients can lead to signal distortion
Wavelet	Spatial information is kept. The width of the analysis window is automatically varied. For best performance, adaptive wavelets should be considered but the optimization methodology can have significant impact on classifier performance	The choice of the mother wavelet is usually difficult

An example of the use of spectral features to perform classification of TPI signals is discussed in Yin et al. [17]. The amplitude and phase at certain key frequency components constitute pairs of feature subsets on which the classification is based. An important advantage of this approach is the small dimensionality of feature vectors. This allows the features to be directly extracted from the pulse responses with relatively low computational complexity. Figure 3.8 shows the phase and amplitude plots in the frequency domain for six different powder samples: sand, talcum, salt, powdered sugar, wheat flour, and baking soda. Each curve is associated with a single pixel sampled from the image data. The spectrum has a cut-off frequency at 3 THz. Sharp changes of amplitude at the second frequency bin may be observed in Fig. 3.8a. It can also be seen that samples have significantly different frequency dependent phase patterns, so that a classifier using this information can be implemented as illustrated in Fig. 3.8b.

The main objective of feature extraction techniques for THz pattern analysis is to isolate the relevant features from the T-ray signals and use these features to improve

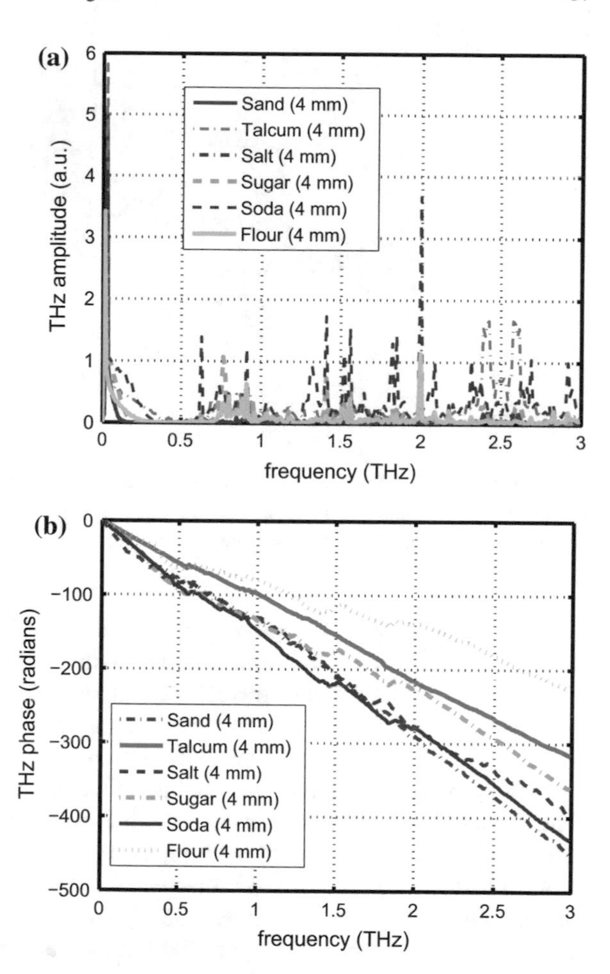

Fig. 3.8 Illustration of Fourier spectrum regarding the THz response of a number of powder samples. **a** Amplitude (attenuation) as a function of THz frequency. **b** Corresponding frequency dependent phase delay (equivalent to chromatic dispersion)

classifier performance. As stated in Chap. 2, WTs complement the traditional Fourier-based techniques in THz signal analysis by providing superior time-frequency localization characteristics. The work by Stephani et al. [351] discussed the use of wavelet coefficients to extract features from hyperspectral THz-RDS datasets. An alternative approach is through the wave atoms transform (WAT) which was first introduced by Fu et al. [352] in the context of THz transient processing of reflectance signatures. This is a multi-resolution technique that has a sparser expansion for oscillatory and oriented sample textures. It can provide improved resolution for pattern identification, when textural artefacts contaminating the THz transient response are concealing the compositional absorbance or reflectance of the sample. An alternative to occasionally generate even more parsimonious feature matrices, reported by Yin et al. [11], assuming AR, MA and ARMA models of different order, may also be considered depending on the data structure. In that approach, the averages of the modelling coefficients, (denoted as DC values in Fig. 3.9), are computed over the three decom-

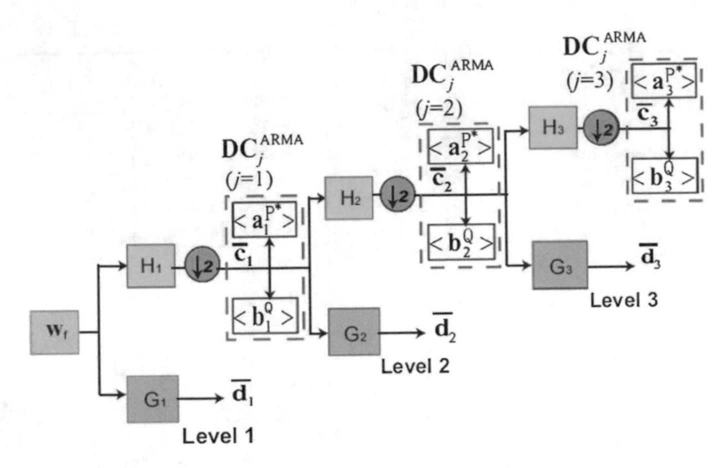

Fig. 3.9 In this modelling, H and G denote the low- and high-pass filters, respectively, w_f is the de-noised T-ray input. The arrow depicts the diadic down-sampling operator. Similar illustration related to DC^{AR} and DC^{MA} feature matrix are assumed

position levels of the WT employed on each data set. The model coefficient averages are then joined to produce feature vectors with a dimension equal to the number of sub-bands in the adopted wavelet decomposition. The feature vectors obtained from two different AR orders, and MA orders may be combined respectively to form the final AR and MA feature matrices. The ARMA feature matrix is obtained by combining two different orders of AR and MA vectors. The extracted AR and MA feature vectors are calculated at each decomposition level j. This approach may be introduced to further suppress the number of features in the input of the classifier so as to further improve its generalization ability. The complete procedure for calculating DC_j^{ARMA} is depicted in Fig. 3.9. The technique is now being superseded as adaptive wavelets, which are optimised at each decomposition level to account for most of the energy in the signal at each sub-band, offer similarly compact support.

A particularly interesting pre-processing methodology for linear system identification in frequency sub-bands by using wavelet packets was pioneered by Galvão's group [353]. The technique uses a wavelet-packet decomposition tree to establish frequency bands where sub-band models are created. An algorithm is then used to adjust the tree structure to achieve a compromise between accuracy and parsimony of the model.

Figure 3.10 illustrates the procedure adopted to identify each subband model $M_{i,j}$. Symbol $\mathbf{u}$ is the input signal for identification. Symbols y and $\check{u}_{i,j}$ are the waveform dynamics and subband model outputs, respectively. Residue $e_{i,j}$ denotes the wavelet-packet coefficients of the difference between y and $\check{u}_{i,j}$, in the frequency band under consideration.

The structure adopted for the subband model is a transfer function of the form

$$M_{i,j}(z) = P_{i,j}(z)Q_{i,j}(z) \tag{3.14}$$

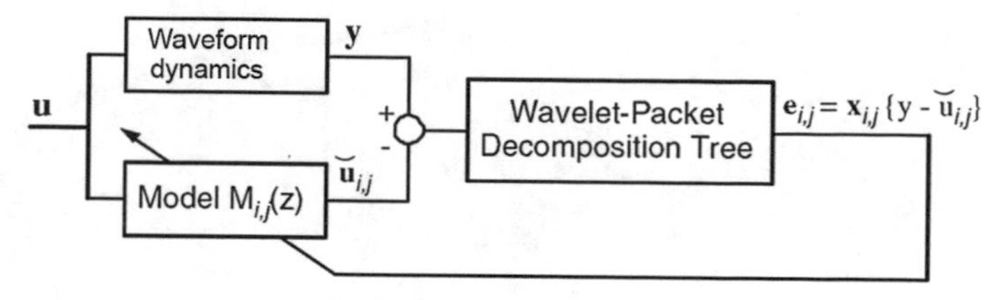

Fig. 3.10 Identification of subband model $M_{i,j}$. After [353]

where

$$P_{i,j}(z) = \left[\frac{1}{1 - z^{-1}}\right]^{s_{i,j}}, s_{i,j} \in z;\ Q_{i,j}(z) = \alpha_{i,j} + \beta_{i,j}z^{-1}, \alpha_{i,j}, \beta_{i,j} \in P \quad (3.15)$$

Function $P_{i,j}(z)$ is aimed at roughly approximating the band-limited frequency response of the waveform dynamics, whereas the FIR term $Q_{i,j}(z)$ provides a fine-tuning for the approximation. The identification procedure could be easily extended to accommodate more filter taps in $Q_{i,j}(z)$. However, since the model (Eq. 3.14) only needs to represent the system on a limited frequency band, only two taps are used in $Q_{i,j}(z)$ in the formulation. Such an over-simplification is compensated by the flexibility of adjusting the structure of the decomposition tree to improve the match between the waveform dynamics and the approximation model.

A least-square adjustment for the parameters of $M_{i,j}$ can be carried out by minimizing the following cost function $J_{i,j} : Z \times P^2 \to P$:

$$J_{i,j}(S_{i,j}, \alpha_{i,j}, \beta_{i,j}) = e_{i,j}(e_{i,j})^T \quad (3.16)$$

where $e_{i,j}$ denotes the row vector of residues for the identification procedure shown in Fig. 3.10.

This algorithm was subsequently adapted to perform the classification of lactose, mandelic acid and dl-mandelic acid, on the basis of their respective THz transient spectra [354]. In this case, a wavelet-packet decomposition tree was used to establish the frequency bands at which the sub-band models of the respective spectra will be created as illustrated in Fig. 3.11. Each leaf node of the decomposition tree was associated with a THz frequency band, and the complete set of leaf nodes composed the entire span of the frequency range covered by the spectrometer. For each frequency band, a sub-band model was therefore created. An optimization of the tree structure was then performed using a generalized cross-validation method in order to achieve a compromise between accuracy and parsimony of the overall model. Such a procedure automatically determined the most appropriate frequency partitioning for the sub-band models. The figure below shows, as an example, the implementation of the algorithm to the processing of the lactose sample. The complex insertion loss function of the sample after ratioing the spectra of the background and sample are shown (an asymmetric Mertz apodization window was used for the FFT calcula-

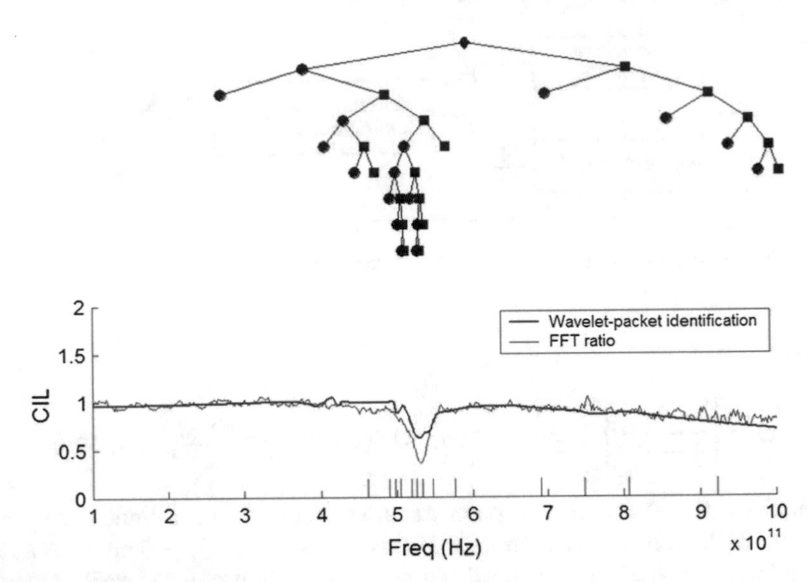

Fig. 3.11 **a** Wavelet-packet tree corresponding to the complex insertion loss of lactose as determined through measurements using a THz transient spectrometer and **b** the FFT result as obtained from conventional processing and the wavelet packet identification routine. The frequency-domain segmentation automatically defined in the identification procedure is indicated by vertical *lines* at the *bottom* of the graph. As can be seen, the segmentation is more refined in the spectral region corresponding to the THz absorption region. After [354]

tions). A db12 wavelet is used in the identification, and a dyadic tree with a depth of 9 (including the root node) was identified by the algorithm. The tree is deeper in a particular frequency range, which actually corresponds to the THz absorption region. It is worth noting that the segmentation is more refined in the frequency region corresponding to deeper levels of the tree. This tree structure was automatically defined by the identification algorithm, with no prior knowledge of the spectral features of the sample under consideration.

Other feature extraction methods include those proposed by Zhang et al. [355] that avoid sample misplacement phase error in terahertz reflection time-domain spectroscopy (THz-RTDS). They showed that the first or second derivative of the phase of the relative sample reflectance (with respect to the background reflectance) can be used to extract the frequency dependent absorption signatures of the materials under study. Ryniec et al. [364] applied decision trees to assist with feature selection demonstrating the effectiveness of decision tree methods in THz spectra classification. Finally, features extracted using the Radon transform have also been considered. This transform has been used extensively for the identification of micro-Doppler motion of a target and has its origins in the high-resolution radar community. Xu et al. [365] suggested a combination of time-frequency analysis with the Radon transform to perform micro-feature extraction. This transform should be carefully applied to datasets because the approach incorporates echo-cancellation that often leads to an undesirable channel spectrum in the frequency domain which, as discussed earlier, is a common source of error in TPI imaging that can seriously compromise classifier performance.

Advantages and shortcomings of some of the more widely used linear transforms can be found in [45]. Generally, Fourier expansions suffer from drawbacks such as the notion of an infinite support in the time domain [31], which compromises the quality of the signal unless apodization routines are adopted [45] to eliminate Gibb's ripple resulting from discontinuities at the edges of the time domain interferogram. This is especially true when fast scan data acquisition is performed in TPI applications where the time domain signals are more truncated.

These drawbacks are more efficiently addressed through the use of windowed FTs that further reduce the number of coefficients needed to describe the transformed dataset in featureless parts of the spectrum as well as through the WT which addresses the issue by successively increasing the resolution (increase in scale) of both the temporal and frequency domain features of the TPI signal.

3.2.2 *Feature Extraction and Selection on the Basis of Cross-correlation Sequences*

Recent work by Siuly et al. [350] explored the use of a cross correlation between the reference and sample time domain signatures from each sample class. In this study, each powder substance is considered to belong to a single class: sand (Class 1), talcum (Class 2), salt (Class 3), powdered sugar (Class 4), wheat flour (Class 5), and baking soda (Class 6). The sample holder response (which should be seen as a free-space equivalent of a cuvette) provides the reference signal used for evaluating the complex insertion loss. Using the reference signal in conjunction with the other sample signal in a class, the cross-correlation sequence is computed on a pixel by pixel basis. Once the characteristic features are extracted from each cross-correlation sequence associated with every class, all features are integrated forming a feature set.

Once cross-correlation features between sample and background are generated, a further 2-D cross-correlation technique [366–368] is used to calculate a spatial cross-correlation sequence (denoted by $CC(k,l)$) across the image. The graphical presentation of a cross-correlation sequence is commonly known as a cross-correlogram. The 2-D cross-correlation of X (M × N matrix) and H (P × Q matrix) is a matrix CC of size $(M+P-1)\times(N+Q-1)$:

$$CC(k,l)=\sum_{m=0}^{M-1}\sum_{n=0}^{N-1}X(m,n)\overline{H}(m-k,n-l); \tag{3.17}$$

where $-(P-1)\leq k\leq M-1$ and $-(Q-1)\leq l\leq N-1$. The symbol X denotes the reference signal and H is regarded as any other signal belonging to a sample class. The bar over H denotes complex conjugation. The output matrix, $CC(k, l)$, has negative and positive row and column indices. A negative row index corresponds to an upward shift of the rows of H and a negative column index corresponds to a leftward shift of the columns of H. A positive row index corresponds to a downward shift of the rows of H. A positive column index corresponds to a rightward shift of the columns. It is worth noting that each of the signals, X and H, consist of a finite number samples S, so the resultant cross-correlation sequence has $2S - 1$ samples.

The THz transient transmission reference signal is considered as noiseless for most parts of the spectrum, so the variance in the noise when ratioing a sample with a background does not get disproportionally amplified [52]. Each powder sample is considered as belonging to a distinct class. Figure 3.12 illustrates how a cross-correlogram is obtained from a reference signal (holder) and any of the other sample signals, on the basis of Eq. 3.17.

The cross-correlogram signals convey greater information than the original powder spectra of the sample and reference signals and thus have superior signal to noise ratio than the original signals. In addition, cross-correlograms contain additional information regarding the spectral coherence of the waveforms. As the cross-correlation sequences still contain a large number of data points, these need to be further compressed into a more parsimonious feature space so as not to overwhelm the classifier.

3.2.2.1 Statistical Feature Extraction from Cross-correlation Sequences

To reduce the dimensions of the cross-correlation sequences, one can consider the following statistical features: mean, standard deviation, skewness, kurtosis, 1st quartile (Q1), 3rd quartile (Q3), inter-quartile range (IQR), median, maximum and minimum as calculated from each cross-correlation sequence. This information can be used to create new feature vector sets. There are several valid reasons for the considerations of these. Mean and standard deviation are particularly informative in describing a distribution [369]. Skewness provides information on the degree of asymmetry of the observed distribution around its mean [367]. Kurtosis provides a measure of flatness relative to a normal distribution. Q1 and Q3, measure how the data are distributed in the two sides of the median. IQR is the difference between Q3 and Q1 and is used in measuring the spread of a data set, such information can be used to exclude outliers [370]. Median, which is associated with the observation encountered most often, is also an additional valuable metric that needs to be retained for classification purposes. Maximum and minimum values are also used to describe the range of observations within the distribution. For the example in Fig. 3.8, subroutines can be run for each cross-correlation sequence associated with each powder substance. All ten statistical features from each cross correlation sequence and each powder substance form the content of a feature set that can finally be associated with each powder material sample.

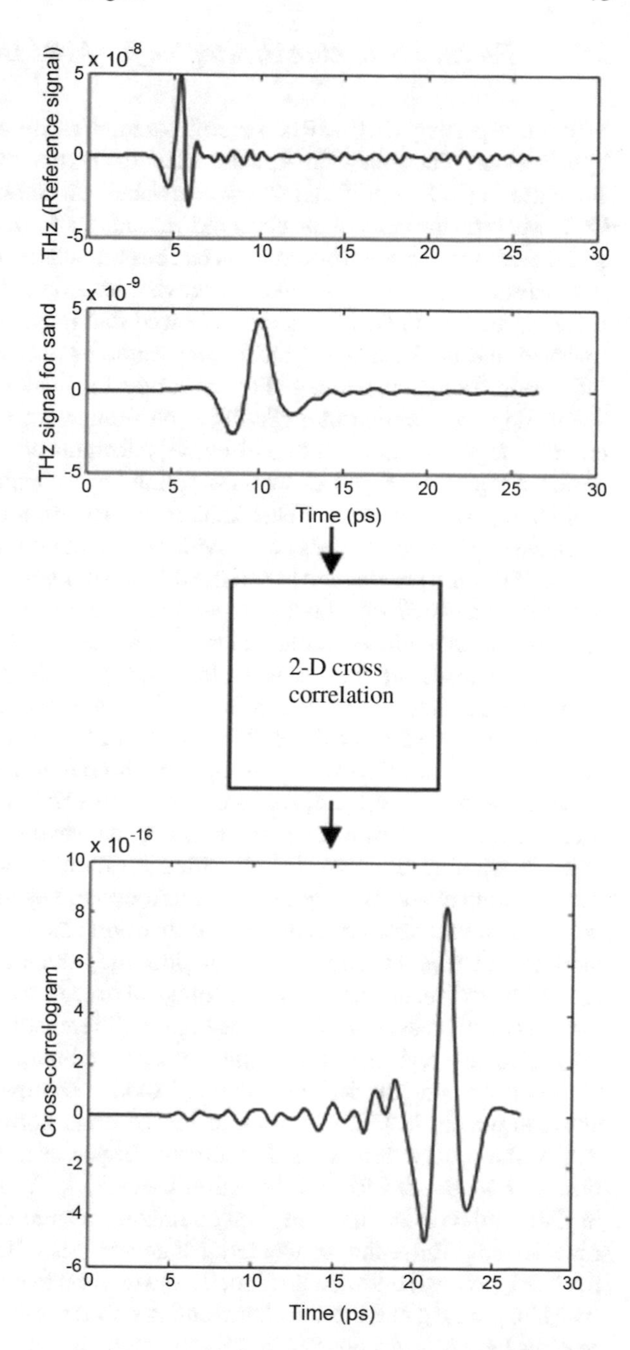

Fig. 3.12 Typical cross-correlogram from THz background and sample time domain signatures. After [350]

3.2.3 Feature Selection Strategies for MRI Datasets

When interpreting DCE-MRIs, several parameters are simultaneously considered by clinicians. These include vascular kinetics, texture, shape, and size of tumour. As stated in [371], significant prognostic value can be obtained from pre-treatment DCE-MRIs on the basis of the observed vascularization as well as the texture, shape, and size of tumours. Such information can be particularly useful to patients diagnosed with advanced breast cancer and can provide important direction for therapy. In the work discussed in [371] the authors showed that multivariate survival analysis has revealed that model-retained DCE-MRI variables provide independent prognostic information complementing traditional survival indicators. Clearly, such parameters are worth incorporating in a classification framework if appropriate robust mathematical representations can be effectively formulated. This is, however, a multi-parametric problem that may not be simplified by a simple reduction of image information in parameter space. There is already concern, for example, that just relying on intensity-time curves does not provide sufficient information for a complete evaluation of disease progression [372]. In addition, it is worth noting that measurements are often associated with a large range of parameters; for example, vascular kinetics reflects both blood flow, vascular density, and vessel permeability.

When considering the vascular kinetics, the pixel-by-pixel nature of the analysis makes possible an assessment of lesion heterogeneity. Interestingly, mean and median kinetics values seem of little prognostic value, and do not sufficiently characterize a tumour [373–378]. It is also worth noting that the above list of features is not exhaustive. For example, as discussed in [379] in the case of breast cancer, there are also other parameters in an image that should be presented to a classifier when developing an automated classification framework, and MR-derived angular second moment and entropy features representing heterogeneity provide important information on tissue composition. Furthermore, as the authors state, entropy features can differentiate between histological and immune-histochemical subtypes of breast cancer (ductal and lobular histological grade cancers). Differing entropy features between breast cancer subtypes implies differences in lesion heterogeneity. The study also acknowledged that texture analysis of breast cancer potentially provides added information for decision making. Another example further strengthening the above argument in [380] shows that higher order correlation analysis might also lead to the observation of additional features that need to be taken into consideration in an automated feature extraction framework. A further suggestion discussed in [381] points at the necessity for optimizing feature selection for mass and non-mass lesions. The author concluded that an analysis of feature importance (through a ranking process) revealed that kinetic and textural features have higher importance weighting among mass lesions than among non-mass lesions, whereas morphologic features have higher importance weighting among non-mass lesions.

A case for textural analysis is conducted when considering triple negative breast cancer (TNBC) where estrogen (ER), progesterone (PR), and human epidermal, growth factor (HER2) are combined to determine a patient's treatment protocol.

Such cancers respond more readily to chemotherapy treatment due to their increased surrounding vasculature. In those cancers, texture analysis is rapidly becoming the preferred diagnostic tool. In its simplest form, texture analysis relates gray-level intensity with spatial variation across the image [382] and extracts features that can characterize the underlying structure of the object under investigation. Textural features have been linked, not only with traditional breast cancer prognostic indicators, but also the initial response to neoadjuvant chemotherapy (NAC) treatment. Quantification of texture is discussed in [383]. Furthermore, in a very comprehensive study taking into consideration 16 texture features (angular second moment, contrast, correlation, variance, inverse difference moment, sum variance, sum entropy, entropy and difference variance, difference entropy, two information measures of correlation, maximal correlation coefficient, cluster shade and cluster prominence) [384], it was concluded that several of those features could provide clinicians with additional information to increase the accuracy of the prediction of an individual response before NAC is started.

Changes in the intensity of imaged tumours in MRIs are common in clinical practice and, as a consequence, this leads to an inherent difficulty in the segmentation of an object of interest. This variation is mainly attributed to intrascan intensity inhomogeneities. Susceptibility artefacts in gradient echo images are known to frequently affect the observed intensities, causing significant intrascan intensity inhomogeneities [640]. Therefore, although MRI images may appear visually uniform, the intrascan inhomogeneities often scramble intensity-based segmentation. A typical example of such an intra-scan intensity inconsistency for a tumorous breast tissue is illustrated in Fig. 3.13a. The image depicts a ductal carcinoma (malignant tumour) in situ. Although the parts depicted by the arrows show the same anatomical structure taken from the same tumour region, the intensity values are different. The intensity indicated by a yellow arrow is higher than the intensity indicated by the red arrows. After conducting intensity based segmentation, i.e. FCM, as illustrated in Fig. 3.13b, the region with low intensity either forms an irregular ring, or forms a gap that separates the image into two disconnected parts. The gap is shown as an area with reduced intensity without well defined edges. In the absence of reconstruction artefacts, this area should be filled-in by voxels of increased intensities.

The unified reconstruction of a volume image from multiple channels [59] is illustrated in Fig. 3.13c. This shows a greatly improved intensity consistency with the tumorous regions colour-coded in blue clearly separated from the red background region. Figure 3.13d illustrates the resultant segment of the tumour after reconstruction. When this is compared with Fig. 3.13b, where the whole tumour region shows intensity inhomogeneity and not well defined edges, the resulting segmentation through the multi-channel reconstruction shows more homogeneous boundaries for the tumours; in addition, the entire tumour shape and tumour position are clearly retrieved. This can be validated further by the overlapping images, shown in Fig. 3.13e, where the yellow region consists of voxels mainly from the reconstructed tumour used to fill in the missing voxels from the classified pre-processed image. As a result, the reconstruction correctly locates tumour boundaries while eliminating inconsistent detection of boundaries in the original enhanced tumour image. The

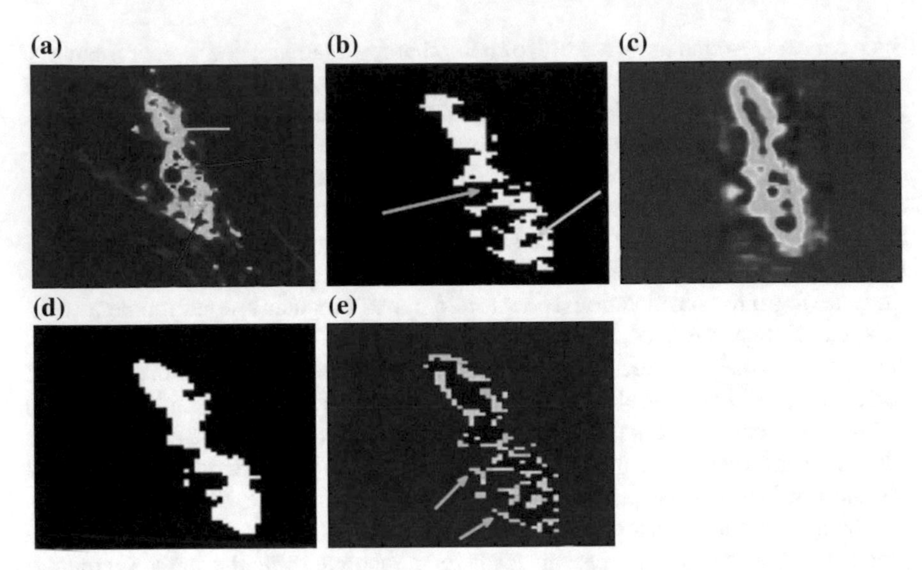

Fig. 3.13 **a** Illustration of intensity inconsistency for breast tumour tissue images. *Yellow arrows* indicate a high intensity and *red arrows* low intensity. **b** Illustration of intensity based segmentation with inhomogeneous boundaries; *yellow arrows* indicate an irregular annular region and the *green arrow* indicates missing areas. **c** Reconstructed volume image from multiple channels. **d** Tumour segment after reconstruction. **e** Overlapped images (*brown*) between original tumour segment (*blue*) and reconstructed tumor segment (*yellow*). The *green arrow* indicates the fuzzy edges associated with the original image. The imaged tumour corresponds to an in situ ductal carcinoma

proposed reconstruction leads to a better segmentation of the enhanced patterns compared to regions where heterogeneous internal enhancement patterns were originally achieved. A unified analysis of MRIs for tumour identification is discussed in [62]. This analysis can be combined with fast dynamic magnetic resonance imaging using the sparse recovery methods discussed in [385]. The use of both methods decreases sampling errors and significantly reduces storage space; furthermore because of the sparsity in the datasets, it has improved computational speed.

Recently, Minkowski functionals (MFs) have been proposed as a novel way of describing image texture [386]. The technique, has been used successfully in computed tomography (CT) and mammography, [387–389] as well as to analyze MRI images to determine malignancy [390] in the breast and measure response to chemotherapy [391, 392]. It is, therefore, important to note that textural analysis can also be placed in a more generic unified topological framework, from which additional features may be extracted for use in a classification context [393]. This is a particularly interesting approach where points in an image forming a point-cloud are associated with elementary blocks such as vertices, edges, triangles, or simplices of higher dimensions (which would potentially account for folds in a tissue). All closed surfaces can be approximated by using triangles after identifying some of their edges in this simplicial complex framework. Čech complexes are generated using a set of points associated with the point-cloud and constructing balls of radius r around each point, and then connecting the vertices by an edge if the balls intersect, adding a triangle. The resulting Čech complexes are an enlargement of the point cloud. If due to folds, a high-dimensional Euclidean space is required to fully describe the dataset, the full embedding information is needed to generate an accurate distance metric for the points in hand. When sufficient information is not available for the generation of complexes, filled-in triangles generating flag complexes are generated, requiring all three edges. The flag complexes are an approximation of the topological space reconstructed.

A Vietoris-Rips complex is another possible construction of a simplicial complex related to the point-cloud. The advantage of this complex is that it is determined from only the distances between the points, without having to know their exact embedding. The construction of a topological invariant for the above mentioned complexes starts with the generation of a vector space whose basis elements are all the vertices, edges and triangles of a given simplicial complex. A linear difference or boundary operator is then defined. This, when applied to an edge, yields a difference in vertices. Higher order boundary operators are similarly defined to act on triangles and other simplices. A matrix representation of these linear operators is then obtained. As further explained in [393], the algebraic structure that is imposed on the basic construction of the spaces makes sequential application of boundary operators possible in any higher dimension. This construction contains information about the holes or bounding areas that are not filled in, thus defining homology spaces where higher-order Laplacian operators are used for identifying higher-order topological properties of any simplicial complex. The discretization of texture traces [394, 395] is still an emergent area in computer vision which should have significant applications within the MRI community, not only for texture analysis, but also in segmentation [396] as well as with motion analysis [397], which can also be associated with MRI scans. The proposed technique could complement other attempts to use computer aided texture analysis in DCE-MRI [398].

Another study that correlates radiomic image phenotyping for identifying triple-negative breast cancers with quantitative texture features (heterogeneity of background parenchymal enhancement) from DCE-MRI considering the tumor as well as its surrounding parenchyma, is discussed in [399]. The aim of the study was to determine the discriminative value of detailed quantitative characterization of background parenchymal enhancement. The technique showed that quantitative texture features provided better differentiation for triple-negative subtype cancers. Both these studies make a strong case for the incorporation of textural features in a feature selection framework. Such efficient feature extraction strategies incorporating texture information can also assist in disease treatment selection. For example, in a recent study [401] it was shown that pre-NAC texture and kinetic parameters help predict treatments of non-benefit to NAC and demonstrated that NAC has advantages compared with adjuvant chemotherapy. In addition, segmentation defining shape and size of lesions is another area where textural information needs to be considered [402].

Finally, there are new studies [403, 404] aiming to identify associations between semi-automatically extracted DCE-MRI features and breast cancer luminal A and luminal B molecular subtypes, taking into consideration imaging information of the volume of the enhancing background parenchyma as a function of the total background parenchyma volume, so as to make a link between morphologic, texture, and dynamic features with radio-genomics. Another study in this context that showed progress towards making an association between a validated gene-expression-based aggressiveness assay (Oncotype Dx RS), morphological image features and texture-based (gray-scale correlation matrix Gray-Level Co-Occurrence Matrix (GLCM) based features in invasive ductal carcinomas (IDCs) is discussed in [405]. These studies also make a strong case for further potential benefits that can be realized through the associations of image features with specific molecular markers. Such benefits could potentially be more easily realized through the further integration of the DCE-MRI and THz-TPI modalities.

At this point it is worth noting that, although independent component analysis (ICA) can also be seen as a very promising feature extraction methodology for both MRI as well as THz-TPI on the basis of the additional degrees of freedom associated with non-orthogonal projections associated with PCA, the current discussion does not provide many examples of this line of work because, in an inaugural article in PNAS, by Daubechies et al. [406], it was shown that the effectiveness of independent component analysis (ICA) of brain fMRI using InfoMax and FastICA algorithms for separating a signal mixture into its components was more linked to their ability to handle effectively sparse components rather than independent components. Their work concluded that future work on the mathematical design of better analysis tools for brain fMRI should emphasize mathematical characteristics other than independence.

A key challenge for cognitive neuroscience is determining how mental representations map onto patterns of neural activity [357]. Structural and functional MRI data are inherently multivariate in nature, since each scan contains information about, for example, tissue structure or brain activation at thousands of measured locations (voxels). Considering that most brain functions are distributed processes involving a wide network of connected neuronal tissue brain regions, it would seem desirable to use the spatially distributed information contained in the data to obtain a better understanding of brain functions in normal and abnormal conditions. This spatially distributed information can be investigated using Multivariate Pattern Analysis (MVPA) in fMRI. The basic MVPA method is a straightforward application of pattern classification techniques, where the patterns to be classified are (typically) vectors of voxel activity values.

The requirement to understand spatiotemporal correlations in datasets from different voxels is currently leading to the development of new multidimensional fMRI datasets. The MVPA approach seeks to boost sensitivity by simultaneously processing datasets across multiple voxels. A study by Haxby et al. [363] illustrates how multi-voxel patterns of activity can be used to distinguish between cognitive states. Subjects viewed faces, houses, and a variety of object categories (e.g. chairs, shoes, bottles). The data were split in half, and the multi-voxel pattern of response to each category in ventral temporal (VT) cortex was characterized separately for each half. By correlating the first-half patterns with the second-half patterns (within a particular subject), Haxby et al. were able to show that each category was associated with a reliable, distinct pattern of activity in the VT cortex (e.g. the first-half 'shoe' pattern matched the second-half 'shoe' pattern more than it matched the patterns associated with other categories). Voxels with particularly high levels of noise (and low levels of signal) can sharply reduce classifier performance. This suggests that classifier performance will benefit from feature selection methods that remove noisy and/or un-informative voxels before classification. One way to select features is to limit the analysis to specific anatomical regions (e.g. in their study of visual object processing, Haxby et al. [363] focused on the ventral temporal cortex). Figure 3.14 provides an example where the use of correlations used as indices of similarity are identified as useful features for multi-voxel pattern analysis.

The above discussion, makes it clear that there are similarities in the structure of both THz TPI and DCE-MRI feature vectors, and developed feature extraction techniques in one imaging modality can benefit the other. Many of the parameters used by the DCE-MRI community have yet to be explored in a THz-TPI context as this is a new modality for biomedical imaging. Nevertheless, some potential synergies for feature extraction on the basis of molecular discrimination offered by THz-TPI should be of significant benefit to the DCE-MRI community.

3.2.4 Spatiotemporal Correlations and Cluster Analysis of Brain Activity Using fMRI

Recent studies on functional connectivity magnetic resonance imaging (fcMRI) [362] are paving the way for the modelling of brain activity as a functional network on the basis of spatio-temporal correlations. Currently, it is possible to distinguish between resting-state and active-state regions in the brain on the basis of the BOLD signal.

This approach detects temporal correlations in neural activity between distant brain regions by monitoring the oscillatory signal associated with blood oxygen while subjects rest quietly in a scanner [407]. These correlations provide an assessment of brain functional connectivity between particular brain regions, making functional neuro-imaging currently a very active area of research. An increasing number of pathologic conditions appear to have specific patterns and thus be well reflected [408] in these scans. FMRI is enabling physicians to provide both a more comprehensive diagnosis of seveal conditions with increased confidence as well as to further explore noninvasively the functional network structure of the human brain [409].

It is convenient to invoke a graph theoretical framework to model neuronal connectivity patterns [410]. A graph or network can be defined by a collection of nodes (vertices), and links (edges) between pairs of nodes. Nodes (neural elements) in large scale brain networks usually represent brain regions, while links represent region-to-region relationships including anatomical, functional, or effective connections, depending on the dataset.

The network structure of a graph is described by the graph's adjacency matrix (or connection matrix) [411, 412]. Rows and columns in these matrices denote nodes,

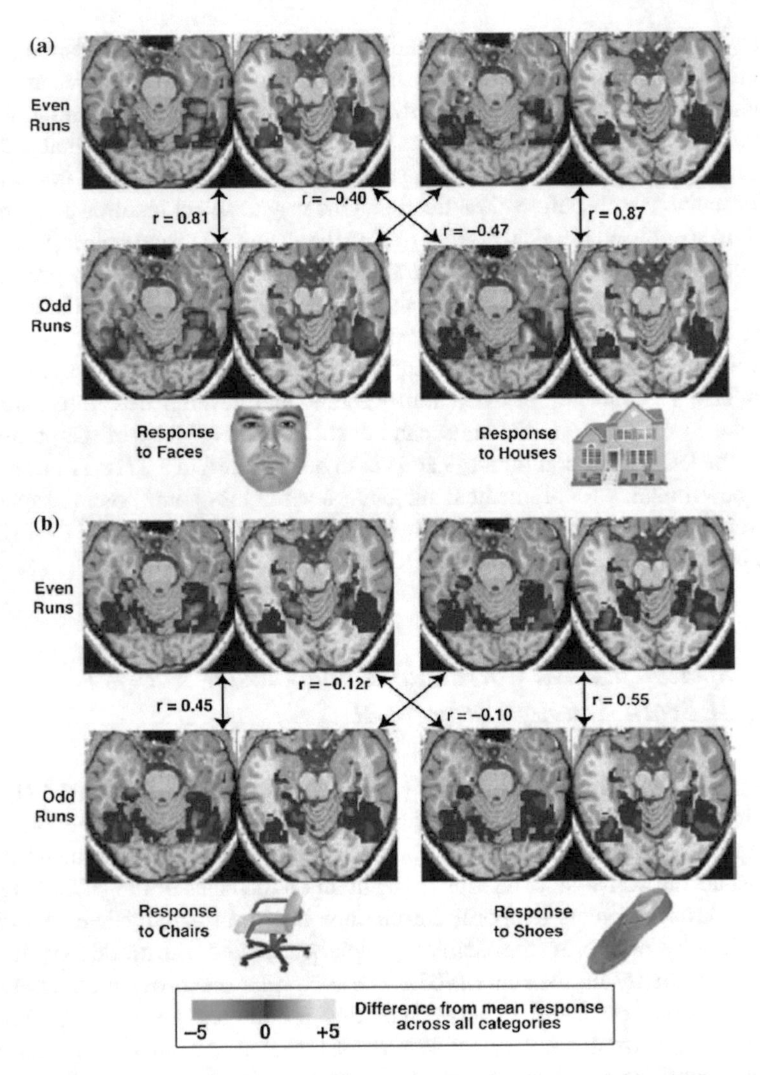

Fig. 3.14 Illustration of recorded fMRI patterns associated with specific stimuli from everyday objects (faces, houses, chairs and shoes), that invoke a known cognitive response. Brain images shown here are the normalized response patterns from two axial slices in a single subject. The responses from the ventral temporal cortex are subsequently compared. The *left* side of the brain corresponds to the *left* side of each image. The pattern of response to each category was measured separately from data obtained on even-numbered and odd-numbered runs in each individual subject. These patterns were normalized and baseline filtered to ensure a zero mean value for each voxel across all categories by subtracting the mean response across all categories. For each pairwise comparison, the within-category correlation is compared with one between-category correlation. **a** Comparisons between response patterns to faces and houses for one subject. The within-category correlations for faces (r = 0.81) and houses (r = 0.87) are both markedly larger than the between-category correlations, confirming that, when the subject correctly identifies each category, a similar response in the MRI scan is invoked. **b** Comparisons between the patterns of response to chairs and shoes from the same subject are shown. The category being viewed was always correctly identified from the MRI scan. After [363]

while matrix entries denote links. A matrix element a_{ij} is nonzero if the connection from j to i is present. In binary adjacent matrices, the link between nodes j and i is represented by 1 whereas when there is no connection, this is represented by 0. The resulting matrix also has an all-zero main diagonal, as shown in Fig. 3.15a. When the adjacency matrix is weighted and normalized, the value of a_{ij} will lie in the interval between 0 and 1, as shown in Fig. 3.15c. Moreover, network links can be classified as un-directed (Fig. 3.15a) or directed (Fig. 3.15b). In an un-directed network, the number of links in a node, k, corresponds to the degree of this node. An un-directed network is represented by a symmetric matrix. In a directed network, the in-degree and the out-degree attributes correspond to the number of in-coming and out-going links, respectively. The average degree of all the nodes defines the degree of the network. A weighted adjacency matrix is used to express the connection strength of an edge between two vertices, and this is given by its entry value. An entry equal to 0 implies that there is no edge between the two vertices i and j. In most of cases, the strength given by the edge weight and the degree of the end vertices k_i and k_j are well correlated. A large weight is attributed when there is a high value to the degree of connectivity between vertices.

In graph theory, a source vertex (or edge) j is linked to a target vertex (or edge) i. If $j = i$ through a path. Paths are all ordered sequences of distinct edges and vertices. When a source vertex is linked to itself, this is called a cycle [413]. A problem that often arises in optimisation theory is that of finding a path between two vertices (or nodes) in a graph such that the sum of the weights of its constituent edges is minimized. A graphical representation of the shortest path length between two nodes is illustrated in Fig. 3.15d.

Assuming parallel flux of information, the efficiency ε of communication between two nodes i and j is defined to be inversely proportional to the shortest path length d, $\varepsilon_{ij} = 1/d_{ij}$ [415]. The efficiency of a set of nodes N is the sum of the efficiencies of all node pairs, normalized by the maximal number of links $N(N-1)/2$.

At this point, it is worth noting that, in any graph representation of a collection of neurons, there will be vertices that are more central than others. The following metrics are defined to identify these vertices. The *Center* of a graph is a descriptive metric that is formed by evaluating the distances between vertices; the associated vertices are chosen so that the distance of each vertex to the most distant vertex is as small as possible. The *Median* of a graph corresponds to the center of a graph so that the total distance from a vertex to all the other vertices is as small as possible. The *Shortest-path betweenness center* of a graph is a metric chosen to solve optimization problems in communication networks where the load at each vertex is of interest. It is defined as the ratio of the number of shortest paths that pass through a vertex to the number of all shortest paths. The shortest-path betweenness can be adapted to find the center of a graph. This metric is more significant if it yields a higher value of shortest-path betweenness than the other vertices [416]. Figure 3.16 is an illustration of establishing nodal characteristics of group-based functional brain networks [400].

Another fundamental characteristic of brain networks is their functional *integration*. This metric indicates how integrated a network is and, thus, how easily information flows across its nodes [410]. The average of the shortest path length

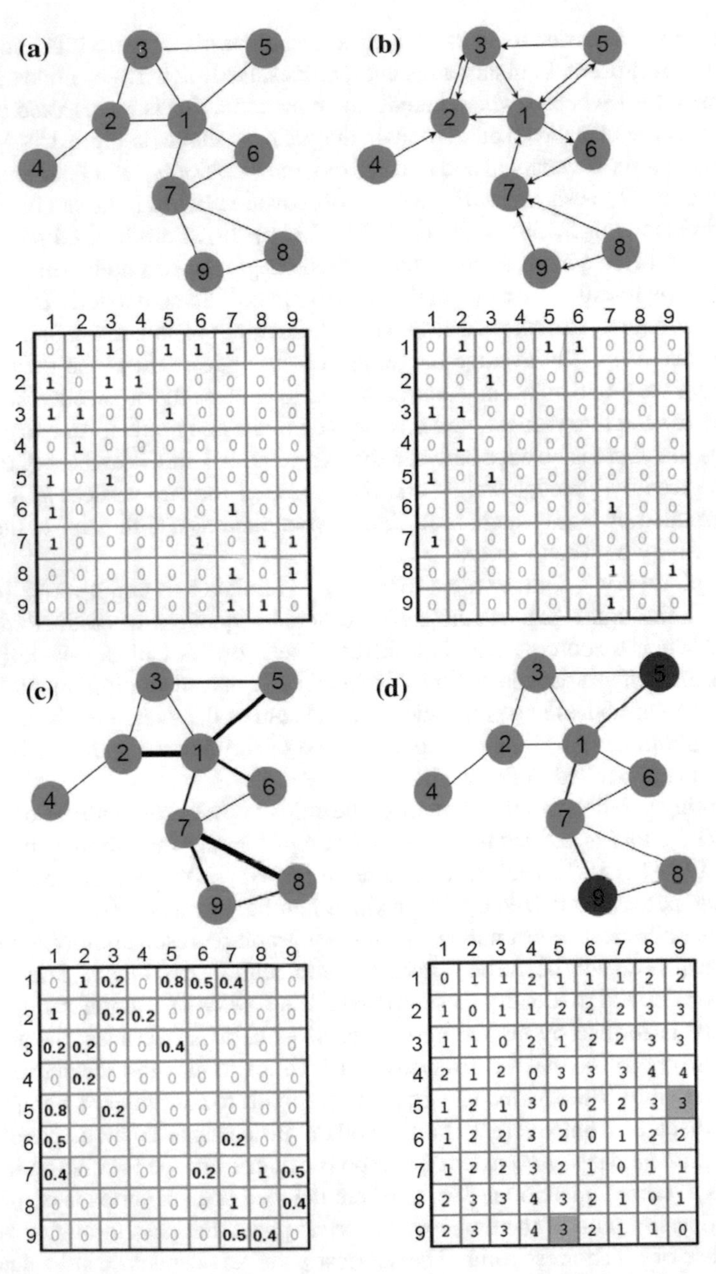

Fig. 3.15 Examples of undirected **a**, directed **b**, and weighted **c** networks and their corresponding adjacency matrices. **d** A graphical representation of shortest path length between nodes 5 and 9 (*thick line*) (*above*) and (*below*) its path length matrix (or distance matrix). After [414]

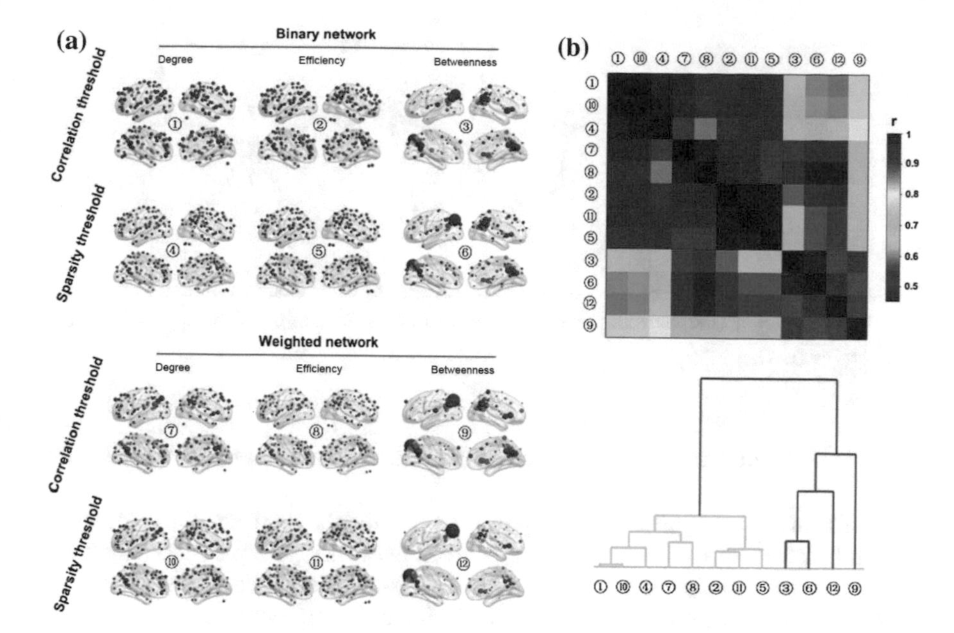

Fig. 3.16 Establishing nodal characteristics of group-based functional brain networks. **a** Nodal degree, efficiency and betweenness for both binary and weighted resting-state fMRI brain networks mapped using both the correlation and sparsity thresholding procedures (only nodes with centralities larger than the mean of the whole brain network are shown). **b** Typical cross-correlogram of observed spatial distributions among the three nodal centrality measures regardless of network type and threshold procedure used; in this case, nodal betweenness revealed unique spatial patterns. These patterns were also correlated to nodal degree and efficiency, identified using hierarchical cluster analysis. After [400]

between all pairs of nodes in a network is called the characteristic path length. A small characteristic path length implies that there is a stronger potential for integration [410].

Prior to topological characterization, a thresholding procedure is typically applied to exclude the confounding effects of spurious relationships between inter-regional connectivity matrices. Two thresholding strategies are normally adopted. These are based on an absolute connectivity strength threshold metric and a relative sparsity threshold metric [417].

The *connectivity strength threshold* is defined in such way that network connections with weights greater than a given threshold are retained, whereas those below the threshold value are ignored. The connectivity strength provides a quantitative description of the overall absolute network organization.

Sparsity is defined as the ratio of the number of actual edges divided by the maximum possible number of edges in the network. For networks with the same number of nodes, the sparsity threshold ensures the same number of edges for each network This is achieved by applying a subject specific connectivity strength threshold. Spar-

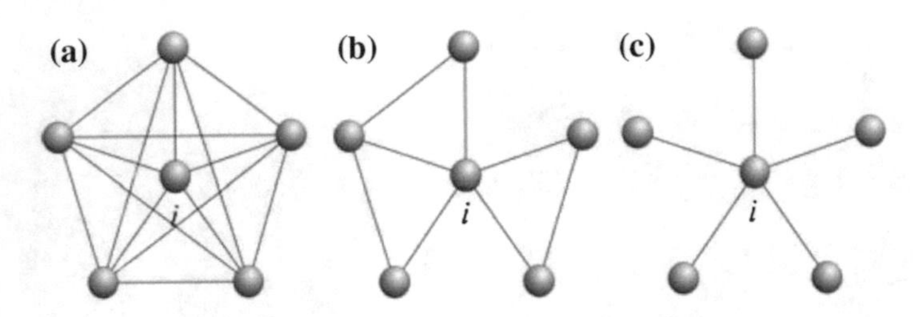

Fig. 3.17 Example of three networks and respective clustering coefficients in undirected networks. In **a**, $C_i = \frac{10(2)}{5(4)} = 1$ (the vertices around node i are fully connected), **b** $C_i = \frac{3(2)}{5(4)} = 0.3$ and **c** $C_i = \frac{0(2)}{5(4)} = 0$. After [419]

sity provides a quantitative description of the overall relative network organization [417].

Cluster analysis is particularly helpful in elucidating how information processing is distributed across different regions in brain networks, and provides functional segregation of the different regions in the brain. The clustering coefficient of a node, C_i, is a measure of the number of edges 'around' the vertex i, which can be calculated as the ratio of the number of links that exist between the nearest neighbours of the chosen node and the maximum number of edges among possible links [418]. The maximum number of edges among the neighbours of vertex i is given by $k_i(k_i - 1)/2$ where k_i denotes the number of the nearest neighbours of i. In undirected networks, the clustering coefficient C_i of a node i is defined as $C_i = \frac{e_i(2)}{k_i(k_i-1)}$, e_i is the number of connected pairs between all neighbors of i. In directed networks, the definition is slightly different: $C_i = \frac{e_i}{k_i(k_i-1)}$. An example of three networks and their respective clustering coefficients in undirected networks is shown in Fig. 3.17.

To illustrate how the hierarchical cluster structure depicting brain connectivity analysis is developed, an example is provided in Fig. 3.18. This shows the modular organization of human cortico-cortical connectivity, as identified from diffusion spectrum imaging [420]. Cortical areas are arranged in a circle so that highly interlinked areas are placed close to each other (Fig. 3.18a). The nodes in the same cluster show a high structural similarity which is also correlated to a similarity in function. The degree of this correlation is used to develop a dendrogram using hierarchical clustering as shown in Fig. 3.18b. The dendrogram, when observed from its base on the left and after following the branching to the right, connects the different objects in the tree. The distance of each branching point on the x-axis is proportional to the structural and functional cross-correlation.

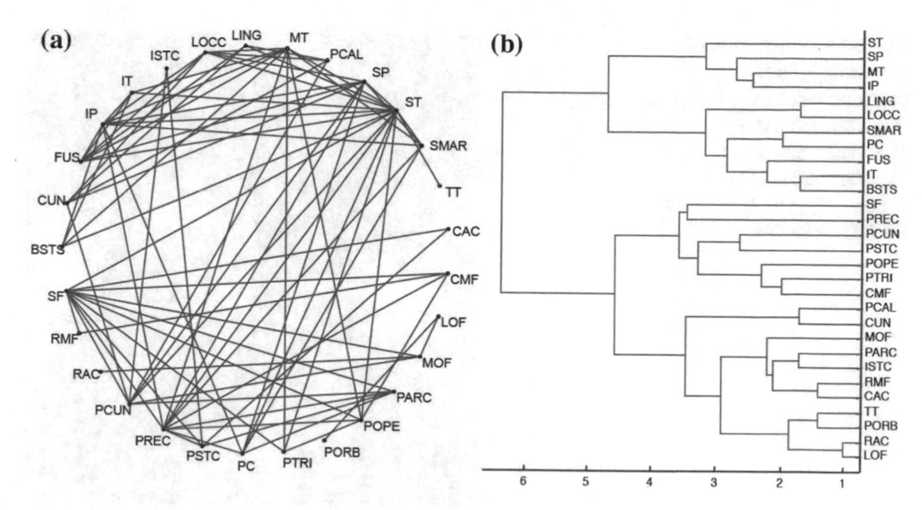

Fig. 3.18 Clusters. **a** Cluster structure of human cortico-cortical connectivity. Cortical areas are arranged in a *circle* using evolutionary optimization, so that highly inter-linked areas are placed close to each other. **b** Dendrogram of the same network using hierarchical clustering. After [420]

3.2.5 *Feature Selection in Retinal Fundus Photography Following Image Enhancement*

As stated in the previous chapter, retinal images acquired using a fundus camera are usually characterized by low level contrast and low dynamic range. This may seriously affect any subsequent automatic segmentation operation aimed at assisting diagnosis. Therefore, it is necessary to carry-out preprocessing before segmentation to improve image contrast effectively. To facilitate segmentation, various kernels (or filters) have been designed to enhance the vessels in an image. Most filtering techniques are based on image intensity (amplitude) and adopt matched filtering techniques [421], amplitude-modified second order Gaussian filtering [422], eigenvalue-based filtering [423], multi-scale linear operators [424], wavelets [425], contourlets [426], Gabor filters [427], or COSFIRE filters [428].

An alternative approach that conducts local curvature analysis of retinal image contrast features using a Hessian matrix, has been suggested by Yin et al. [226]. Feature extraction and segmentation is then performed using morphological operators following a maximum entropy binarization step.

3.2.5.1 Eigenvalue Analysis of the Hessian Matrix of a Fundus Image

The first step of the algorithm requires an eigenvalue analysis of the image Hessian matrix at a single scale. This is a simplification of the multiscale algorithm that Frangi et al. proposed [423]. The fundus photograph is once again pre-processed using a

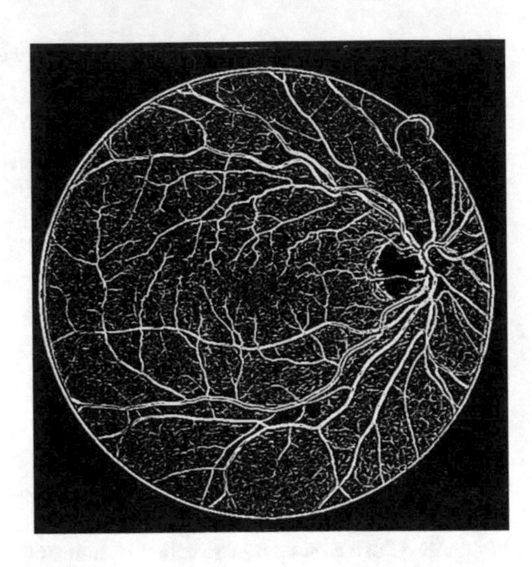

Fig. 3.19 Illustration of a curvature based enhancement of the image of the retina from the eigenvalue analysis of the Hessian matrix. The image used is `02_test` from the DRIVE database

top-hat transformation to produce $\mathbf{I}_T$. The local behaviour of each point in the pre-processed image $I_T(l,k)$ is then determined from a second order Taylor's series expansion in the neighbourhood of each point (l_0,k_0). For convenience, simplified point coordinates are adopted $I_T(l,k)$ to $I_T(x)$ and (l_0,k_0) to (x_0). The second order Taylor's series expansion corresponds to the associated second order directional derivative given from:

$$(\delta x_0)^T \mathcal{H}_0 \delta x_0 = (\frac{\partial}{\partial \delta x_0})(\frac{\partial}{\partial \delta x_0}) I_T(x_0). \tag{3.18}$$

The main idea behind eigenvalue analysis of the Hessian matrix $\mathcal{H}_0$ is to extract the principal directions in which the local second order structure of the image can be decomposed [423]. In this case, the direction of smallest curvature along the vessel can be computed directly. This is achieved by finding the eigenvectors corresponding to the smallest eigenvalues. Figure 3.19 shows the resulting enhancement following eigenvalue analysis.

3.2.5.2 Threshold Binarization Using Maximization of Entropy Criteria

When a grayscale image is binarised, a threshold value must be specified. In our approach, the optimum threshold value is determined according to the pixel intensity from the histogram of the image that exhibits the maximum entropy over the entire image. To represent spatial structural information of an image, a co-occurrence matrix is generated from the pre-processed image. It is a mapping of the pixel to pixel greyscale transitions (i.e. the gray level i follows the gray level j) in the image between the neighbouring pixel to the right and below each pixel in the image. The co-occurrence matrix of the pre-processed image $I_T(l,k)$ is a $P \times Q$ dimensional matrix $\mathscr{C} = [c_{ij}]_{P \times Q}$, where the elements c_{ij} are defined as:

$$c_{ij} = \sum_{l=1}^{P} \sum_{k=1}^{Q} \delta_{lk}, \quad (3.19)$$

where $\delta_{lk} = 1$, if

$$\begin{cases} I_T(l,k) = i, & I_T(l,k+1) = j \\ I_T(l,k) = i, & I_T(l+1,k) = j \end{cases},$$

and otherwise, $\delta_{lk} = 0$.

The probability of co-occurrence satisfies the equation, $p_{ij} = \frac{c_{ij}}{\sum_i \sum_j c_{ij}}$. The candidate threshold $0 \leq s \leq L-1$ co-occurrence matrix that may be split into four regions representing class transitions within object (P_A), within background (P_C), object to background (P_B), and background to object (P_D). Let L be the maximum intensity value of the image to be analysed. The second-order entropy of the object ($H_A^{(2)}(s)$) and background ($H_C^{(2)}(s)$) are defined as:

$$H_A^{(2)}(s) = -\frac{1}{2} \sum_{i=0}^{s} \sum_{j=0}^{s} (P_{ij}/P_A) \log_2(P_{ij}/P_A)$$

$$H_C^{(2)}(s) = -\frac{1}{2} \sum_{i=s+1}^{L-1} \sum_{j=s+1}^{L-1} (P_{ij}/P_C) \log_2(P_{ij}/P_C).$$

Finally, the total second-order entropy of the object and the background are calculated, and the optimal threshold is estimated by maximizing the associated entropies as a function of the threshold. Using the proposed entropy based binarisation algorithm, one can obtain the threshold surface $\bar{s}(x,y)$ to be used with $s(x,y)$. An analysis of the entropy based filtered output shows that the response magnitude of the vessel pixels is larger near the centreline than near the vessel edges. Therefore binarisation is performed as follows:

$$\text{Out}(x,y) = \begin{cases} 1, & \bar{s}(x,y) \leq s(x,y) \\ 0, & \text{otherwise} \end{cases}$$

where $\text{Out}(\cdot)$ stands for the finally segmented binary mask of the vessel image. To obtain the initial mask of retinal vessels, a smaller magnitude of the threshold at vessel pixels near the vessel edges is selected. Finally, the eigenvalue based enhanced image (after threshold) shown in Fig. 3.19, is convolved with the entropy based mask shown in Fig. 3.20a. The resulting image is shown in Fig. 3.20b. The method performs well in extracting the enhanced retinal vessels from the background with significantly reduced noise compared to other unsupervised mask or segmentation techniques.

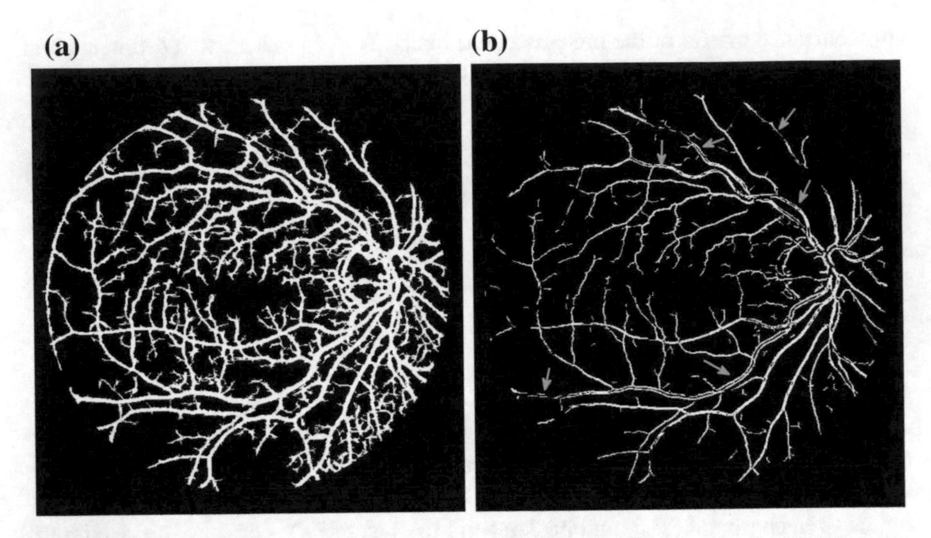

Fig. 3.20 Multiplication of images with an original image named `02_test` extracted from the DRIVE database. **a** Illustration of the resulting mask used for extraction of the enhanced retinal vessels through entropy based binarisation. **b** The resulting global thresholded image after combining (a) and the information in Fig. 3.19

3.2.5.3 Performing Segmentation on the Basis of Curvature Analysis

Segmentation using the proposed curvature analysis method often shows obvious signs of central light reflex. According to Spencer, the normal light reflex of the retinal vasculature is formed by reflection from the interface between the blood column and the vessel walls, and the thicker these vessel walls are, the more diffuse the light reflex becomes. This phenomenon is also accompanied by an overall decrease in the observed intensity [429–431]. In order to eliminate the undesirable effects of the central light reflex, the binarisation procedure using the top-hat pre-processing step of the images is repeated, this time using a larger threshold at the vessel pixels near the related centre-line of the retina vessels mostly affected by the central light reflex. The thresholds are manually adjusted and the ideal segments of the central light reflex vessels are re-calculated. The final segmentation is the result of a superposition of the segmentation from the extracted enhanced image, shown in Fig. 3.20b and the image binarisation step that was performed on the basis of the entropy criterion discussed earlier. This is shown in Fig. 3.21a, where the effect of the central light reflex, indicated by green arrows in Fig. 3.20b, has been removed in the resultant image, as shown in Fig. 3.21b. The proposed method is now known as the dual-threshold entropy approach, to differentiate it from the other retina vessel segmentation methods discussed in the literature, e.g. [434] (Fig. 3.21).

To achieve a clearer segmentation of blood vessels in the images of the retina, it is advisable to conduct additional morphology post-processing. This requires the use of morphological connectivity constraint operations which are applied on the

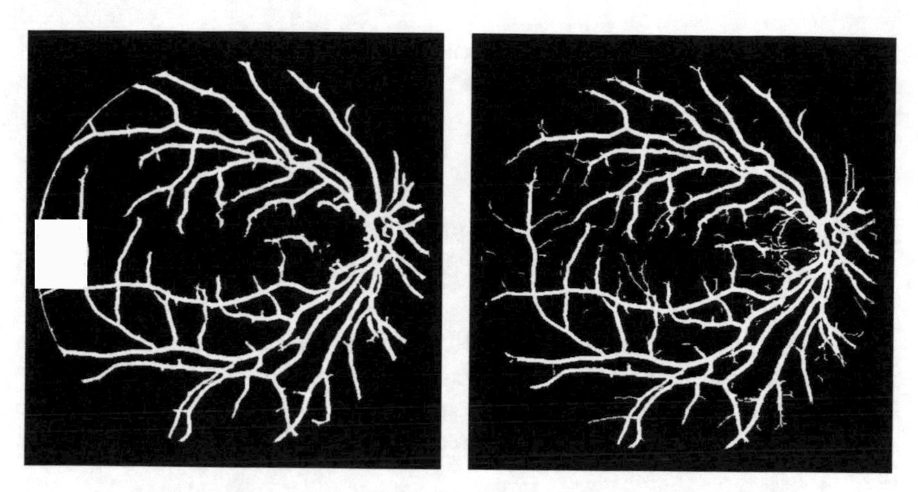

Fig. 3.21 Outputs of interim processing steps. The *left panel* is an illustration of binarisation with threshold selected to maximise entropy. The *right panel* is an illustration of the final segmentation, where the effect of central light reflex, indicated by *green arrows* in Fig. 3.20b has been removed in the resultant image

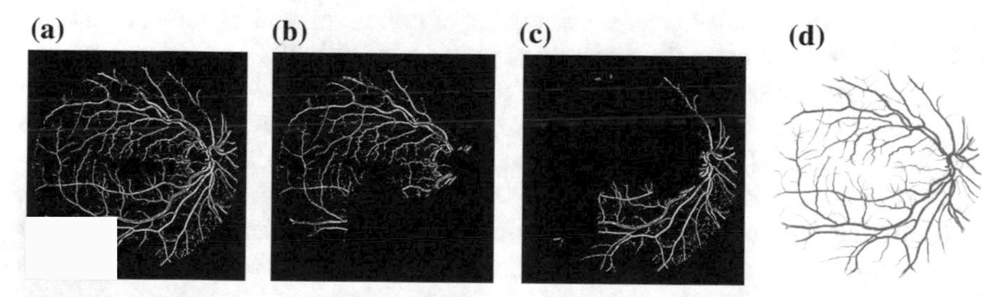

Fig. 3.22 Overview of the main steps in the proposed algorithm when processing a fundus image. **a** Illustration of globally thresholded image after multiplication between Figs. 3.19 and 3.20a. **b** and **c** Illustration of two partitions using segmentation of (**a**) on the basis of color coded mapping in Fig. 3.5b. **d** Illustration of good overlap (*blue*) between the resultant segment (*yellow*) and a gold standard segment (*green*)

extracted curvature based enhanced images. The connectivity constraint is determined according to the features present in the different textural regions. When the images display non-uniform illumination they can be partitioned into two regions by taking into consideration both variation in illumination as well as vessel size. For example, the extracted enhanced image illustrated in Fig. 3.22a, consists of two regions: one where small vessels are dominant Fig. 3.22b, where it is reasonable to select the smaller connectivity constraint and regions that consist mainly of larger vessels Fig. 3.22c. The vessel segments corresponding to different image textures are then linearly combined to produce the final segmentation of the curvature-based enhanced image. A similar method may be used to provide segmentation for a retinal image with tissue that depicts a pathological condition; in this case, the resulting segmented image differentiates well the two regions showing the presence or absence of pathology.

3.2.6 *Feature Extraction and Pattern Identification of Pathology Distortion in SD-OCT Imaging*

As discussed in Chap. 1, spectroscopic OCT provides additional information on the spectral content of backscattered light obtained by detection and processing of the interferometric OCT signal. The spectrum of backscattered light over the entire available optical bandwidth can be measured simultaneously in a single measurement [245].

Research carried out in [241], discusses current automatic methods of retinal SD-OCT image analysis by broadly separating them into four categories: (1) retinal layer tracking, (2) optic disc segmentation (3) vessel tracking and (4) pathology quantification [119, 432]. The layer tracking methods can be classified further into the following two groups: layer segmentation of normal or healthy subjects' images and layer segmentation in the presence of pathology [119, 432].

For clinical purposes, retinal SD-OCT image analysis should be capable of identifying and extracting the associated pathological features present in the image. This is discussed further in [241] where a method for automatic identification of the boundary of different layers captured in an SD-OCT image in the presence of pathology is presented. The approach first establishes an approximate location of three reference layers, and then uses these to bound the search space for the actual layers. This is achieved by representing the problem as a graph model and applying Dijkstra's shortest path algorithm so that the most likely order of the layers can be de-embedded. This work showed that the proposed method clearly identified retinal ILM-RNFL, ISLEZ,IZ-RPE and RBC boundaries from retinal SD-OCT B-scan images even in the presence of pathology.

The different steps involved in the implementation of the algorithm are shown in Fig. 3.23. In the first step, additive and speckle noise in the image are reduced by applying Wiener and Anisotropic Diffusion (AD) filters. Their function is to remove the associated impulse noise in the image while preserving the boundary position in all layers captured in the image. The second step computes the approximate locations of three reference (aprxTR) layers using their relative positions and pixel intensities. Following this procedure, the aprxTR layers are used as reference layers to detect the ILM-RNFL boundary. Due to its high contrast, the ILM-RNFL boundary is easily identifiable compared to other boundaries. This forms the basis for a reduced search space for computing the other boundaries. In step 4, the location of aprxTR layers is further refined to increase the accuracy of identification of other layer boundaries. In step 5, the RBC boundary is identified using the refined aprxTR layers. Through this procedure, the search region is further reduced to within the ILM-RNFL and

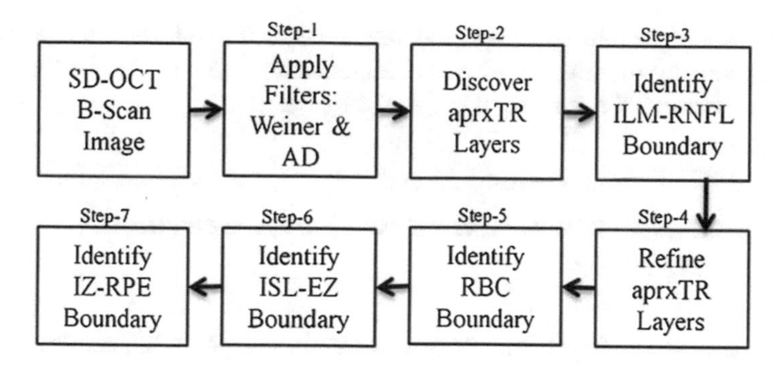

Fig. 3.23 Flow diagram of the proposed method by Hussain et al. [241] for automatic identification of pathology distorted retinal layer boundaries via SD-OCT imaging

RBC boundaries. This further reduced search space is used to identify the ISL-EZ boundary more accurately, in step 6. In the final step of the algorithm, the IZ-RPE boundary is identified by searching between the ISL-EZ and RBC boundaries.

It should be noted that IZ-RPE and RBC are the most difficult boundaries of the retina to be identified due to their low contrast and potential distortion by drusen (yellow deposits under the retina) as well as OCT identified atrophy. The boundary-confined search provides excellent accuracy even in the presence of pathology and displays superior performance over other methods discussed in the literature. A stochastic optimization method, Simulated Annealing (SA) [433], is used for approximating the global optimum which is used for finding each constant parameter.

Of particular note to the discussion above is that the algorithms developed for the identification of different layers in an image as developed by the SD-OCT community, may be further adapted to the identification of layered tissues in THz reflection tomography. In THz transient spectroscopy, it is currently not possible to identify different layers in an image when the layer thickness is smaller than the width of a pulse. Although in principle one could start with a very narrow pulse at the emitter port of the instrument, it is often the case that most samples will be quite dispersive so that, upon reflection on the sample, the pulse would have broadened too much for individual layers to be de-embedded by the gated echoes. The proposed methodology may thus provide a way for super-resolving the individual signatures from multiple layers if additional features in the image can be identified as discussed by the work in [241].

In a similar manner, the THz time-domain spectroscopy community has also developed their own super-resolution algorithms [274] which may be adopted by the OCT community. For continuous wave OCT methods, the work discussed in [44] may be adapted by developing specialized polarimetric fibre optic hardware to perform the reflectometric measurements using a null-balance de-embedding procedure. Alternatively, one could adapt to the optical part of the spectrum, the methodology discussed in [275], although the technique requires a more complex data acquisition procedure where the illumination would have to be performed over a range of angles (by systematically rotating the source at increments of one degree with respect to normal incidence to the eye over a range of angles).

3.2.7 Statistical Analysis Based on Feature Selection Strategies

Finally, it is worth noting that in medical research, data are often collected serially on subjects. The statistical analysis of such data is often inadequate in two ways: it may fail to settle clinically relevant questions and it may be statistically invalid. A commonly used method which compares groups at a series of time points, possibly with 't' tests, is flawed on both counts. As discussed by Matthews et al., (1990), however, [300] there may, be a remedy, which takes the form of a two stage method that uses summary measures. In the first stage a suitable summary of the response corresponding to an individual metric, such as a rate of change or an area under a curve, is identified and calculated for each subject. In the second stage these summary measures discussed in Sects. 3.2.2 and 3.2.3 are analysed by simple statistical techniques as though they were raw data. The method is statistically valid and likely to be more relevant to the study questions. If this type of analysis is borne in mind when the experiment is being planned it should promote studies with enough subjects and sufficient observations at critical times to enable useful conclusions to be drawn. Use of summary measures to analyse serial measurements, though not new, is potentially a useful and simple tool in medical research which could also be adopted when evaluating the performance of AI classifiers.

Chapter 4
Pattern Classification

This chapter discusses pattern classification of high dimensional medical datasets of breast, brain, and retinal tissue on the basis of their extracted features. The extracted features can show linear or non-linear separability, furthermore, they may also be multi-modal or highly correlated. Different algorithms that can be used to generate decision boundaries associated with the observed features are considered. Each feature is presented to a feature vector as a separate entry. The entire set or a subset of feature vectors is then used to perform the classification task. Statistical techniques commonly used for classification include those based on similarity measures (e.g. template matching, k-nearest neighbor), or those based on probabilistic assumptions (e.g. Bayes rule), definition of boundaries (e.g. decision trees, neural networks), and clustering (e.g. k-means, or hierarchical). In addition, this chapter discusses recent advances in complex support vector machine and extreme learning machine classifiers. An extension to multidimensional extreme learning machine classifiers is also provided. Examples of binary as well as multiclass classification tasks using THz datasets are presented. The performance of other classifiers such as multimodal logistic regression, and nave Bayesian, in classifying THz datasets is also compared. In addition, some recent advances in clustering and segmentation techniques for THz datasets as well as for fundus images are also discussed. Current methods for automatic retinal vessel classification are also highlighted, as it is envisaged that the improved edge detection algorithms discussed in the previous chapters in conjunction with the proposed classification methodologies can lead to better discrimination between arteries and veins. Finally, this chapter discusses some recent advances in automated image classification using performance criteria directly developed by clinicians.

4.1 Introduction to Pattern Classification

Following the discussions in the previous chapter regarding feature extraction, the quantitative features extracted from each object are organized into a fixed length feature vector. Each feature is represented within the vector (i.e. the first feature describes

X. Yin et al., *Pattern Classification of Medical Images: Computer Aided Diagnosis*, Health Information Science, DOI 10.1007/978-3-319-57027-3_4

a particular characteristic of the data, the second feature describes another characteristic, and so on). The collection of feature vectors generated by the description task are then passed on to perform the classification task. Statistical techniques used for the classification task include those based on similarity measures (e.g. template matching, k-nearest neighbor), or can be based on probabilistic assumptions (e.g. Bayes rule), or on the definition of boundaries (e.g. decision trees, neural networks), and clustering (e.g. k-means, hierarchical, multi-channel reconstruction [89]).

The quantitative nature of statistical pattern recognition makes it difficult to discriminate across different groups based solely on the morphological (i.e. shape based or structural) sub-patterns and their interrelationships embedded within the data. This limitation provided the impetus for the development of a structural approach to pattern recognition that is supported by psychological evidence pertaining to the functioning of human perception and cognition. Object recognition in humans has been demonstrated to involve mental representations of explicit, structure-oriented characteristics of objects, and human classification decisions have been shown to be made on the basis of the degree of similarity between the extracted features and those of a prototype developed for each group. For instance, the recognition by components theory explains the process of pattern recognition in humans: (1) the object is segmented into separate regions according to edges defined by differences in surface characteristics (e.g. luminance, texture, and color), (2) each segmented region is approximated by a simple geometric shape, and (3) the object is identified based on the similarity in composition between its geometric representation and the main characteristic features of each group. This theorized functioning of human perception and cognition serves as the foundation for the structural approach to pattern recognition.

The classification scheme is usually based on training sets that have already been successfully classified (supervised learning strategies) [31]. Learning can also be unsupervised, but such approaches usually fall short from a biomedical software certification perspective. The following sections discuss several schemes that have been successfully implemented for the imaging modalities considered such as statistical (or decision-theoretic) approaches using a Mahalanobis distance classifier [11, 12, 18], an Euclidean discrimination matrix, Support Vector Machines (SVMs) [17], Extreme Learning Machine [226, 447] (ELM) classifiers, ridge estimators, k-nearest neighbours (KNN), and naïve Bayes (NB) [350]. An overview of the adopted algorithms is also provided.

4.2 Feature Based Mahalanobis Distance Classifiers

The Mahalanobis distance classifier [435] is a type of minimum distance classifier that is optimal for normally distributed classes with equal covariance matrices (linear discriminant) and equal *a priori* probabilities. Such a classifier is often chosen because it is simple to implement and provides reasonable results for a variety of biomedical waveforms.

One possible approach is to formulate the Mahalanobis classification scheme on a set of feature matrices of Auto Regressive Moving Average (ARMA) modelled datasets after signal decomposition in wavelet subbands [11]. For a given class, m, the distance from a feature matrix $\mathbf{DC_j^{\mathit{l}}}$ to the class mean $\mathscr{A}_m$, is defined as

$$\rho_m(X) = \sqrt{(\mathbf{DC_j^{\mathit{l}}} - \mathscr{A}_m)^{\mathrm{T}} \mathbf{C}_m^{-1} (\mathbf{DC_j^{\mathit{l}}} - \mathscr{A}_m)} \tag{4.1}$$

where $\mathbf{C}_m$ is the covariance matrix of the feature vectors regarding class m, $\mathbf{DC_j^{\mathit{l}}}$ with $l = 1, 2, 3$ represents the averaged coefficients matrix related to AR ($l = 1$), MA ($l = 2$), and ARMA ($l = 3$) modeling of wavelet approximation coefficients at three decomposition levels $\mathbf{j}$, that is, $\mathbf{DC_j^1}$ being $\mathbf{DC_j^{AR}}$, $\mathbf{DC_j^2}$ being $\mathbf{DC_j^{MA}}$, $\mathbf{DC_j^3}$ being $\mathbf{DC_j^{ARMA}}$. In practice, the covariance matrix is estimated from the training vectors. During classification, the minimum Mahalanobis distance from the feature matrix $\mathbf{DC_j^{\mathit{l}}}$ to each class centre $\mathscr{A}_m$, is used to assign the appropriate class label.

4.3 Support Vector Machine Classifiers (SVMs)

Recent advances in statistical learning theory [451] have led to a wide proliferation of an important class of machine learning algorithms known as Support Vector Machines. (SVM) These algorithms perform a mapping of lower-dimensional datasets into a high-dimensional feature space where a separating hyperplane, which maximizes the boundary margin between two classes, can be established. Although originally SVMs have been used for binary classification tasks, recent extensions have extended their use to multiclass classification problems. Both of these algorithms are discussed in the following sections.

4.3.1 Binary Classification of SVMs

In their simplest implementation, support vector machines are binary classifiers, which classify data on the basis of a set of support vectors [452]. The training data sets are obtained from a set of labelled samples called learning vectors. We denote such a set of learning vectors as $(\mathbf{x_i}, y_i) \in R^N \times \{\pm 1\}, i = 1, \ldots, l$, and y_i denote the class label corresponding to each input vector $\mathbf{x}_i$. The support vectors are subsets of the training data sets and are used to construct an l-dimensional hyperplane in feature space, which acts as a boundary separating the different classes. A decision function $f(\alpha) : R^N \rightarrow \pm 1$ is calculated based on a given class function $f(\alpha) : \alpha \in \Lambda$, and the aim is to correctly assign class labels to test unclassified samples $\mathbf{x}$. The Vapnik-Chervonenkis (VC) dimension [451, 453] is a property of a set of functions $f(\alpha)$, which is defined as the maximum number of training points that can be segmented by $f(\alpha)$. Note that α corresponds to the weights and biases, which can be adjusted to label the output $f(\mathbf{x}, \alpha)$ based on the input $\mathbf{x}$. The expectation of the test error for a learning machine is:

$$R(\alpha) = \int \frac{1}{2}|y - f(\mathbf{x}, \alpha)| \mathrm{d}P(\mathbf{x}, y) \tag{4.2}$$

where, $R(\alpha)$ is called the expected risk. It is the quantity associated with density $p(\mathbf{x}, y)$ that the user is ultimately interested in. The 'empirical risk' $R_{\mathrm{emp}}(\alpha)$ is defined to be the measured mean training error for a fixed, finite number of observations:

$$R_{\mathrm{emp}}(\alpha) = \frac{1}{2l} \sum_{i=1}^{l} |y_i - f(\mathbf{x}_i, \alpha)|. \tag{4.3}$$

The quantity $\frac{1}{2}|y_i - f(\mathbf{x}_i, \alpha)|$, which is called the loss, and may have two values, 0 or 1. When the user sets the probability to $1 - \eta$, the following bound is observed for the classification task:

$$R(\alpha) \leq R_{\mathrm{emp}}(\alpha) + \sqrt{\left(\frac{h(\log(2l/h)+1)-\log(\eta/4)}{l}\right)}. \tag{4.4}$$

The non-negative integer h is called the VC dimension, and provides a measure of the *capacity* of multiple hypotheses that can be considered on the basis of the available training data. When a sufficiently small η is selected, the right hand side of the equation is minimized, and the $f(\mathbf{x}, \alpha)$ functions provide the lowest upper bound of the actual classification risk. This is the reason SVMs are often associated with structural risk minimization.

As minimizing the training error (the computation of VC-dimension) does not guarantee a small test error, to make the decision function f perform well on previously unseen patterns, the principle of structural risk minimization needs to be applied to minimize the test error and achieve a capacity that is suitable for the amount of available training data sets.

The learning algorithm is designed to allow the computation of support vectors by implicitly performing structure risk minimization. In other words, a VC-dimension bound is calculated to identify the optimal hyperplane that maximizes the margin of the nearest learning vectors. The decision hyperplane is calculated based on the following equation:

$$f(\mathbf{x}) = \mathrm{sgn}\left(\sum_{i=1}^{s} y_i \alpha_i (\mathbf{x}_i \cdot \mathbf{x}) + b\right) \tag{4.5}$$

where $\mathbf{x}_i$, $(i = 1, \ldots, s)$ are support vectors, which are the closest points from the training vectors (learning vectors) to the separate hyperplane where sgn is the signum function. The solution of this large-scale quadratic programming problem is used to calculate the coefficients α_i and b. The procedure requires the solving of the well known dual problem, which is to maximize

$$L(\alpha) = \sum_{i=1}^{l} \alpha_i - \frac{1}{2} \sum_{i,j=1}^{l} \alpha_i \alpha_j y_i y_j (\mathbf{x}_i \cdot \mathbf{x}_j) \tag{4.6}$$

subject to $\sum_{i=1}^{l} \alpha_i y_i = 0$ and $0 \leq \alpha_i \leq C$ for $i = 1, \ldots, l$.

The penalty parameter C is selected by the user. This should be viewed as a regularization parameter for the linearly inseparable learning vectors aiming to accept the possible misclassifications.

Note that SVMs use a kernel function [349, 454], which allows the fitting of the hyperplane to the data. Instead of a linear classifier, which is limited to producing linear decision surfaces, the hyperplane [455] may also need to be modified to fit nonlinear decision surfaces. In order to generate such non-linear decision surface, a dot product space is constructed by re-mapping the data, this is realised by performing a nonlinear mapping operation $\phi : R^N \rightarrow F$. The above linear algorithm then can be applied in the new feature space F. The solution satisfies the following expression:

$$f(\mathbf{x}) = \mathrm{sgn}(\sum_{i=1}^{s} y_i \alpha_i \phi(\mathbf{x}_i) \cdot \phi(\mathbf{x}) + b). \tag{4.7}$$

This is a nonlinear transformation of the original input vectors $\mathbf{x}$.

According to Cover's theorem [456], a new feature space F can be defined in a multidimensional space, where the dimensionality of the feature space is high enough to allow the target patterns to be linearly separable with a high probability. The inner products (dot products) enable the high dimensional space to be identified through the mapping of function ϕ. Accordingly, the kernel function K is defined as:

$$K(\mathbf{x}, \mathbf{y}) = \phi(\mathbf{x}) \cdot \phi(\mathbf{y}). \tag{4.8}$$

There are four popular kernel functions:

- linear Kernel:

$$K(\mathbf{x}, \mathbf{y}) = \mathbf{x}^{\mathrm{T}}\mathbf{y} \tag{4.9}$$

- polynomial kernel:

$$K(\mathbf{x}, \mathbf{y}) = (\gamma \mathbf{x}^{\mathrm{T}}\mathbf{y} + r)^p, \gamma > 0 \tag{4.10}$$

- RBF (Gaussian) kernel:

$$K(\mathbf{x}, \mathbf{y}) = \exp(-\lambda \left\| \mathbf{x} - \mathbf{y} \right\|^2), \lambda > 0 \tag{4.11}$$

- Hyperbolic tangent kernel:

$$K(\mathbf{x}, \mathbf{y}) = \tanh(\gamma \mathbf{x}^{\mathrm{T}}\mathbf{y} + r), \gamma > 0 \tag{4.12}$$

where $\mathbf{x}$, $\mathbf{y}$ are SVM data vectors, T denotes vector transpose, γ and r denote the scale and offset of the corresponding kernels respectively (they are normally set to 1), p denotes the degree of polynomial kernel, and λ denotes the width parameter of the Gaussian kernel.

In the instance of identifying RNA samples, presented in Fig. 4.6, the RBF kernel function is used as the preferred choice, and it was found to give good classification performance. Meanwhile, it was found that polynomial kernels were best suited to achieve multiclass classification of powdered samples.

4.3.2 Pairwise SVM Classification of Multiple Classes

The previous section described a SVM for two-class THz pulse signal classification. This type of binary hypothesis is addressed by *dichotomy* (from Greek 'τομη', or sectioning), classifiers. This is appropriate for simple two-class classification problems where, say, different objects from T-ray pulses need to be discriminated. However, the majority of object recognition problems require the simultaneous classification of several objects. The optimal choice of design parameters of multiclass SVM classifiers is still an area of active research. One frequently adopted method is to use a pairwise classifier, based on one-against-one decomposition, and a decision function, f_{kl}. Here, kl indicates each pair of classes selected from separated target classes. One can write $f_{kl} = -f_{kl}$, where f_{kl} satisfies the following equation:

$$f_{kl}(\mathbf{x}) = \mathbf{w}_{kl}\mathbf{x} + b_{kl} \tag{4.13}$$

where $\mathbf{w}$ is normal to the hyperplane between class k and class l, $|b|/||\mathbf{w}||$ is the perpendicular distance from the hyperplane to the origin, and $||\mathbf{w}||$ is the Euclidean norm of $\mathbf{w}$ with a vector dimension of M.

The signum function is used for the hard threshold decisions:

$$\mathrm{sgn}(f_{kl}(\mathbf{x})) = \begin{cases} 1, & f_{kl}(\mathbf{x}) > 0 \\ -1, & f_{kl}(\mathbf{x}) \leq 0. \end{cases} \tag{4.14}$$

The class decision can be achieved by summing up the pairwise decision functions according to:

$$f_k(\mathbf{x}) = \sum_{k \neq l, l=1}^{n} \mathrm{sgn}(f_{kl}(\mathbf{x})) \tag{4.15}$$

where n is the number of the separated target classes.

The pairwise classifier proceeds as follows: assign a label to the class, $\{\text{argmax}\, f_k(\mathbf{x}), (k = 1, \ldots, n)\}$. The max number of votes for k classes holds $\{\max k \rightarrow f_k = (k-1)\}$. If Eq. (4.15) is satisfied for $\{\max k \rightarrow f_k < (k-1)\}$, $\mathbf{x}$ is unclassifiable. The pairwise classification procedure, iteratively converts the n-class classification problem into $n(n-1)/2$ two-class problems which cover all pairs of classes.

4.3.3 Application of SVM Classifiers to THz-TPI Measurements

Kernel based learning and SVM methodologies reside at the core of a range of interdisciplinary challenges. Their formulation shares concepts from different disciplines such as: linear algebra, mathematics, statistics, signal processing, systems and control theory, optimization, machine learning, pattern recognition, data mining and neural networks. As stated earlier, the idea of the SVM is to map data from the input space into a high-dimensional feature space, in which an optimal separating hyperplane that maximizes the boundary margin between two classes can be established. At its core, SVMs are two-class classifiers. Recently, SVMs have been extended to solve multi-class classification problems from noisy biomedical measurements. Furthermore, there are several reports discussing the use of SVMs for THz material identification. Pan et al. [436] used SVMs to classify THz absorption spectra for the purpose of illicit drug identification. They successfully identified seven pure illicit drugs establishing this methodology for drug identification. Fitzgerald et al. [166] applied the SVM approaches combined with a radial basis function to discriminate normal from malignant breast tissue from THz-TPI. Yin et al. [17] applied SVMs to perform multi-class classification of THz powder spectra for six types of powder materials with similar optical properties. Figure 4.1 illustrates the multi-class separation for these six types of powder substances using SVMs, after adopting according to a pair wise-strategy. One real Gaussian kernel with $C = 1000$ and $\sigma = 1 \times 10^{-7}$ is used to map the input data into a 2D Fourier feature space for visualisation purposes. The support vectors indicated by cyan circles are subsets of the training data sets and are used to construct a two-dimensional hyperplane in feature space that acts as a boundary separating each class of different powder materials.

Within the MRI community, SVM is also quickly being established as an important emergent classification modality. Examples of early adoption of the technique include the work by Selvaraj et al. who used linear as well as nonlinear Radial Basis Function (RBF) kernels and compared those with other classifiers like SVM with linear and nonlinear RBF kernels, an RBF classifier, a Multi Layer Perceptron (MLP) classifier and a K-NN classifier to identify normal and abnormal slices of brain MRI data [437]. Their work showed promising results using least-squares (LSSVM) classifiers. Other examples include SVM based meta-analysis combining information from magnetic resonance imaging (MRI) and fluorodeoxyglucose positron emission tomography (FDG-PET) for improved detection and differentiation of Alzheimer's

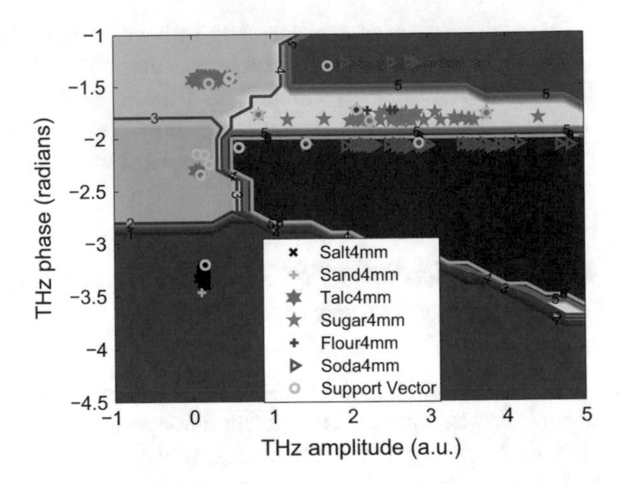

Fig. 4.1 Learning vectors for the powder data sets plotted to illustrate the linear decision function between the pairs of classes after applying a Gaussian kernel for mapping. There are 49 pixels randomly selected from each of the six powder samples. Background colour clearly shows the contour shape of the decision surface. The small *yellow* region on the *bottom* of the *right* hand side denotes undecided classification

disease, dementia and frontotemporal lobar degeneration [438]. Singh and Kaur discussed the possibility of performing classification of abnormalities in brain MRI images using GLCM, PCA and SVM [439]. Zacharaki et al. provided preliminary results on MRI data classification of brain tumour types and grades [440]. This work was followed by another study [440] combining textural (Gabor texture) and shape information using a ranking based criterion for feature selection (RFE) before presenting the sub-features to SVM-RFE, LDA, and k-NN classifiers. Zhang et al. [441] proposed multi-kernel SVM integrated with a fusion process, to segment brain tumor from multi-sequence MRI (T2, PD, FLAIR) images. Ortiz et al. [442] discussed MRI image segmentation using SOM and CONN linkage and subsequent feature reduction based on Fisher Discriminant Ratio (FDR) and Learning Vector Quantization (LVQ) using a hybrid (LVQ-SVM) algorithm for the diagnosis of the Alzheimer's Disease (AD). There have also been examples of deep learning based feature representation such as the work in [443] which proposed computer-aided diagnosis of AD at early stages of mild cognitive impairment. The comprehensive study by Aguilar et al. [444] that used four supervised learning methods to classify AD patients: controls orthogonal projections to latent structures (OPLS), decision trees (Trees), artificial neural networks (ANN) and LIBSVM implementation of SVM also paves the way for the adoption of deep learning techniques in the future. Another study by Akselrod-Ballin et al. [445] that combines a multiscale multi-channel three dimensional segmentation algorithm with an SVM classifier for the automatic identification of anatomical brain structures in MRI, can also be placed in a deep learning context. Feature selection in that work is also biased using an MRI probabilistic atlas. As discussed in a following section, the above studies make artificial intelligence algorithms based on deep architectures, a focal point for future research. Recent multispectral MRI studies [446] are also pointing towards a need to consider a multi-parametric input classifier space. So in the following section an extreme learning machine (ELM) classifier is discussed as it has been recently extended to higher dimensional spaces.

4.4 Real-Valued Extreme Learning Machine Classifier

The real-valued extreme learning machine is a generalised single-hidden-layer feed-forward network (SLFN). It maps the training data $\mathbf{X}$ from input space to feature space using a feature map $\boldsymbol{\psi}(\mathbf{X})$ with output weights ω. In contrast to SVMs, ELM theory [448, 449] shows that the item bias b should not be given in the ELM learning. Therefore, in this feature space, a linear decision function f_L is constructed as $\mathrm{f}_L(\mathbf{X}) = \boldsymbol{\psi}(\mathbf{X})\omega^v$ where $\omega^v = [\omega_1, \ldots, \omega_L]^T$ is the vector of the output weights between the hidden layer of L nodes and the output node and $\boldsymbol{\psi}(\mathbf{X}) = [\varphi_1(\mathbf{X}), \ldots, \varphi_L(\mathbf{X})]$ is the output feature vector of the hidden layer with respect to the input $\mathbf{X}$. The latter maps the data from the λ dimensional input space to the L-dimensional hidden-layer feature space or ELM feature space $\mathscr{H}$.

Given a set of training data (x_i, ϑ_i^v), and $\boldsymbol{\theta} = [\vartheta_1^v, \ldots, \vartheta_N^v]^T$ with ϑ_i^v $(i \in 1, \ldots, N)$ real-valued known label matrix corresponding to m classes, the function of the ELM algorithm is to minimize the training error $\| \boldsymbol{\psi}\boldsymbol{\omega} - \boldsymbol{\theta} \|^2$ and the norm of the output weights $\|\boldsymbol{\omega}\|$. The hidden-layer feature mapping matrix ψ is represented as:

$$\psi = \begin{bmatrix} \varphi_1(x_1) & \cdots & \varphi_L(x_1) \\ \vdots & \vdots & \vdots \\ \varphi_1(x_N) & \cdots & \varphi_L(x_N) \end{bmatrix} \tag{4.16}$$

where the size of ψ is only decided by the numbers of training samples N and the number of hidden nodes L, which is irrelevant to the number of output nodes (number of classes), and $x_1, \ldots, x_n \in \mathbf{X}$.

For an m class classifier with m output nodes where $m > 1$, the classification problem (denoted by $\hbar_P$) using the ELM classifier can be formulated as

$$\min : \hbar_P = \frac{1}{2}\|\boldsymbol{\omega}\|^2 + C\frac{1}{2}\sum_{i=1}^{N} \|\xi_i^v\|^2 \tag{4.17}$$

where $\xi_i^{vT} = \vartheta_i^{vT} - \boldsymbol{\psi}(x_i)\boldsymbol{\omega}$, $i = 1, \ldots, N$, $\vartheta_i^v = \vartheta_{i,1}, \ldots, \vartheta_{i,N}$, $\boldsymbol{\omega} = [\omega_1^v, \ldots, \omega_m^v]$, and the training error vector $\xi_i^v = [\xi_{i,1}, \ldots, \xi_{i,m}]^T$. Symbol C is a penalty variable, which is a user-specific parameter and provides a trade-off between the distance of the separating margin and the training errors. When the Sth element $\vartheta_{i,S}$ is one and the remaining of ϑ_i^v are zero, that means the original class label is S.

The Karush-Khun-Tuker (KKT) theorem is used to solve the dual optimization problem (denoted by $\hbar_D$) in order to train the ELM classifier:

$$\hbar_D = \frac{1}{2}\|\boldsymbol{\omega}\|^2 + C\frac{1}{2}\sum_{i=1}^{N}\|\xi_i^{\nu}\|^2$$
$$-\sum_{i=1}^{N}\sum_{\iota=1}^{m} a_{i,\iota}(\psi(x_i)\omega_\iota - \vartheta_{i,\iota} - \xi_{i,\iota}) \tag{4.18}$$

where ω_ι^ν is the vector of the weights linking the hidden layer to the ιth output node, and $\boldsymbol{\omega} = [\omega_1^\nu, \ldots, \omega_m^\nu]$. The Lagrange multiplier $\mathbf{A} = [\mathbf{a}_1, \ldots, \mathbf{a}_N]^T$ is used with each element $\mathbf{a}_i = [a_{i,1}, \ldots, a_{i,m}]$ to be a vector. The rules of Wirtinger's Calculus are employed to compute the respective gradients:

$$\frac{\partial \hbar_D}{\partial \omega_\iota^\nu} = 0 \rightarrow \boldsymbol{\omega} = \boldsymbol{\psi}^T\mathbf{A} \tag{4.19}$$

$$\frac{\partial \hbar_D}{\partial \xi_i^\nu} = 0 \rightarrow \mathbf{a}_i = C\xi_i^\nu, \quad i = 1, \ldots, N \tag{4.20}$$

$$\frac{\partial \hbar_D}{\partial \mathbf{a}_i} = 0 \rightarrow \boldsymbol{\psi}(x_i)\boldsymbol{\omega} - \vartheta_i^{\nu T} + \xi_i^{\nu T} = 0, \quad i = 1, \ldots, N \tag{4.21}$$

According to the aforementioned equations, for the case where the number of training samples is not too large ($L >> N$) the output function of the ELM classifier is:

$$\mathrm{f}(\mathbf{X}) = \boldsymbol{\psi}(\mathbf{X})\omega = \boldsymbol{\psi}(\mathbf{X})\boldsymbol{\psi}^T(\frac{\mathbf{I}}{C} + \boldsymbol{\psi}\boldsymbol{\psi}^T)^{-1}\boldsymbol{\theta} \tag{4.22}$$

where $\mathbf{I} = [1, 1, \ldots, 1]^T$.

With $\mathrm{f}_\iota(\mathbf{X})$ denoting the output function of the ιth output node and $\mathrm{f}(\mathbf{X}) = [\mathrm{f}_1(\mathbf{X}), \ldots, \mathrm{f}_m(\mathbf{X})]$, the predicted class label of sample $\mathbf{X}$ is

$$\mathrm{label}(\mathbf{X}) = \arg_{i \in 1,\ldots,m} \max \mathrm{f}_i(\mathbf{X}). \tag{4.23}$$

In this case where the number of training samples is very large ($N >> L$), the output function of the ELM classifier is given from:

$$\mathrm{f}(\mathbf{X}) = \boldsymbol{\psi}(\mathbf{X})\omega = \boldsymbol{\psi}(\mathbf{X})(\frac{\mathbf{I}}{C} + \boldsymbol{\psi}^T\boldsymbol{\psi})^{-1}\boldsymbol{\psi}^T\boldsymbol{\theta} \tag{4.24}$$

4.5 Complex Valued ELMs for Classification

Another important direction for feature classification is discussed in the recent work by Yin et al. [447], where they discussed the application of extended Extreme Learning Machines (ELMs) [448, 449] to complex valued problems. The motivation for the proposed extension stems from the fact that the real valued ELM has shown some of the lowest training errors among machine learning algorithms and in particular SVM classifiers [17, 31, 450, 451]. Furthermore, existing machine learning techniques are focused on real valued datasets.

Traditional amplitude only based pattern mining approaches of spatio-temporal images has classification limitations in samples that display highly correlated time-frequency or time-space features. The complex-valued ELMs (CELMs) adopt induced complex RKHS kernels [458] to map inputs from complex-valued non-linear spaces to other real valued higher dimensional linear spaces. This permits us to classify the inputs with linear complex valued feature vectors, for example, preserving the information in the phase of the signal (dispersion). This approach is based on concepts developed for complex or quaternion variable classification, through the introduction of two complex-coupled hyperplanes [459]. A widely linear estimation processing approach is adopted and the argument composed of the sum of the two parts (real and imaginary) is employed to relate the input feature space to the output feature space through the hidden layer of the classifier. This approach enables us to define a kernel function specific for the separation of the data in high dimensional complex coupled hyperplanes. The approach is also compatible with the processing of datasets in tensorial format which enable additional image features (hyperspectral, amplitude, phase, polarization or spatiotemporal components) to be simultaneously retained.

4.5.1 *Review of Complex-Valued RKHS and Wirtinger's Calculus*

Kernel based methods have been used as popular tools to solve non-linear classification problems in machine learning, among which Reproducing Kernel Hilbert Spaces (RKHS) algorithms play a central role. Recently, a novel class of complex-valued RKHS (CRKHS) algorithms was introduced aimed at mapping the inputs to the primal and dual Hilbert space [459]. The general class of CRKHS algorithms develop kernel algorithms in the widely linear sense [459] that are suitable for the processing of complex-valued data, i.e. higher dimensional datasets which are often associated with separable features in both space and time. Throughout this section, we denote the sets of all integers, real and complex numbers by $\mathscr{N}$, $\mathscr{R}$, and $\mathscr{C}$ respectively. We use $\Re$ and $\Im$ to denote the real and imaginary parts. The imaginary operator is denoted by $\mathscr{J}$. Complex-valued quantities are denoted using the caret symbol and matrix and vector valued quantities are labelled by boldfaced symbols.

The CRKHS algorithm performs a nonlinear estimation via mapping the input space to an infinite dimensional feature space, where the output is a linear combination of the feature maps. The presented methods build upon kernel matrices of the form $(\hat{\boldsymbol{\psi}}(\hat{z}_1), \ldots, \hat{\boldsymbol{\psi}}(\hat{z}_N))$, $N \in \mathscr{N}$, and $\hat{z}_n$ $(n = 1, 2, \ldots, N)$ denotes the nth set of complex valued input data with $\hat{z}_n \in \mathscr{C}^{(\varpi)}$ and ϖ denoting the number of dimensions of $\hat{z}_n$. The complex data $\hat{\mathbf{Z}} = \hat{z}_1, \hat{z}_2, \ldots, \hat{z}_N$ are mapped to the feature space $\hat{\mathscr{H}}$ such that $\hat{\boldsymbol{\psi}} : \mathscr{C}^n \rightarrow \hat{\mathscr{H}} : \hat{\boldsymbol{\psi}}(\hat{\mathbf{Z}}) = \hat{\kappa}(\cdot, \hat{\mathbf{Z}})$, where $\hat{\mathscr{H}}$ is also called complex-valued Hilbert spaces and is the complex-valued RKHS induced by the complex kernel function $\hat{\kappa} : \hat{\chi} \times \hat{\chi} \rightarrow \hat{\mathrm{f}}$ with $\hat{\mathbf{Z}} = \mathbf{X} + \mathscr{J}\mathbf{Y} \in \hat{\chi}$, and $\hat{\mathrm{f}}$ is a complex decision function. We call $\hat{\boldsymbol{\psi}}$, the feature map of $\hat{\mathscr{H}}$. An important complex kernel that may be used is the complex Gaussian kernel. This is defined as follows:

$$\kappa^{j}_{\sigma_j, \mathscr{C}^d}(\hat{\mathbf{Z}}, \hat{\boldsymbol{\omega}}) := \exp\left(- \frac{\sum_{k=1}^{d} (\hat{z}_k - \hat{\boldsymbol{\omega}}_k^*)^2}{\sigma_j^2} \right), \tag{4.25}$$

where $\hat{\mathbf{Z}}, \hat{\boldsymbol{\omega}} \in \mathscr{C}^d$, $d \in \mathscr{N}$ or infinite, and $\hat{\boldsymbol{\omega}}$ labels complex weight (margin), with the symbol $*$ denoting a Hermitian matrix, $\hat{z}_k$ denoting the k-th component of the complex vector $\hat{\mathbf{Z}} \in \mathscr{C}^d$ and $\exp(\cdot)$ denotes the extended exponential function in the complex domain. Here, κ^j indicates the j-th kernel function, depending on the value of kernel parameter σ_j, which in our case can be varied to account for different input requirements. A simpler method is to fix the value of kernel parameter σ_j to σ for all kernels in order to simplify computation [457].

The inner product of a complex kernel function $\hat{\kappa}$ is defined so that it satisfies the following equations:

$$\hat{\kappa}(\hat{\mathbf{Z}}, \hat{\mathbf{Z}}') = (\langle \hat{\kappa}(\cdot, \hat{\mathbf{Z}}), \hat{\kappa}(\cdot, \hat{\mathbf{Z}}') \rangle_{\hat{\mathscr{H}}})^* \tag{4.26}$$

This equation shows that the inner product of the complex kernel function $\hat{\kappa}$ is Hermitian, indicated by $*$. We define the spaces $\mathscr{X}^2 \equiv \mathscr{X} \times \mathscr{X} \subseteq \mathscr{R}^{2n}$ and $\hat{\mathbf{Z}}, \hat{\mathbf{Z}}' \in \hat{\chi} \subseteq \mathscr{C}^n$ (two complex inputs to be classified on the basis of $\hat{\mathbf{Z}}$ and $\hat{\mathbf{Z}}'$). Then every $\hat{\mathrm{f}} \in \hat{\mathscr{H}}$ can be viewed as a function defined on either $\mathscr{X}^2$ or $\hat{\chi}$ such that

$$\hat{\mathrm{f}}(\hat{\mathbf{Z}}) = \hat{\mathrm{f}}(\mathbf{X} + \mathscr{J}\mathbf{Y}) = \hat{\mathrm{f}}(\mathbf{X}, \mathbf{Y}). \tag{4.27}$$

According to [458], the complexity of Hilbert space $\hat{\mathscr{H}} = \hat{\mathrm{f}}^{\Re} + \mathscr{J}\hat{\mathrm{f}}^{\Im}; \hat{\mathrm{f}}^{\Re}, \hat{\mathrm{f}}^{\Im} \in \mathscr{H}$ is a doubled real space $\mathscr{H}$, and satisfies $\hat{\mathscr{H}} = \mathscr{H} \times \mathscr{H} = \mathscr{H}^2$. The complexified space $\hat{\mathscr{H}}$ is a complex RKHS with complex kernel $\hat{\kappa}$, which can be represented by its respective real kernel with corresponding imaginary part of zero. The complex feature map $\hat{\boldsymbol{\psi}}(\hat{\mathbf{Z}})$ of the sampled data from the complex input space to the complexified RKHS $\hat{\mathscr{H}}$ follows the equation:

$$\hat{\boldsymbol{\psi}}(\hat{\mathbf{Z}}) = \hat{\boldsymbol{\psi}}(\mathbf{X} + \mathscr{J}\mathbf{Y}) = \hat{\boldsymbol{\psi}}(\mathbf{X}, \mathbf{Y}) = \boldsymbol{\psi}(\mathbf{X}, \mathbf{Y}) + \mathscr{J}\boldsymbol{\psi}(\mathbf{X}, \mathbf{Y}) \tag{4.28}$$

where $\psi \in \mathscr{R}$ is the feature map of the real reproducing kernel $\kappa \in \mathscr{R}$ and satisfying $\psi(\mathbf{X}, \mathbf{Y}) = \kappa(\cdot, (\mathbf{X}, \mathbf{Y}))$.

We deduce the following equation:

$$\begin{aligned}\langle \hat{\psi}(\hat{\mathbf{Z}}), \hat{\psi}(\hat{\mathbf{Z}}')\rangle_{\hat{\mathscr{H}}} &= 2\langle \psi(\mathbf{X}, \mathbf{Y}), \psi(\mathbf{X}', \mathbf{Y}')\rangle_{\mathscr{H}} \\ &= 2\kappa\langle (\mathbf{X}', \mathbf{Y})', (\mathbf{X}, \mathbf{Y})\rangle \end{aligned} \tag{4.29}$$

We can extend the two-dimensional complex inner product to three dimensions. This can be described as

$$\begin{aligned}&\langle \hat{\psi}(\hat{\mathbf{Z}}), \hat{\psi}(\hat{\mathbf{Z}}')\rangle_{\hat{\mathscr{H}}} = \langle \psi(\mathbf{X}, \mathbf{Y}, \mathbf{V}), \psi(\mathbf{X}', \mathbf{Y}', \mathbf{V}')\rangle_{\mathscr{H}^3} \\ &= 2\langle [\mathbf{e}_1', \mathbf{e}_2'], [\mathbf{e}_1, \mathbf{e}_2]\rangle + 2\langle [\mathbf{e}_2', \mathbf{e}_3'], [\mathbf{e}_2, \mathbf{e}_3]\rangle + 2\langle [\mathbf{e}_1', \mathbf{e}_3'], [\mathbf{e}_1, \mathbf{e}_3]\rangle \end{aligned} \tag{4.30}$$

where $[\mathbf{e}_1, \mathbf{e}_2] = \psi(\mathbf{X}, \mathbf{Y}) = \psi(\mathbf{Y}, \mathbf{X}) = [\mathbf{X}, \mathbf{Y}]$ with $\mathbf{X}, \mathbf{Y} \in \mathscr{R}$, and similar to $[\mathbf{e}_1, \mathbf{e}_3]$, $[\mathbf{e}_2, \mathbf{e}_3]$, $[\mathbf{e}_1', \mathbf{e}_2']$, $[\mathbf{e}_1', \mathbf{e}_3']$, and $[\mathbf{e}_2', \mathbf{e}_3']$. The bivectors $\mathbf{e}_\upsilon$ and $\mathbf{e}_\upsilon'$, $\upsilon = 1, 2, 3$ are the orthonormal basis (planes) of the two complex inputs $\hat{\mathbf{Z}}$ and $\hat{\mathbf{Z}}' = \mathscr{R}\mathbf{X}' + \mathscr{J}\mathbf{Y}' + \mathscr{K}\mathbf{V}'$, respectively, where the quantities $\mathscr{R}$, $\mathscr{J}$ and $\mathscr{K}$ are the scalar parts of a hypercomplex-like inner product structure; the kernel function with the equation $\kappa(,) = \langle , \rangle$ reproduces a Hilbert space $\mathscr{H}$. By following Eq. 4.30, we can easily deduce that the dual of the 3D complexified ELM task is equivalent to six real ELM tasks employing the kernel 2κ.

4.5.2 *Defining Higher-Dimension Hyprplanes Using Quaternion and Other Division Algebras for Classification*

An important aspect in machine learning is to find hyperplanes that separate the associated input and output vector spaces according to different target classes. Using a binary classification for example, as shown in Fig. 4.2, a hyperplane can be defined

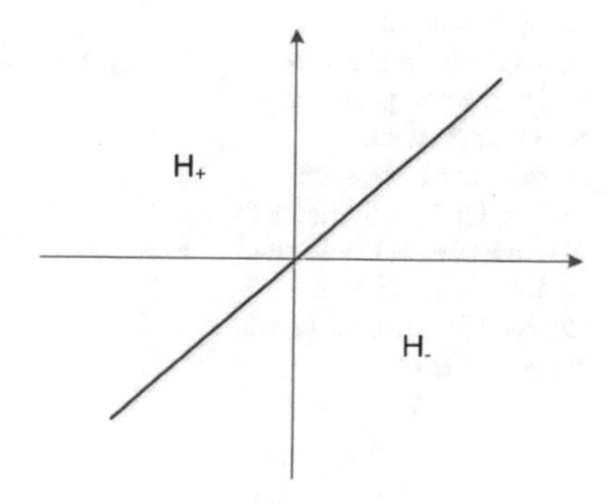

Fig. 4.2 Illustration of a hyperplane in EML to separate the space $\mathscr{H}$ into two parts, $\mathscr{H}_+$ and $\mathscr{H}_-$

for the Extreme Learning Machine to separate the space $\mathscr{H}$ into two parts, $\mathscr{H}_+$ and $\mathscr{H}_-$.

Recall that in any real Hilbert space $\mathscr{H}$, a hyperplane may be defined, containing all the elements $\mathrm{f} \in \mathscr{H}$ that satisfy

$$\langle \mathrm{f}, \boldsymbol{\omega} \rangle_{\mathscr{H}} = 0, \tag{4.31}$$

for some $\boldsymbol{\omega} \in \mathscr{H}$. In contrast to real-valued SVM algorithms, in the real-valued ELM algorithms, the offset of the hyperplane from the origin has been removed. As shown in Fig. 4.2, where ELM is used to obtain binary classification of inputs, any hyperplane of $\mathscr{H}$ divides the space into two parts, $\mathscr{H}_+ = \mathrm{f} \in \mathscr{H}; \langle \mathrm{f}, \boldsymbol{\omega} \rangle_{\mathscr{H}} > 0$ and $\mathscr{H}_- = \mathrm{f} \in H; \langle \mathrm{f}, \boldsymbol{\omega} \rangle_{\mathscr{H}} < 0$. The goal of the ELM classifiers is to separate distinct classes of data via minimising the norm of output weights $\|\boldsymbol{\omega}\|$ that actually leads to a maximum margin hyperplane [457]. To generalize the ELM classifier to operate in a complex space, we adopt the method proposed in [458], and define a complex hyperplane that divides the complex space $\hat{\mathscr{H}}$ into four parts by introducing a Hermitian matrix, label $*$. This approach enables the classification of objects into four classes (instead of two), as shown in Fig. 4.3. In imaging applications, spatial features in adjacent pixels can be retained, i.e. we have real and imaginary components in x and y directions. According to [458], we have $\langle \hat{\mathrm{f}}, \hat{\boldsymbol{\omega}} \rangle_{\hat{\mathscr{H}}} = \langle \hat{\mathrm{f}}^{\mathfrak{R}}, \hat{\boldsymbol{\nu}}^{\mathfrak{R}} \rangle_{\mathscr{H}} + \langle \hat{\mathrm{f}}^{\mathfrak{I}}, \hat{\boldsymbol{\omega}}^{\mathfrak{I}} \rangle_{\mathscr{H}} + \mathscr{I}(\langle \hat{\mathrm{f}}^{\mathfrak{I}}, \hat{\boldsymbol{\omega}}^{\mathfrak{R}} \rangle_{\mathscr{H}} - \langle \hat{\mathrm{f}}^{\mathfrak{R}}, \hat{\boldsymbol{\omega}}^{\mathfrak{I}} \rangle_{\mathscr{H}})$ where $\hat{\mathscr{H}} = \mathscr{H}^2$, $\hat{\mathrm{f}}, \hat{\boldsymbol{\omega}}$ indicates a complex decision function and the corresponding margin of the hyperplane $\hat{\mathscr{H}}$. The symbol of $\langle \cdot \rangle_{\mathscr{H}}$ denotes the inner product in the corresponding real-valued input space. It can be represented by its respective real kernel with corresponding imaginary part of zero. It satisfies the equation:

$$\begin{aligned} \kappa(\mathbf{X}, \mathbf{Y}) &= \langle \kappa(\cdot, \mathbf{X}), \kappa(\cdot, \mathbf{Y}) \rangle_{\mathscr{H}} \\ &= \kappa \langle (\cdot, \mathbf{Y}), \kappa(\cdot, \mathbf{X}) \rangle_{\mathscr{H}} = \kappa^*(\mathbf{X}, \mathbf{Y}) \end{aligned} \tag{4.32}$$

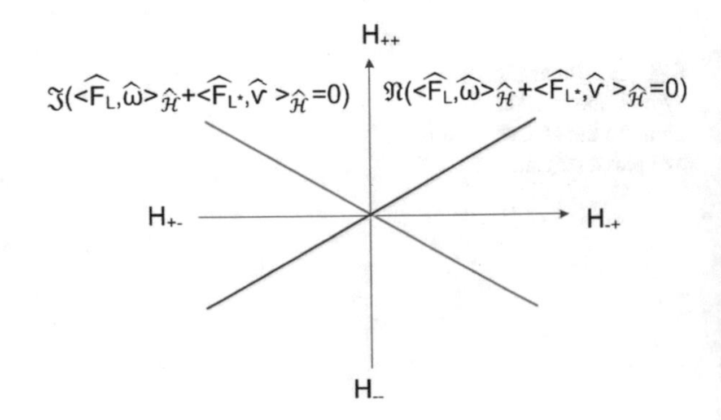

Fig. 4.3 Illustration of a complex couple of hyperplanes in ELM to divide the complex space $\hat{\mathscr{H}}$ into four parts via introducing Hermitian matrix, label $*$. Symbols of $\hat{\boldsymbol{\omega}}$ and $\hat{\boldsymbol{\nu}}$ denote the output weights in relation to decision function of $\hat{\mathrm{f}}_L$ and its couple $\hat{\mathrm{f}}_{L*}$

The Hermitian matrix, indicated by $*$, is a matrix with complex entries and is equal to its own conjugate transpose. The kernel $\kappa(\cdot, \mathbf{X})$ is used for a feature map of real-valued input space $\mathscr{H}$, labelled by $\psi(\mathbf{X})$. The corresponding complex kernel $\hat{\kappa}(\cdot, \hat{\mathbf{Z}})$ is a linear combination of real value kernels. We use symbols $\hat{\boldsymbol{\psi}}(\hat{\mathbf{Z}})$ to denote complex feature mapping in the context. In this, as well as in the following section, in addition to the bold-faced symbols used for the vector and matrix valued quantities, we use the symbol caret above all the complex-valued quantities that are related to matrices, with specific subscripts to denote the corresponding row and/or column of the complex-valued entries.

Let $\hat{\mathscr{H}}$ be a complex Hilbert space. The complex couple of hyperplanes is defined as the set of all $\mathrm{f} \in \hat{\mathscr{H}}$ that satisfy one of the following relations

$$\Re(\langle \hat{\mathrm{f}}_L, \hat{\boldsymbol{\omega}} \rangle_{\hat{\mathscr{H}}} + \langle \hat{\mathrm{f}}_{L^*}, \hat{\boldsymbol{\nu}} \rangle_{\hat{\mathscr{H}}}) = 0 \tag{4.33a}$$

$$\Im(\langle \hat{\mathrm{f}}_L, \hat{\boldsymbol{\omega}} \rangle_{\hat{\mathscr{H}}} + \langle \hat{\mathrm{f}}_{L^*}, \hat{\boldsymbol{\nu}} \rangle_{\hat{\mathscr{H}}}) = 0 \tag{4.33b}$$

for some $\hat{\boldsymbol{\omega}}, \hat{\boldsymbol{\nu}} \in \hat{\mathscr{H}}$, where $\hat{\mathrm{f}}_L \in \hat{\mathscr{H}}$ represents two hyperplanes of the doubled real space, $\mathscr{H}^2$.

The input space is divided into four portions which are associated with the complex couple of hyperplanes as shown below:

$$\mathscr{H}_{++} = \begin{cases} \Re(\langle \hat{\mathrm{f}}_L, \hat{\boldsymbol{\omega}} \rangle_{\hat{\mathscr{H}}} + \langle \hat{\mathrm{f}}_{L^*}, \hat{\boldsymbol{\nu}} \rangle_{\hat{\mathscr{H}}}) > 0 \\ \Im(\langle \hat{\mathrm{f}}_L, \hat{\boldsymbol{\omega}} \rangle_{\hat{\mathscr{H}}} + \langle \hat{\mathrm{f}}_{L^*}, \hat{\boldsymbol{\nu}} \rangle_{\hat{\mathscr{H}}}) > 0 \end{cases} \tag{4.34a}$$

$$\mathscr{H}_{+-} = \begin{cases} \Re(\langle \hat{\mathrm{f}}_L, \hat{\boldsymbol{\omega}} \rangle_{\hat{\mathscr{H}}} + \langle \hat{\mathrm{f}}_{L^*}, \hat{\boldsymbol{\nu}} \rangle_{\hat{\mathscr{H}}}) > 0 \\ \Im(\langle \hat{\mathrm{f}}_L, \hat{\boldsymbol{\omega}} \rangle_{\hat{\mathscr{H}}} + \langle \hat{\mathrm{f}}_{L^*}, \hat{\boldsymbol{\nu}} \rangle_{\hat{\mathscr{H}}}) < 0 \end{cases} \tag{4.34b}$$

$$\mathscr{H}_{-+} = \begin{cases} \Re(\langle \hat{\mathrm{f}}_L, \hat{\boldsymbol{\omega}} \rangle_{\hat{\mathscr{H}}} + \langle \hat{\mathrm{f}}_{L^*}, \hat{\boldsymbol{\nu}} \rangle_{\hat{\mathscr{H}}}) < 0 \\ \Im(\langle \hat{\mathrm{f}}_L, \hat{\boldsymbol{\omega}} \rangle_{\hat{\mathscr{H}}} + \langle \hat{\mathrm{f}}_{L^*}, \hat{\boldsymbol{\nu}} \rangle_{\hat{\mathscr{H}}}) > 0 \end{cases} \tag{4.34c}$$

$$\mathscr{H}_{--} = \begin{cases} \Re(\langle \hat{\mathrm{f}}_L, \hat{\boldsymbol{\omega}} \rangle_{\hat{\mathscr{H}}} + \langle \hat{\mathrm{f}}_{L^*}, \hat{\boldsymbol{\nu}} \rangle_{\hat{\mathscr{H}}}) < 0 \\ \Im(\langle \hat{\mathrm{f}}_L, \hat{\boldsymbol{\omega}} \rangle_{\hat{\mathscr{H}}} + \langle \hat{\mathrm{f}}_{L^*}, \hat{\boldsymbol{\nu}} \rangle_{\hat{\mathscr{H}}}) < 0 \end{cases} \tag{4.34d}$$

We now extend the formulation to 3D complex inputs. The 3D complex inputs are orthogonally projected into three 2D complex input spaces along horizontal ($\mathbf{e}_1$), vertical ($\mathbf{e}_2$) and frontal ($\mathbf{e}_3$) directions. As a result, we obtain three decision functions: $\hat{\mathrm{f}}_{Le_1}, \hat{\mathrm{f}}_{Le_2}, \hat{\mathrm{f}}_{Le_3}$ and the associated output weights $\hat{\boldsymbol{\omega}}_{e_1}, \hat{\boldsymbol{\omega}}_{e_2}, \hat{\boldsymbol{\omega}}_{e_3}$. The three decision functions span the subspace of the three real hyperplanes $\mathscr{H}_{\mathbf{E}}$, $E = \mathbf{e}_1, \mathbf{e}_2, \mathbf{e}_3$. That

Fig. 4.4 Illustration of a rational complex hyperpspace consisting of three complex couples of hyperplanes calculated via ELMs

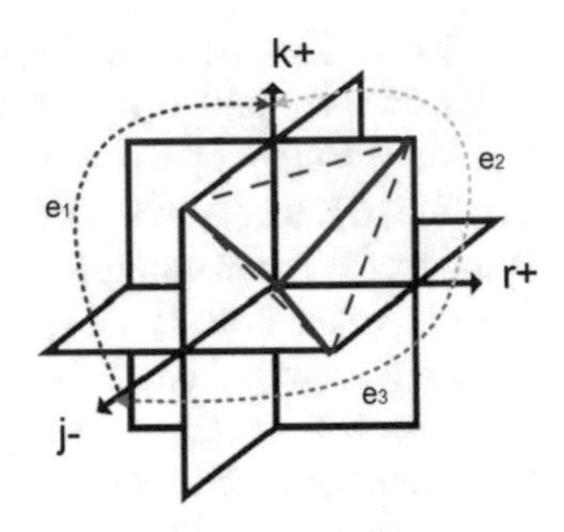

is, $\hat{\mathrm{f}}_{Le_1} \in \mathscr{H}_{\mathbf{e}_1}$, $\hat{\mathrm{f}}_{Le_2} \in \mathscr{H}_{\mathbf{e}_2}$, $\hat{\mathrm{f}}_{Le_3} \in \mathscr{H}_{\mathbf{e}_3}$. As the three coupled hyperplanes form 3D hyperspaces, in the following equations, we use Ω instead of $\mathscr{H}$ to represent the real hyperspace in three dimensions. The complexified hyperspace $\hat{\boldsymbol{\omega}}$ in three dimensions is equivalent to triple $\mathscr{H}$. The coupled parts consist of $\hat{\mathrm{f}}^*_{Le_1}, \hat{\mathrm{f}}^*_{Le_2}, \hat{\mathrm{f}}^*_{Le_3}$ and $\hat{\ddot{\boldsymbol{\omega}}}_{e_1}, \hat{\ddot{\boldsymbol{\omega}}}_{e_2}, \hat{\ddot{\boldsymbol{\omega}}}_{e_3}$. As shown in Fig. 4.4, we label the coordinate planes of $x - y$, $x - z$ and $y - z$ with $\mathbf{e}_1$, $\mathbf{e}_2$, $\mathbf{e}_3$, respectively. We use r, j, k instead of $-$, $+$ to label the 3D complex hyperspaces $\hat{\boldsymbol{\omega}}$ split into eight quadrants. The symbols of r, j, k are associated with the x-axis, y-axis, z-axis, respectively, and satisfy the functions: $r = \mathbf{e}_2\mathbf{e}_3$, $j = \mathbf{e}_3\mathbf{e}_1$, and $k = \mathbf{e}_1\mathbf{e}_2$. These complex hyper-spaces are represented as follows:

$$\Omega_{rrj} = \begin{cases} \mathscr{R}(\langle \hat{\mathrm{f}}_{Le_1}, \hat{\boldsymbol{\omega}}_{e_1} \rangle_{\hat{\mathscr{H}}_{\mathbf{e}_1}} + \langle \hat{\mathrm{f}}^*_{Le_1}, \hat{\ddot{\boldsymbol{\omega}}}_{e_1} \rangle_{\hat{\mathscr{H}}_{\mathbf{e}_1}}) > 0 \\ \mathscr{R}(\langle \hat{\mathrm{f}}_{Le_2}, \hat{\boldsymbol{\omega}}_{e_2} \rangle_{\hat{\mathscr{H}}_{\mathbf{e}_1}} + \langle \hat{\mathrm{f}}^*_{Le_2}, \hat{\ddot{\boldsymbol{\omega}}}_{e_2} \rangle_{\hat{\mathscr{H}}_{\mathbf{e}_2}}) > 0 \\ \mathscr{J}(\langle \hat{\mathrm{f}}_{Le_3}, \hat{\boldsymbol{\omega}}_{e_3} \rangle_{\hat{\mathscr{H}}_{\mathbf{e}_1}} + \langle \hat{\mathrm{f}}^*_{Le_3}, \hat{\ddot{\boldsymbol{\omega}}}_{e_3} \rangle_{\hat{\mathscr{H}}_{\mathbf{e}_3}}) > 0 \end{cases} \tag{4.35a}$$

$$\Omega_{jrk} = \begin{cases} \mathscr{J}(\langle \hat{\mathrm{f}}_{Le_1}, \hat{\boldsymbol{\omega}}_{e_1} \rangle_{\hat{\mathscr{H}}_{\mathbf{e}_1}} + \langle \hat{\mathrm{f}}^*_{Le_1}, \hat{\ddot{\boldsymbol{\omega}}}_{e_1} \rangle_{\hat{\mathscr{H}}_{\mathbf{e}_1}}) > 0 \\ \mathscr{R}(\langle \hat{\mathrm{f}}_{Le_2}, \hat{\boldsymbol{\omega}}_{e_2} \rangle_{\hat{\mathscr{H}}_{\mathbf{e}_1}} + \langle \hat{\mathrm{f}}^*_{Le_2}, \hat{\ddot{\boldsymbol{\omega}}}_{e_2} \rangle_{\hat{\mathscr{H}}_{\mathbf{e}_2}}) > 0 \\ \mathscr{K}(\langle \hat{\mathrm{f}}_{Le_3}, \hat{\boldsymbol{\omega}}_{e_3} \rangle_{\hat{\mathscr{H}}_{\mathbf{e}_1}} + \langle \hat{\mathrm{f}}^*_{Le_3}, \hat{\ddot{\boldsymbol{\omega}}}_{e_3} \rangle_{\hat{\mathscr{H}}_{\mathbf{e}_3}}) > 0 \end{cases} \tag{4.35b}$$

$$\Omega_{rkk} = \begin{cases} \mathscr{R}(\langle \hat{\mathrm{f}}_{Le_1}, \hat{\boldsymbol{\omega}}_{e_1} \rangle_{\hat{\mathscr{H}}_{\mathbf{e}_1}} + \langle \hat{\mathrm{f}}^*_{Le_1}, \hat{\ddot{\boldsymbol{\omega}}}_{e_1} \rangle_{\hat{\mathscr{H}}_{\mathbf{e}_1}}) < 0 \\ \mathscr{K}(\langle \hat{\mathrm{f}}_{Le_2}, \hat{\boldsymbol{\omega}}_{e_2} \rangle_{\hat{\mathscr{H}}_{\mathbf{e}_1}} + \langle \hat{\mathrm{f}}^*_{Le_2}, \hat{\ddot{\boldsymbol{\omega}}}_{e_2} \rangle_{\hat{\mathscr{H}}_{\mathbf{e}_2}}) > 0 \\ \mathscr{K}(\langle \hat{\mathrm{f}}_{Le_3}, \hat{\boldsymbol{\omega}}_{e_3} \rangle_{\hat{\mathscr{H}}_{\mathbf{e}_1}} + \langle \hat{\mathrm{f}}^*_{Le_3}, \hat{\ddot{\boldsymbol{\omega}}}_{e_3} \rangle_{\hat{\mathscr{H}}_{\mathbf{e}_3}}) > 0 \end{cases} \tag{4.35c}$$

$$\Omega_{jkj} = \begin{cases} \mathscr{J}(\langle \hat{\mathrm{f}}_{Le_1}, \hat{\boldsymbol{\omega}}_{e_1} \rangle_{\hat{\mathscr{H}}_{\mathrm{e}_1}} + \langle \hat{\mathrm{f}}^*_{Le_1}, \hat{\hat{\boldsymbol{\omega}}}_{e_1} \rangle_{\hat{\mathscr{H}}_{\mathrm{e}_1}}) < 0 \\ \mathscr{K}(\langle \hat{\mathrm{f}}_{Le_2}, \hat{\boldsymbol{\omega}}_{e_2} \rangle_{\hat{\mathscr{H}}_{\mathrm{e}_1}} + \langle \hat{\mathrm{f}}^*_{Le_2}, \hat{\hat{\boldsymbol{\omega}}}_{e_2} \rangle_{\hat{\mathscr{H}}_{\mathrm{e}_2}}) > 0 \\ \mathscr{J}(\langle \hat{\mathrm{f}}_{Le_3}, \hat{\boldsymbol{\omega}}_{e_3} \rangle_{\hat{\mathscr{H}}_{\mathrm{e}_1}} + \langle \hat{\mathrm{f}}^*_{Le_3}, \hat{\hat{\boldsymbol{\omega}}}_{e_3} \rangle_{\hat{\mathscr{H}}_{\mathrm{e}_3}}) > 0 \end{cases} \tag{4.35d}$$

$$\Omega_{-rkk} = \begin{cases} \mathscr{R}(\langle \hat{\mathrm{f}}_{Le_1}, \hat{\boldsymbol{\omega}}_{e_1} \rangle_{\hat{\mathscr{H}}_{\mathrm{e}_1}} + \langle \hat{\mathrm{f}}^*_{Le_1}, \hat{\hat{\boldsymbol{\omega}}}_{e_1} \rangle_{\hat{\mathscr{H}}_{\mathrm{e}_1}}) > 0 \\ \mathscr{K}(\langle \hat{\mathrm{f}}_{Le_2}, \hat{\boldsymbol{\omega}}_{e_2} \rangle_{\hat{\mathscr{H}}_{\mathrm{e}_1}} + \langle \hat{\mathrm{f}}^*_{Le_2}, \hat{\hat{\boldsymbol{\omega}}}_{e_2} \rangle_{\hat{\mathscr{H}}_{\mathrm{e}_2}}) < 0 \\ \mathscr{K}(\langle \hat{\mathrm{f}}_{Le_3}, \hat{\boldsymbol{\omega}}_{e_3} \rangle_{\hat{\mathscr{H}}_{\mathrm{e}_1}} + \langle \hat{\mathrm{f}}^*_{Le_3}, \hat{\hat{\boldsymbol{\omega}}}_{e_3} \rangle_{\hat{\mathscr{H}}_{\mathrm{e}_3}}) < 0 \end{cases} \tag{4.35e}$$

$$\Omega_{-jkj} = \begin{cases} \mathscr{J}(\langle \hat{\mathrm{f}}_{Le_1}, \hat{\boldsymbol{\omega}}_{e_1} \rangle_{\hat{\mathscr{H}}_{\mathrm{e}_1}} + \langle \hat{\mathrm{f}}^*_{Le_1}, \hat{\hat{\boldsymbol{\omega}}}_{e_1} \rangle_{\hat{\mathscr{H}}_{\mathrm{e}_1}}) > 0 \\ \mathscr{K}(\langle \hat{\mathrm{f}}_{Le_2}, \hat{\boldsymbol{\omega}}_{e_2} \rangle_{\hat{\mathscr{H}}_{\mathrm{e}_1}} + \langle \hat{\mathrm{f}}^*_{Le_2}, \hat{\hat{\boldsymbol{\omega}}}_{e_2} \rangle_{\hat{\mathscr{H}}_{\mathrm{e}_2}}) < 0 \\ \mathscr{J}(\langle \hat{\mathrm{f}}_{Le_3}, \hat{\boldsymbol{\omega}}_{e_3} \rangle_{\hat{\mathscr{H}}_{\mathrm{e}_1}} + \langle \hat{\mathrm{f}}^*_{Le_3}, \hat{\hat{\boldsymbol{\omega}}}_{e_3} \rangle_{\hat{\mathscr{H}}_{\mathrm{e}_3}}) < 0 \end{cases} \tag{4.35f}$$

$$\Omega_{-rrj} = \begin{cases} \mathscr{R}(\langle \hat{\mathrm{f}}_{Le_1}, \hat{\boldsymbol{\omega}}_{e_1} \rangle_{\hat{\mathscr{H}}_{\mathrm{e}_1}} + \langle \hat{\mathrm{f}}^*_{Le_1}, \hat{\hat{\boldsymbol{\omega}}}_{e_1} \rangle_{\hat{\mathscr{H}}_{\mathrm{e}_1}}) < 0 \\ \mathscr{R}(\langle \hat{\mathrm{f}}_{Le_2}, \hat{\boldsymbol{\omega}}_{e_2} \rangle_{\hat{\mathscr{H}}_{\mathrm{e}_1}} + \langle \hat{\mathrm{f}}^*_{Le_2}, \hat{\hat{\boldsymbol{\omega}}}_{e_2} \rangle_{\hat{\mathscr{H}}_{\mathrm{e}_2}}) < 0 \\ \mathscr{J}(\langle \hat{\mathrm{f}}_{Le_3}, \hat{\boldsymbol{\omega}}_{e_3} \rangle_{\hat{\mathscr{H}}_{\mathrm{e}_1}} + \langle \hat{\mathrm{f}}^*_{Le_3}, \hat{\hat{\boldsymbol{\omega}}}_{e_3} \rangle_{\hat{\mathscr{H}}_{\mathrm{e}_3}}) < 0 \end{cases} \tag{4.35g}$$

$$\Omega_{-jrk} = \begin{cases} \mathscr{J}(\langle \hat{\mathrm{f}}_{Le_1}, \hat{\boldsymbol{\omega}}_{e_1} \rangle_{\hat{\mathscr{H}}_{\mathrm{e}_1}} + \langle \hat{\mathrm{f}}^*_{Le_1}, \hat{\hat{\boldsymbol{\omega}}}_{e_1} \rangle_{\hat{\mathscr{H}}_{\mathrm{e}_1}}) < 0 \\ \mathscr{R}(\langle \hat{\mathrm{f}}_{Le_2}, \hat{\boldsymbol{\omega}}_{e_2} \rangle_{\hat{\mathscr{H}}_{\mathrm{e}_1}} + \langle \hat{\mathrm{f}}^*_{Le_2}, \hat{\hat{\boldsymbol{\omega}}}_{e_2} \rangle_{\hat{\mathscr{H}}_{\mathrm{e}_2}}) < 0 \\ \mathscr{K}(\langle \hat{\mathrm{f}}_{Le_3}, \hat{\boldsymbol{\omega}}_{e_3} \rangle_{\hat{\mathscr{H}}_{\mathrm{e}_1}} + \langle \hat{\mathrm{f}}^*_{Le_3}, \hat{\hat{\boldsymbol{\omega}}}_{e_3} \rangle_{\hat{\mathscr{H}}_{\mathrm{e}_3}}) < 0 \end{cases} \tag{4.35h}$$

Here, $\mathscr{H}_-$ denotes the opposite site associated with the complex hyperplane surfaces $\mathscr{H}$. The decision functions $\hat{\mathrm{f}}$, $\hat{\mathrm{g}}$, $\hat{\mathrm{d}}$ are implemented using the same kernel with different coordinates. As shown in Fig. 4.4, the three complex couples (indicated by three red solid lines) of hyperplanes in the fourth quadrant form a rational complex hyperplane (a 3D rational complex hyper-space). The complex hyper-spaces divide the 3D complex entries into eight parts. For classification of $m > 1$ classes, these inputs will be further grouped with total $2^{3-1} \times m$ classes via ELM.

We formulate the complex ELM classification task as follows. The given complex-valued training samples consist of eight separate classes Λ_{rrj}, Λ_{jrk}, Λ_{rkk}, Λ_{jkj}, Λ_{-rkk}, Λ_{-jkj}, Λ_{-rrj}, Λ_{jrk} such as $\{(\hat{z}_n, \vartheta_n); n = 1, \ldots, N\} \subset \Psi \times \{\pm \mathrm{r} \pm \mathrm{j} \pm \mathrm{k}\}$. That is: if $\vartheta_n = +\mathscr{R} + \mathscr{R} + \mathscr{J}$, then $\hat{z}_n \in \Lambda_{rrj}$; If $\vartheta_n = +\mathscr{J} + \mathscr{R} + \mathscr{K}$, then $\hat{z}_n \in \Lambda jrk$; If $\vartheta_n = -\mathscr{R} + \mathscr{K} + \mathscr{K}$, then $\hat{z}_n \in \Lambda_{rkk}$; If $\vartheta_n = -\mathscr{J} + \mathscr{K} + \mathscr{J}$, then $\hat{z}_n \in \Lambda_{jkj}$; If $\vartheta_n = +\mathscr{R} - \mathscr{K} - \mathscr{K}$, then $\hat{z}_n \in \Lambda_{-rkk}$; If $\vartheta_n = +\mathscr{J} - \mathscr{K} - \mathscr{J}$, then $\hat{z}_n \in \Lambda_{-jkj}$; If $\vartheta_n = -\mathscr{R} - \mathscr{R} - \mathscr{J}$, then $\hat{z}_n \in \Lambda_{-rrj}$; If $\vartheta_n = -\mathscr{J} - \mathscr{R} - \mathscr{K}$, then $\hat{z}_n \in \Lambda_{-jrk}$. Here, $\hat{z}_n = \mathbf{X} + \mathscr{J}\mathbf{Y} + \mathscr{K}\mathbf{Z}$, $\Lambda^- + \Lambda = \mathbf{0}$, and $\Lambda, \Psi \in \hat{\boldsymbol{\omega}}$.

4.5.3 Determination of the Maximum-Margin Hyperplanes of CELM

The goal of the complex machine learning task is to estimate a complex couple of maximum margin hyperplanes. According to the work in [458], for a 2D simple case, the aim is to minimise

$$\left\| \begin{matrix} \hat{\boldsymbol{\omega}}^r + \hat{\boldsymbol{\nu}}^r \\ \hat{\boldsymbol{\omega}}^j - \hat{\boldsymbol{\nu}}^j \end{matrix} \right\|^2_{\mathscr{H}^2} + \left\| \begin{matrix} -(\hat{\boldsymbol{\omega}}^j + \hat{\boldsymbol{\nu}}^j) \\ \hat{\boldsymbol{\omega}}^r - \hat{\boldsymbol{\nu}}^r \end{matrix} \right\|^2_{\mathscr{H}^2} = 2(\|\hat{\omega}\|^2_{\mathscr{H}} + \|\hat{\boldsymbol{\nu}}\|^2_{\mathscr{H}}).$$

In a similar manner to the ELM algorithm, for the classification task, CELM is used to minimize the training error $\hat{\delta} = \|\psi\hat{\boldsymbol{\omega}} + \psi^*\hat{\boldsymbol{\nu}} - \hat{\theta}\|^2$ with $\hat{\theta} = [\hat{\vartheta}_1, \ldots, \hat{\vartheta}_N]^T$ being a known complex-valued label matrix corresponding to m classes, as well as the norm of the output margins (weights). Therefore, the primal complex ELM optimization problem can be formulated as

$$\min_{(\hat{\omega},\hat{\nu},C)} = \left(\frac{1}{2} \parallel \hat{\boldsymbol{\omega}} \parallel^2_{\hat{\mathscr{H}}} + \frac{1}{2} \parallel \hat{\boldsymbol{\nu}} \parallel^2_{\hat{\mathscr{H}}} + \frac{C}{N} \sum_{n=1}^{N} (\hat{\delta_n}^2) \right), \tag{4.36}$$

Subject to:

$$\begin{cases} \Re(\langle \hat{\boldsymbol{\psi}}_{\hat{\mathscr{H}}}(\hat{z}_n), \hat{\boldsymbol{\omega}} \rangle + \langle \hat{\boldsymbol{\psi}}^*_{\hat{\mathscr{H}}}(\hat{z}_n), \hat{\boldsymbol{\nu}} \rangle) \geq \hat{\vartheta}^r_n - \hat{\delta}^r_n \\ \Im(\langle \hat{\boldsymbol{\psi}}_{\hat{\mathscr{H}}}(\hat{z}_n), \hat{\boldsymbol{\omega}} \rangle + \langle \hat{\boldsymbol{\psi}}^*_{\hat{\mathscr{H}}}(\hat{z}_n), \hat{\boldsymbol{\nu}} \rangle) \geq \hat{\vartheta}^j_n - \hat{\delta}^j_n \end{cases} \tag{4.37}$$

where C is a parameter given by users aiming to trade-off the distance to the separating margin with the training error. Using positive Lagrangian multipliers **a** and **b**, the Lagrangian function becomes:

$$\begin{aligned} \mathrm{L}(\hat{\boldsymbol{\omega}}, \hat{\boldsymbol{\nu}}, \mathbf{a}, \mathbf{b}) &= \frac{1}{2} \parallel \hat{\boldsymbol{\omega}} \parallel^2_{\hat{\mathscr{H}}} + \frac{1}{2} \parallel \hat{\boldsymbol{\nu}} \parallel^2_{\hat{\mathscr{H}}} + \frac{C}{N} \parallel \hat{\delta}^r_{n,\rho} + \hat{\delta}^j_{n,\rho} \parallel^2 \\ &- \sum_{n=1}^{N} \sum_{\rho=1}^{m} a_{n,\rho} \\ &\left(\Re(\langle \hat{\boldsymbol{\psi}}_{\hat{\mathscr{H}}}(\hat{z}_n), \hat{\boldsymbol{\omega}}_\rho \rangle + \langle \hat{\boldsymbol{\psi}}^*_{\hat{\mathscr{H}}}(\hat{z}_n), \hat{\boldsymbol{\nu}}_\rho \rangle) - \hat{\vartheta}^r_{n,\rho} + \hat{\delta}^r_{n,\rho} \right) \\ &- \sum_{n=1}^{N} \sum_{\rho=1}^{m} b_{n,\rho} \\ &\left(\Im(\langle \hat{\boldsymbol{\psi}}_{\hat{\mathscr{H}}}(\hat{z}_n), \hat{\boldsymbol{\omega}}_\rho \rangle + \langle \hat{\boldsymbol{\psi}}^*_{\hat{\mathscr{H}}}(\hat{z}_n), \hat{\boldsymbol{\nu}}_\rho \rangle) - \hat{\vartheta}^j_{n,\rho} + \hat{\delta}^j_{n,\rho} \right) \end{aligned} \tag{4.38}$$

Here, $\hat{\theta}_n = \{\hat{\vartheta}_{n,\rho}\}$ with $\rho = 1, \ldots, m$ and $n \in 1, \ldots, N$, where $\{\hat{\vartheta}_{n,\rho}\}$ denotes the output value of the ρth output node for the training data $\hat{z}_n$ and m labels the number of the classes of the output. When both the real and imaginary parts of the Sth element $\hat{\vartheta}_{n,S}$ are one and the remaining elements of $\hat{\vartheta}_n$ are zero, the original class label is $S + \mathscr{J} S$. According to Wirtinger's Calculus to compute the respective gradients, we have

$$\frac{\partial \mathrm{L}}{\hat{\boldsymbol{\omega}}_\rho^*} = \frac{1}{2}\hat{\boldsymbol{\omega}}_\rho - \frac{1}{2}\sum_{n=1}^{N} a_{n,\rho}\hat{\boldsymbol{\psi}}^T_{\mathscr{H}}(\hat{z}_n) + \frac{\mathscr{J}}{2}\sum_{n=1}^{N} b_{n,\rho}\hat{\boldsymbol{\psi}}^T_{\mathscr{H}}(\hat{z}_n) = 0$$
$$\Rightarrow \hat{\boldsymbol{\omega}}_\rho = \sum_{n=1}^{N}\left(\alpha_{n,\rho} - \mathscr{J} b_{n,\rho}\right)\hat{\boldsymbol{\psi}}^T_{\mathscr{H}}(\hat{z}_n) \quad (4.39)$$

$$\frac{\partial \mathrm{L}}{\hat{\boldsymbol{v}}_\rho^*} = \frac{1}{2}\hat{\boldsymbol{v}}_\rho - \frac{1}{2}\sum_{n=1}^{N} a_{n,\rho}\hat{\boldsymbol{\psi}}^{*T}_{\mathscr{H}}(\hat{z}_n) + \frac{\mathscr{J}}{2}\sum_{n=1}^{N} b_{n,\rho}\hat{\boldsymbol{\psi}}^{*T}_{\mathscr{H}}(\hat{z}_n) = 0$$
$$\Rightarrow \hat{\boldsymbol{v}}_\rho = \sum_{n=1}^{N}\left(a_{n,\rho} - \mathscr{J} b_{n,\rho}\right)\hat{\boldsymbol{\psi}}^{*T}_{\mathscr{H}}(\hat{z}_n) \quad (4.40)$$

$$\begin{aligned}\frac{\partial \mathrm{L}}{\hat{\delta}^r_{n,\rho}} &= \frac{2C}{N}\hat{\delta}^r_{n,\rho} - a_{n,\rho} = 0 \Rightarrow \hat{\delta}^r_{n,\rho} = \frac{N}{2C}a_{n,\rho}\\ \frac{\partial \mathrm{L}}{\hat{\delta}^j_{n,\rho}} &= \frac{2C}{N}\hat{\delta}^j_{n,\rho} - b_{n,\rho} = 0 \Rightarrow \hat{\delta}^j_{n,\rho} = \frac{N}{2C}b_{n,\rho}\end{aligned} \quad (4.41)$$

$$\frac{\partial \mathrm{L}}{a_{n,\rho}} = -\frac{1}{2}\left(\Re\left(\langle\hat{\boldsymbol{\psi}}_{\mathscr{H}}(\hat{z}_n), \hat{\boldsymbol{\omega}}_\rho\rangle + \langle\hat{\boldsymbol{\psi}}^*_{\mathscr{H}}(\hat{z}_n), \hat{\boldsymbol{v}}_\rho\rangle\right)\right)$$
$$-\frac{1}{2}\left(-\hat{\vartheta}^r_{n,\rho} + \hat{\delta}^r_{n,\rho}\right) = 0 \quad (4.42)$$

$$\frac{\partial \mathrm{L}}{b_{n,\rho}} = -\frac{1}{2}\left(\Im\left(\langle\hat{\boldsymbol{\psi}}_{\mathscr{H}}(\hat{z}_n), \hat{\boldsymbol{\omega}}_\rho\rangle + \langle\hat{\boldsymbol{\psi}}^*_{\mathscr{H}}(\hat{z}_n), \hat{\boldsymbol{v}}_\rho\rangle\right)\right)$$
$$-\frac{1}{2}\left(-\hat{\vartheta}^j_{n,\rho} + \hat{\delta}^j_{n,\rho}\right) = 0 \quad (4.43)$$

According to the last two equations,

$$\langle \hat{\boldsymbol{\psi}}_{\mathscr{H}}(\hat{z}_n), \hat{\boldsymbol{\omega}}_\rho \rangle + \langle \hat{\boldsymbol{\psi}}^*_{\mathscr{H}}(\hat{z}_n), \hat{\boldsymbol{\nu}}_\rho \rangle - \hat{\vartheta}_{n,\rho} + \hat{\delta}_{n,\rho} = 0 \tag{4.44}$$

By substituting Eqs. 4.39–4.41 and 4.44 can be written as

$$\begin{aligned}(\mathbf{a} - \mathscr{J}\mathbf{b}) \left(\hat{\boldsymbol{\psi}}_{\mathscr{H}}(\hat{z}_n) \hat{\boldsymbol{\psi}}^T_{\mathscr{H}}(\hat{z}_n) + \hat{\boldsymbol{\psi}}^*_{\mathscr{H}}(\hat{z}_n) \hat{\boldsymbol{\psi}}^{*T}_{\mathscr{H}}(\hat{z}_n) \right) \\ + \frac{N}{2C}(\mathbf{a} + \mathscr{J}\mathbf{b}) = \hat{\boldsymbol{\theta}}\end{aligned} \tag{4.45}$$

The output decision functions of the CELM classifier are:

$$\begin{aligned}\Re(\hat{\mathrm{f}}_L(\hat{\mathbf{Z}})) &= \Re\left(\hat{\boldsymbol{\psi}}_{\mathscr{H}}(\hat{\mathbf{Z}}), \hat{\boldsymbol{\omega}} \right) \\ &= \Re\left(\hat{\boldsymbol{\psi}}_{\mathscr{H}}(\hat{\mathbf{Z}}) \hat{\boldsymbol{\psi}}^T_{\mathscr{H}} \left(\left(\hat{\boldsymbol{\psi}}_{\mathscr{H}} \hat{\boldsymbol{\psi}}^T_{\mathscr{H}} + \hat{\boldsymbol{\psi}}^*_{\mathscr{H}} \hat{\boldsymbol{\psi}}^{*T}_{\mathscr{H}} \right) + \frac{N}{2C}\mathbf{I} \right)^{-1} \hat{\boldsymbol{\theta}} \right)\end{aligned} \tag{4.46a}$$

$$\begin{aligned}\Im(\hat{\mathrm{f}}_L(\hat{\mathbf{Z}})) &= \Im\left(\hat{\boldsymbol{\psi}}_{\mathscr{H}}(\hat{\mathbf{Z}}), \hat{\boldsymbol{\omega}} \right) \\ &= -\Im\left(\hat{\boldsymbol{\psi}}_{\mathscr{H}}(\hat{\mathbf{Z}}) \hat{\boldsymbol{\psi}}^T_{\mathscr{H}} \left(\left(\hat{\boldsymbol{\psi}}_{\mathscr{H}} \hat{\boldsymbol{\psi}}^T_{\mathscr{H}} + \hat{\boldsymbol{\psi}}^*_{\mathscr{H}} \hat{\boldsymbol{\psi}}^{*T}_{\mathscr{H}} \right) + \frac{N}{2C}\mathbf{I} \right)^{-1} \hat{\boldsymbol{\theta}} \right)\end{aligned} \tag{4.46b}$$

$$\begin{aligned}\Re(\hat{\mathrm{f}}_{L^*}(\hat{\mathbf{Z}})) &= \Re\left(\hat{\boldsymbol{\psi}}^*_{\mathscr{H}}(\hat{\mathbf{Z}}), \hat{\boldsymbol{\nu}} \right) \\ &= \Re\left(\hat{\boldsymbol{\psi}}^*_{\mathscr{H}}(\hat{\mathbf{Z}}) \hat{\boldsymbol{\psi}}^{*T}_{\mathscr{H}} \left(\left(\hat{\boldsymbol{\psi}}_{\mathscr{H}} \hat{\boldsymbol{\psi}}^T_{\mathscr{H}} + \hat{\boldsymbol{\psi}}^*_{\mathscr{H}} \hat{\boldsymbol{\psi}}^{*T}_{\mathscr{H}} \right) + \frac{N}{2C}\mathbf{I} \right)^{-1} \hat{\boldsymbol{\theta}} \right)\end{aligned} \tag{4.46c}$$

$$\begin{aligned}\Im(\hat{\mathrm{f}}_{L^*}(\hat{\mathbf{Z}})) &= \Im\left(\hat{\boldsymbol{\psi}}^*_{\mathscr{H}}(\hat{\mathbf{Z}}), \hat{\boldsymbol{\nu}} \right) \\ &= -\Im\left(\hat{\boldsymbol{\psi}}^*_{\mathscr{H}}(\hat{\mathbf{Z}}) \hat{\boldsymbol{\psi}}^{*T}_{\mathscr{H}} \left(\left(\hat{\boldsymbol{\psi}}_{\mathscr{H}} \hat{\boldsymbol{\psi}}^T_{\mathscr{H}} + \hat{\boldsymbol{\psi}}^*_{\mathscr{H}} \hat{\boldsymbol{\psi}}^{*T}_{\mathscr{H}} \right) + \frac{N}{2C}\mathbf{I} \right)^{-1} \hat{\boldsymbol{\theta}} \right)\end{aligned} \tag{4.46d}$$

where $\hat{\boldsymbol{\psi}}_{\mathscr{H}} \hat{\boldsymbol{\psi}}^T_{\mathscr{H}}$ and $\hat{\boldsymbol{\psi}}^*_{\mathscr{H}} \hat{\boldsymbol{\psi}}^{*T}_{\mathscr{H}}$ are $N \times N$ or $L \times L$ matrices, according to the size of the inputs. The predicted class label of sample $\hat{\mathbf{Z}}$:

$$\mathrm{label}(\hat{\mathbf{Z}}) = \arg \max_{n=1,\ldots,m} (\langle \hat{\boldsymbol{\psi}}_{\mathscr{H}}(\hat{\mathbf{Z}}), \hat{\boldsymbol{\omega}} \rangle + \langle \hat{\boldsymbol{\psi}}^*_{\mathscr{H}}(\hat{\mathbf{Z}}), \hat{\boldsymbol{\nu}} \rangle) \tag{4.47}$$

where $\text{label}(\hat{\mathbf{Z}}) = \text{label}(\Re(\hat{\mathbf{Z}})) + \mathscr{J}\,\text{label}(\Im(\hat{\mathbf{Z}}))$. Here, we employ the induced real kernel $2\hat{\kappa}^r$ instead of the complex kernel $\hat{\kappa}$ for the solution of the complex labelling function.

For the 3D multiclass classification, the complex labelling function can be written as the linear combination of 2D multiclass classification tasks along three orthogonal coordinate planes. It satisfies the following expression:

$$\begin{aligned}\text{label}(\hat{\mathbf{Z}}) = \arg \max_{n=1,\ldots,m} \; & \langle \hat{\boldsymbol{\psi}}(\hat{\mathbf{Z}}), \hat{\omega}_{e_1} \rangle_{\hat{\mathscr{H}}_{e_1}} + \langle \hat{\boldsymbol{\psi}}^*(\hat{\mathbf{Z}}), \hat{\hat{\omega}}_{e_1} \rangle_{\hat{\mathscr{H}}_{e_1}} \\ & + \langle \hat{\boldsymbol{\psi}}(\hat{\mathbf{Z}}), \hat{\omega}_{e_2} \rangle_{\hat{\mathscr{H}}_{e_2}} + \langle \hat{\boldsymbol{\psi}}^*(\hat{\mathbf{Z}}), \hat{\hat{\omega}}_{e_2} \rangle_{\hat{\mathscr{H}}_{e_2}} \\ & + \langle \hat{\boldsymbol{\psi}}(\hat{\mathbf{Z}}), \hat{\omega}_{e_3} \rangle_{\hat{\mathscr{H}}_{e_3}} + \langle \hat{\boldsymbol{\psi}}^*(\hat{\mathbf{Z}}), \hat{\hat{\omega}}_{e_3} \rangle_{\hat{\mathscr{H}}_{e_3}} \end{aligned} \tag{4.48}$$

This is consistent with Sect. 4.5.2.

The block diagram of the proposed algorithm is illustrated in Fig. 4.5. The complex extreme learning machine enables multi-class classification when both the input and output variables, as well as the optimisation variables, are all complex-valued. The label for a given testing sample from multi-class is complex-valued and has the highest output value of the complex-coupled output decision functions $\hat{\mathrm{f}}_L$ and $\hat{\mathrm{f}}_{L^*}$ for the given testing sample.

The CELM classifier approach has a very broad applications domain across the biomedical community, encompassing all types of research associated with the study of the interaction of matter with waves, and in particular spectroscopy (acoustic, dielectric, optical, THz, infrared, electron-spin resonance, nuclear magnetic or paramagnetic resonance, etc.), as well as imaging and tomography modalities encountered across the physical, chemical and biomedical disciplines. It is thus fundamental, both from a machine learning, as well as from a chemometrics perspective [460]. Because the above relations are also analogous to the blurring function (relating amplitude and phase) developed by Bode [461] to describe the dynamics of physical

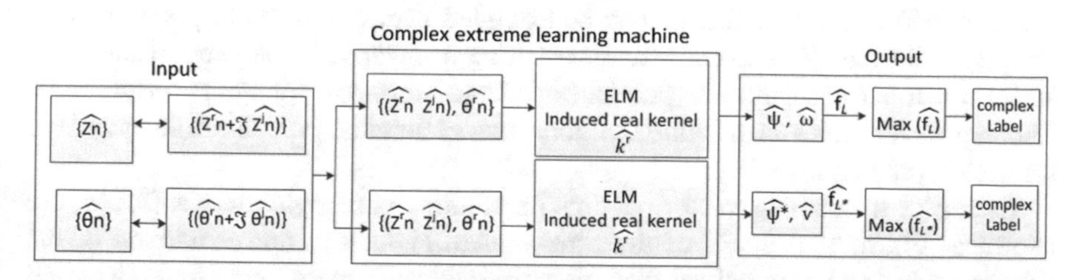

Fig. 4.5 Illustration of the procedure for 2D complex-valued learning via complex extreme learning machine. The system facilitates multi-class classification when both input and output variables are complex-valued. The approach also uses optimisation variables that are complex-valued. The label for a given testing sample from the multi-class is a complex-valued entity which has the highest output value associated with the complex-coupled output decision functions $\hat{\mathrm{f}}_L$ and $\hat{\mathrm{f}}_{L^*}$ for the given testing sample

systems, CELMs have a wide range of applications across all physical sciences. A typical example of the proposed approach is the recent study [226] which focused on the use of CELM to perform binary and multi-class classification of RNA and powder samples respectively, on the basis of images acquired by THz-TPI. The analysis was performed on large data sets as would be the case in a typical biomedical or quality control setting. Classification was performed on the basis of discernible features in the measured THz spectra.

Examples of learning vector patterns for two-class recognition via CELM, and a comparison with SVM classification are shown in Fig. 4.6. Figure 4.6a, b depict 36 training vectors for illustration purposes. The background colour shows the shape of the decision surface. Figure 4.6a illustrates a SVMs classification scheme, where dark blue regions represent the class belonging to the poly-C sample labelled by 1, and light blue regions indicate the class related to poly-A sample labelled by -1. Separating hyperplanes for two classes are indicated by 0. The circles represent the calculated support vectors. Compared with the training vectors, the number of support vectors are reduced, thus enabling quick derivation of the optimal hyperplane shape and speeding up the overall classification time. In both cases, the machine learning for two-class samples—poly-A and poly-C respectively, denoted by white "$+$" and black "$\times$", are approximately separated by their own boundary lines though there is a little overlapping. Detailed results on classification accuracy are described in the following section, where 200 random selections of training vectors are fed to the classifiers.

In Fig. 4.6b, red regions represent the class belonging to the poly-C sample labelled by 1, and blue regions indicate the class related to poly-A sample labelled by -1. Contrary to real-valued machine learning, the labels of CELMs are complex valued. The numbered labels to be output are shown in Fig. 4.6b. These values are calculated as the sum of a doubled value of the real part ($\mathbf{R}$) and the value of the complex part (J), in relation to the complex valued labels, with zero indicating non-classified data. Therefore, each of the numbered labels ($\mathbf{Y}$) satisfies the equation: $\mathbf{Y} = 2 \times \mathbf{R} + \mathbf{J}(\Im)^2$ with $(\Im)^2 = -1$. Specifically, we set the classification label belonging to poly-A as $\mathbf{I} + \Im(\mathbf{I})$, and that belonging to poly-C as $\mathbf{-I} + \Im(\mathbf{-I})$. The $\mathbf{I}$ indicates an identity matrix. As discussed in [447], CELMs may be extended naturally to multi-pixel or voxel images for the classification of features resulting from tensorial decomposition using additional input and output hyperplanes designed through orthogonal projections. The approach enables us to define additional kernel functions which can be optimized for each input class.

Examples of learning vector patterns for multiclass recognition via CELM, are shown in Fig. 4.7a after FT of the time-domain signatures and extraction of the corresponding complex valued features in frequency domain, regarding phase and amplitude. We used 49 input vectors related to each powder sample for training the classifier. Two real RKHS kernels were used for mapping. The optimal Gaussian parameter σ was set to 100 and the penalty parameter C was set to 0.1. The labels were complex-valued and produced 12 output classes. Background colour shows the contour shape of the decision surface (these are numbered from 2–12), and these correspond to the amplitude calculations derived from the sum of real and imaginary

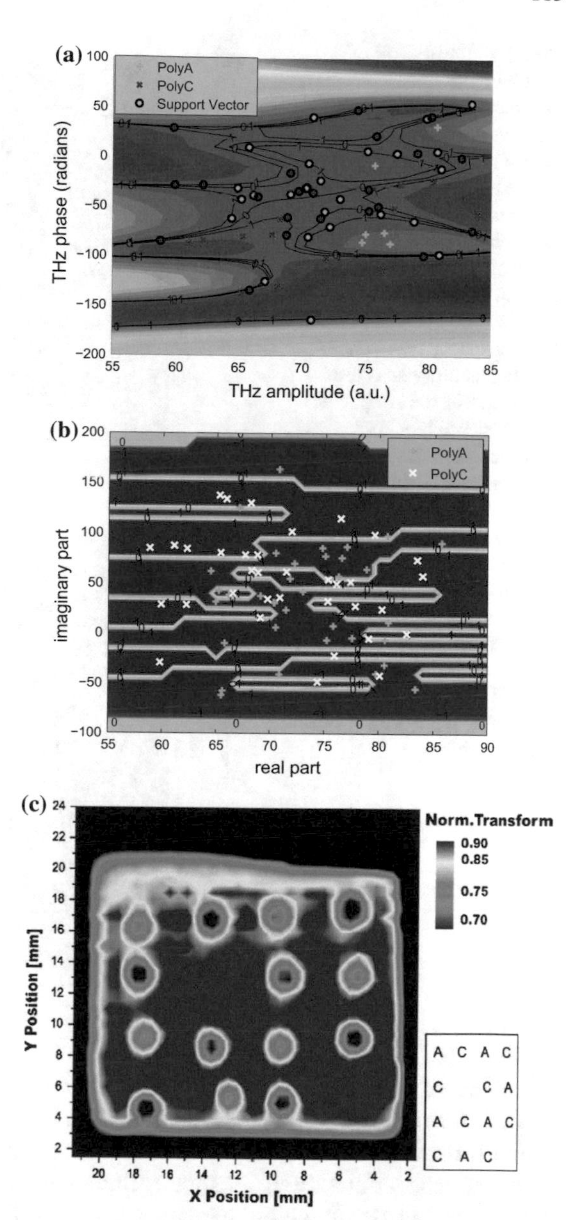

Fig. 4.6 Illustration of binary classification for the recognition of RNA samples consisting of 36 training vectors for each. **a** Illustration of a CELM classification scheme, using two real Gaussian kernels to map the training vectors to a 2-D complex-valued feature space, with the penalty parameter $C = 0.5$ and $\sigma = 1$. **b** Illustration of a real SVM classification scheme, using a real Gaussian kernel to map the training vectors to a 2-D complex-valued feature space. The penalty parameter C is set to infinity and the width parameter of the Gaussian kernel σ is set to $1 \times e^{-5}$. **c** T-ray transmission image of the poly-A and poly-C,showing stronger absorption in poly-C compared with poly-A. Each spot contained 200 μg of either poly-A or poly-C in alternating order, as indicated in the diagram on the *right*. The colour scale indicates the normalized peak values of the two RNA samples

values of the respective complex labels. It can be observed that THz measurements of powder samples of salt, sand, talcum, are grouped more tightly than the powder samples of flour, soda and sugar. The labelled contours that correspond to different real and imaginary parts (the real and imaginary parts label the different classes) are illustrated in Fig. 4.7b. These regions are undecided in the classification process and are therefore excluded to avoid over-fitting problems.

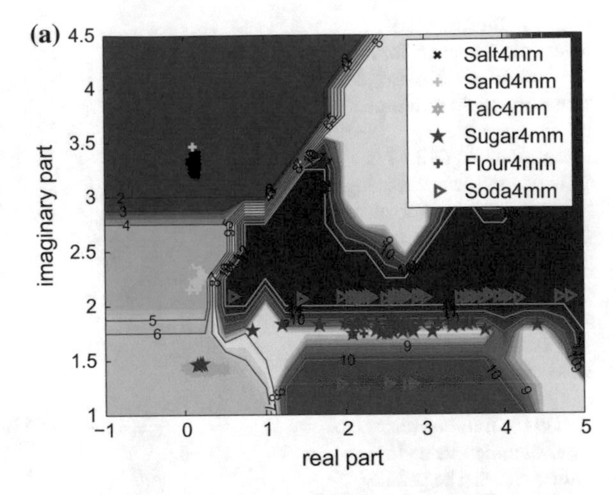

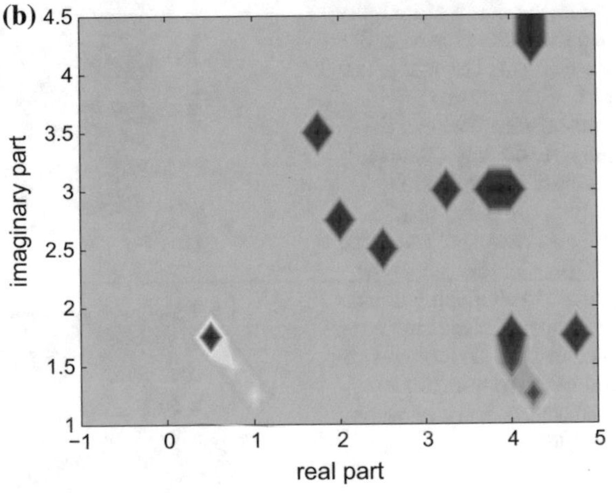

Fig. 4.7 Illustration of CELM multi-class classification scheme. **a** Complex valued learning vectors for the six samples plotted to illustrate the linear decision function among each class by applying induced real RKHS kernels to map the complex input data into 2D complex valued feature space. There are 49 pixels randomly selected from each of the six powder samples. The labels are complex valued, generating 12 classes. **b** Illustration of the colour coded regions with non-zeros indicated by the colour bar. The colour regions with non-zero value indicate that the multi-class powder sample classification process remains undecided by CELM as the real and imaginary parts are not equal to each other

The CELMs may be naturally extended to multi-pixel or voxel images. This aims to achieve complex valued learning of 3D inputs of complex valued features, i.e. to classify the complex valued input data selected from a tensor. The proposed approach could further be extended to address aspects of quaternary classification within a tensor algebra context. For 3D inputs, three pairs of complex coupled hyperplanes may be designed through orthogonal projections. The approach enables us to define a kernel function specific for the calculation of high dimensional complex coupled hyperplanes. It allows effective classification with a more natural representation of the data in a tensor format. The approach is also extendable to hierarchical clustering as discussed in the following section.

4.5.4 *Multinomial Logistic Regression Classifier with Ridge Estimators (MLR)*

Ridge estimators are used in multinomial logistic regression to improve the parameter estimation and to diminish the error associated with further prediction when the application of maximum likelihood estimators (MLE) is inappropriate, because of the non-uniqueness of the solution in the data fitting process. When the number of explanatory variables is relatively large and/or when the explanatory variables are highly correlated, the estimates of the parameters become unstable, and are not uniquely defined (some are infinite) so the maximum of the log-likelihood is achieved at 0 value [462, 463]. In this situation, ridge estimators are used to ensure finiteness and uniqueness of the MLE to overcome such problems. The above rationale provides the necessary justification for considering the use of such classifier to the current task. For a response variable $Y \in \{1, 2, \ldots, k\}$ with k possible values (categories), there are k classes for n instances with m attributes (explanatory variables), and the parameter matrix B that requires to be calculated will have dimension $m \times (k-1)$. In this case, the probability for Class j with the exception of the last class is given from:

$$P_j(X_i) = \frac{\exp(X_i B_j)}{(\sum_{j=1}^{k} \exp(X_i B_j)) + 1} \tag{4.49}$$

The last class has a probability of occurring given by:

$$1 - \sum_{j-1}^{k-1} P_j(X_i) = \frac{1}{\sum_{j-1}^{k-1} \exp(X_i B_j) + 1} \tag{4.50}$$

and the (negative) multinomial log-likelihood is given from:

$$L = -\sum_{i=1}^{n}\{\sum_{j=1}^{k-1}(Y_{ij} \times \ln(P_j(X_i))) + (1 - \sum j = 1^{k-1} Y_{ij} \times \ln(1 - \sum_{j=1}^{k-1} P_j(X_i))\} + \text{ridge} \times B^2 \tag{4.51}$$

In order to find the matrix B for which L is minimized, a Quasi-Newton method is used to search for the optimized values of the $m \times (k-1)$ variables [462]. At this stage it is worth noting that in the current implementation of the algorithm, before we use the optimization procedure, we 'squeeze' the matrix B into an $m \times (k-1)$ matrix. A more detailed description of the MLR adopted can be found in [462, 463]. With reference to the example shown in Fig. 4.1, X relates to the feature set associated with the six powder substances and Y denotes the different categories.

4.5.5 Naive Bayesian (NB) Classifier

The NB classifier is chosen for the study shown in Fig. 4.1, as it is straightforward in its implementation. Furthermore, this is a frequently used probabilistic classifier based on applying Bayes' theorem with strong (naive) independence assumptions [464]. The NB classifier assumes that the presence (or absence) of a particular feature of a class is unrelated to the presence (or absence) of any other feature. Depending on the precise nature of the adopted probability model, the NB classifier can be trained very efficiently in a supervised learning setting. In practical applications, parameter estimation for naive Bayes models uses the maximum likelihood method, where each class with the highest post-probability is labelled as the resulting class.

Suppose, $X = \{X_1, X_2, X3, \ldots, X_n\}$ is a feature vector set that contains $C_k (k = 1, 2, \ldots, m)$ classes of data to be classified. Each class is associated with a probability $P(C_k)$ that represents the prior probability of identifying a feature into C_k and the values of $P(C_k)$ can be estimated from the training dataset. For the n feature values of X, the goal of classification is clearly to find the conditional probability $P(C_k|X_1, X_2, X_3, \ldots, X_n)$. By Bayes's rule, this probability is equivalent to

$$P(C_k|X_1, X_2, X_3, \ldots, X_n) = \frac{P(C_k)P(X_1, X_2, X_3, \ldots, X_n|C_k)}{\sum P(C_k)P(X_1, X_2, X_3, \ldots, X_n|C_k)} \tag{4.52}$$

The final decision rule for the NB classifier is:

$$\mathrm{classify}(\mathrm{X_1, X_2, X_3, \ldots, X_n}) = \arg\max \mathrm{P(C_k)} \prod_{\mathrm{i=1}}^{\mathrm{n}} \mathrm{P(X_i|C_k)} \tag{4.53}$$

For the example shown in Fig. 4.1, we used the extracted feature vector set as the input in Eq. 4.53 and C_k $(k = 1, 2, \ldots, 6)$ indicates the number of the six powder classes within which the unknown samples had to be classified. In the training stage, $P(X_i|C_k)$ is estimated with respect to the training data. In the testing stage, based on the posterior probability $P(C_k|X_i)$, a decision whether a test sample belongs to a particular class C_k or not is made.

4.5.6 Performance Evaluation of Several Different Classifiers

Cross-validation, sometimes called rotation estimation, [4, 30, 465] is a model validation technique for assessing how the results of a statistical analysis will generalize to an independent data set. To reduce any bias of training and test data, a k-fold cross-validation technique is employed [466, 467] by setting $k = 10$ for the example shown in Fig. 4.1. This technique is implemented to create the training set and testing set for evaluation. Generally, with k-fold cross validation, the feature vector set is divided into k subsets of (approximately) equal size. The proposed classifiers are trained and tested k times. Each time, one of the subsets from the training set is left out. One of the subsets (folds) is used as a test set and the other $k-1$ subsets (folds) are put together to form a new training set. Then the average accuracy across all k trials is computed to assess the performance of the classifier.

Subsequently, the individual feature sets from each powder class are combined to form a composite feature set that contains all the features from all T-ray pulse signals associated with all powder substances, i.e. on the basis of the statistical feature extraction process using the cross-correlation sequences. We assess the performance of the proposed classifiers using widely accepted metrics such as accuracy, true positive rate (TPR) (also called sensitivity or recall), false positive rate (FPR) (also called false alarm rate or (1-specificity)), precision (also called positive predictive value), F-measure, mean absolute error (MAE) and kappa statistics. All these criteria were considered when assessing all extracted feature data. The evaluation metric adopted is accuracy rate as a percentage of correct prediction [368]. The TPR provides the fraction of positive cases that are classified as positive [468, 469]. The FPR is the percentage of false positives predicted as positive from samples belonging to the negative class. The FPR usually refers to the expectancy of the false positive ratio. Precision is a measure which is used to estimate the probability that a positive prediction is correct. The F-measure is a metric that provides a combined measure for precision and recall calculated as 2 $\times$ Precision $\times$ Recall/(Precision + Recall) [468]. Mean absolute error (MAE) is used to measure how close predictions are to the eventual outcomes [468]. The Kappa statistic is a chance-corrected measure of agreement between the classifications and the true classes [470]. It is calculated by subtracting the agreement expected by chance from the observed agreement, and dividing it by the maximum possible agreement.

Figure 4.8 represents the classification outcomes for the mixture of 2, 3 and 4 mm thickness samples for all six powder substances with spectra shown in Fig. 3.8 [350]. This classification task is set up as a three class problem. Here, the 2 mm thickness powder substance is considered as belonging to the first class, the 3 mm thickness powder substance is considered as belonging to the second class and the 4 mm thickness powder substance is considered as belonging to the third class. As can be seen from this table, the overall accuracy for the MLR classifier is 99.56% for all the powder samples while this value is 99.35% for the KNN classifier, 91.83% for the SVM classifier and 91.82% for the NB classifier respectively. Similarly to the classification results discussed in the previous sections, in most of the cases, the MLR classifier consistently yields the highest performance whereas NB classifier shows the lowest performance. As shown in Fig. 4.9, good classification performance and classification consistency of the 2D cross correlation based feature extraction approach shows successful denoising, while at the same time enables us to resolve useful features in the time domain signals associated with each pixel in the image in a consistent manner. This is significant bearing in mind that classification tasks that were difficult to perform in the past, due to the presence of some unquantifiable scattering, become now possible. It is also worth noting that although in analytical sciences, cross-correlation techniques have mainly been explored within a de-noising con-

Powder types	Powder thickness	Classifier types			
		MLR (%)	KNN (%)	SVM (%)	NB (%)
Sand	2mm	98.04	100	100	90.19
	3mm	98.04	96.08	98.04	96.08
	4mm	98.04	100	92.16	94.12
Talc	2mm	100	100	96.08	86.27
	3mm	100	100	98.04	84.31
	4mm	100	100	96.08	78.43
Salt	2mm	100	100	100	88.24
	3mm	100	96.08	43.14	80.39
	4mm	100	98.04	100	90.19
Sugar	2mm	98.04	100	80.39	90.19
	3mm	100	100	62.75	86.27
	4mm	100	100	100	94.12
Flour	2mm	100	100	100	96.08
	3mm	100	100	96.1	74.51
	4mm	100	100	94.1	96.08
Soda	2mm	100	100	100	92.16
	3mm	100	98.04	96.08	82.35
	4mm	100	100	100	74.51

Fig. 4.8 Classification performance in three thickness: 2, 3 and 4 mm of each powder

text, the proposed methodology places these algorithms within a machine learning context.

It may also be concluded that the MLR is a powerful and less complex algorithm for THz pulse signals classification. The proposed technique should extend the use of classification algorithms to experiments where samples are not placed in a cuvette, a sample holder or compressed in pellet form in order to perform the spectroscopic investigations, and points towards a new way of performing industrial quality control using THz imaging systems 'in situ' when samples are still in powder form where a different degree of scattering may also be present in the measurement process across the different spectral bands. The proposed methodology therefore, has the potential to significantly extend the applications domain of classifiers for material characterization. This has important applications in high value manufacturing such as the pharmaceutical industry as well as for tissue differentiation and characterization in biomedical imaging.

Figure 4.9 displays kappa statistics for all classifiers assuming a 10 feature input. The aim of the kappa statistics test is to evaluate the consistency of the classifiers. Consistency is considered mild if kappa values are less than 0.2 (20%), fair if they lie between 0.21–0.40 (21–40%), moderate if they lie between 0.41–0.60 (41–60%),

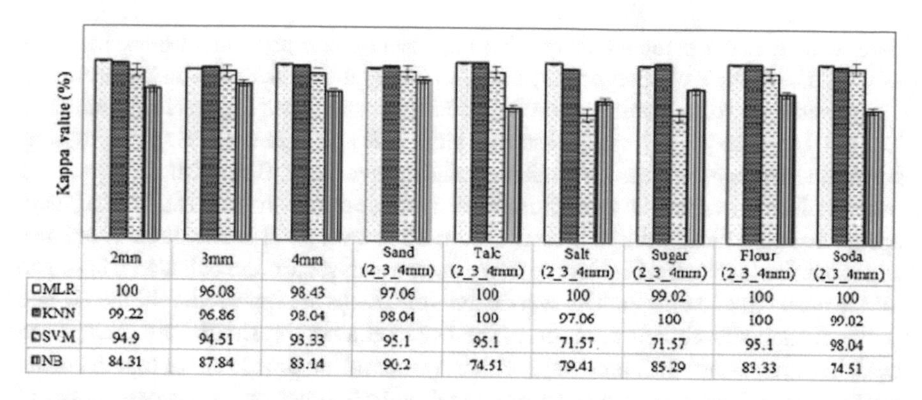

	2mm	3mm	4mm	Sand (2_3_4mm)	Talc (2_3_4mm)	Salt (2_3_4mm)	Sugar (2_3_4mm)	Flour (2_3_4mm)	Soda (2_3_4mm)
MLR	100	96.08	98.43	97.06	100	100	99.02	100	100
KNN	99.22	96.86	98.04	98.04	100	97.06	100	100	99.02
SVM	94.9	94.51	93.33	95.1	95.1	71.57	71.57	95.1	98.04
NB	84.31	87.84	83.14	90.2	74.51	79.41	85.29	83.33	74.51

Fig. 4.9 Kappa statistics values for the MLR, KNN, SVM and NB classifiers for datasets associated with different powder thickness samples

good if it is between 0.61–0.80 (61–80%), and excellent if it is greater than 0.81 (81%). As shown in Fig. 4.9, the highest kappa values are obtained by the MLR on both 2 mm thickness sample datasets (100%), as well as 4 mm (98.43%) datasets. In addition, highest kappa values are obtained for the mixture of 2, 3 and 4 mm samples of talc (100%), salt (100%), flour (100%) and soda (100%). The KNN algorithm also demonstrated very good performance (second best overall) as can be seen in the case of the 3 mm thickness sample datasets (96.86%), and the mixtures of 2, 3 and 4 mm sand (98.04%), talc (100%), sugar (100%) and flour (100%). The kappa values of the other two classifiers (SVM and NB) are systematically lower compared to those achieved by the MLR and KNN irrespective of sample type, furthermore, the values are consistently lowest for the NB classifier. In this figure, the error bars indicate the associated kappa value standard error. In most of the cases, the highest kappa values are obtained using the MLR algorithm.

In another classification example, Eadie et al. [471] carried out multi-dimensional THz imaging analysis for colon cancer diagnosis. Their research uses decision trees to find important parameters of relevance to classification; these are subsequently used with neural networks (NN) and SVMs to classify the THz datasets thus identifying normal and abnormal samples. Their work reports sensitivity values of 90–100% and specificity values of 86–90%. This is a good example where THz reflection imaging is combined with an optimized feature extraction and classification methodology to identify colon cancer.

4.5.7 Clustering Techniques to Segment THz Images

Clustering, also termed *cluster analysis*, is the formal study of algorithms and methods for grouping unlabelled data into subsets (called clusters) according to measured or perceived intrinsic characteristics or degree of similarity. Clustering deals with data without using category labels that tag objects with prior identifiers, i.e. class labels. The absence of category information distinguishes data clustering (unsupervised learning) from classification or discriminant analysis (supervised learning). The two most frequently used clustering techniques that are used in spatial clustering are the k-means and the ISODATA clustering algorithm. Both of these algorithms use iterative procedures in their cluster estimation process. In general, both of them assign first an arbitrary initial cluster vector. Then each pixel is classified as belonging to the closest cluster. Finally the new cluster mean vectors are calculated based on all the pixels in one cluster. The second and third steps are repeated until the change between each subsequent iteration is smaller than a set threshold. The change can be defined in several different ways, either by measuring the distances that the mean cluster vector have changed from one iteration to another or by the percentage of pixels that have changed between iterations. The ISODATA algorithm incorporates some further refinements such as the option of splitting and merging of clusters [472]. Clusters are merged if either the number of members (pixel) in a cluster is less than a certain threshold, or if the centers of two clusters are closer than a certain threshold. Clusters are split into parts (thus forming additional clusters) if the cluster standard deviation exceeds a predefined value and the number of members (pixels) is twice the threshold for the minimum number of members.

Currently, several papers report clustering techniques to segment THz images. Brun et al. [473] reported on THz-TDS imaging of 10 μm thick histological sections, where clustering methods were used in THz spectral images that are produced on the basis of the extracted refractive index data. His study showed that THz spectral differences exist, not only between tumor and healthy tissues, but also within tumors. Ayech and Ziou [474] also discussed k-means clustering methods for segmentation of THz imaging. They used a combination of an autoregressive (AR) model and PCA to extract effective temporal/spectral features from TPI before carrying out soft decision thresholding of the associated k-harmonic-means (KHM). Their method outperform the algorithms based on hard decision thresholding of traditional k-means methods. In [475, 476], a novel approach of segmentation in THz images is also proposed, where the k-means technique is reformulated using a ranked set sample principle. This approach consists of estimating the expected cluster centers, selecting the relevant features and their scores, and classifying the observed pixels of THz images. In another recent study [477], a two-step partitioning clustering approach was used to segment THz measurements of the inner structure of teeth which were extracted from cave bears so as to identify evolutionary traits, life spans and feeding habits. The tomographic measurements with the imaging system showed that the layer-like structures are discernable within the material, giving a more detailed image of the inner structure of the tooth. A k-nearest neighbor graph that is built on the reduced channel information [478] was also used to further assign the observed spatial features in the images into segments, it was achieved by using a minimum edge cut bi-sectioning method.

The use of the ISODATA algorithm to cluster THz spectra and perform image segmentation was first suggested by Berry et al. [479]. In their work, two types of specimens were examined, the first one was of a basal cell carcinoma and the second of a melanoma. Unsupervised ISODATA classification was then compared qualitatively with k-means classification that was performed using the information from the entire time domain sequence for each pixel. In addition, classification was then correlated with conventional stained microscope slides. There was good qualitative agreement between the two classifications methods. Classification results were consistent and preserved the observed characteristics. The results point toward the use of a small number of features to perform classification. If this line of work can be further validated through additional studies, this could lead to considerably reduced acquisition times. In addition, the ISODATA algorithm is particularly useful in further developing convolution network classification approaches, a technique well established within the machine learning community.

4.6 Retinal Fundus Image Analysis via Supervised and Non-supervised Learning

The motivation for using classifiers in fundus photography is to identify specific anatomical structures in the retina. Structures of interest include the optic disk and macula [227]. Identification of abnormal structures, such as retinal vasculature, are also of interest as they can be used to diagnose the presence and severity of diseases such as diabetic retinopathy, occlusion, glaucoma etc. [226, 345].

Features in the optic disk also include the start of optic nerve head (white stock) which connects the eye to the brain as it is also a entry point for major blood vessels to the eye. In the presence of disease, a tree-like structure called blood vasculature (which contains very high frequency components from an image processing perspective) spanning across the fundus image is also likely to change as is the distribution and thickness which is seen in the blood vessels present in the retina. Most diseases in the retina cause substantial changes in the vasculature network characteristics, and if they aren't detected at an early stage, they can lead to vision loss.

4.6.1 Fundus Image Vessel Segmentation

Machine learning classification approaches are perhaps the simplest to adopt for fundus image vessel segmentation. Two distinct categories of pattern classification techniques for vessel segmentation may be considered, and these can be based on supervised [360] and unsupervised training [480]. Training of the classifier is usually performed using datasets of manually labelled vessel images. The aim is usually to allow the classifier to recognise retinal vessel regions from the background. Such techniques have been employed by Staale et al. [481] and Soares et al. [427], among others. In contrast, unsupervised classifiers attempt to find, directly, inherent differences between blood vessels and the background in images of the retina; examples include fuzzy C-means clustering [358] and Bayesian classification. It is generally accepted [434] that supervised classification has improved performance over unsupervised schemes, although performance is affected by issues such as non-uniform illumination. Vessel segmentation can also be used as part of a pre-processing step for the further identification of other retinal structures like optic disc, fovea, location of microaneurisms etc.

Pixel feature classification of retinal blood vessels is performed using the numerical values of individual pixels in combination with their surrounding pixels using a supervised approach. Originally, pixel intensity was used as the sole feature for the classification task. More recently however, n-dimensional multi-feature vectors are utilized; features include pixel contrast with the surrounding region, its proximity to an edge, and similarity metrics. In addition, some other multi-feature vectors calculated for each pixel, including local convolutions with multiple Gaussian derivative, Gabor, or other wavelet kernels [119] have also been proposed. The image is thus transformed into an n-dimensional feature space and pixels are classified according to their position in that feature space. The resulting hard (categorical) or soft (probabilistic) classification is then used to either assign labels to each pixel (for example vessel or nonvessel in the case of hard classification), or to construct class-specific likelihood maps (e.g. a map of the degree of vessel vasculature for soft classification).

4.6.2 Algorithmic Detection of the Optic Disk

Locating and segmenting the optic disc (OD) is important in retinal image analysis, since all the vessels emerge from the OD in the retina. In order to segment vessels or perform an identification of a Region of Interest (ROI) for vessels classification, analysis of OD swelling, in conjunction with OD localization is necessary. There have been several studies in the literature on the automatic detection and segmentation of OD. Usually, the candidate regions for OD are first detected using template-matching, then the accurate candidate region is selected on the basis of a 'vessel-pattern' property inside the OD, and finally the OD boundary segmentation is analysed by making use of local gradient information.

The proposed method has been tested on the publically available MESSIDOR dataset and achieved 99% accuracy. There have been some additional studies using morphological operations for OD detection. Choukikar et al. [482] located the OD position by applying histogram equalization on original RGB fundus images, this was followed by the application of closing and opening morphological operations. Furthermore, Aquino et al. [484] suggested a new template-based methodology for segmenting the OD from digital retinal images. This methodology uses morphological and edge detection techniques followed by the Circular Hough Transform to obtain a circular OD boundary approximation. A drawback of the technique is that it requires the identification of a pixel located within the OD, this seeding process is formed using a voting-type algorithm which can be somehow arbitrary. Figure 4.10

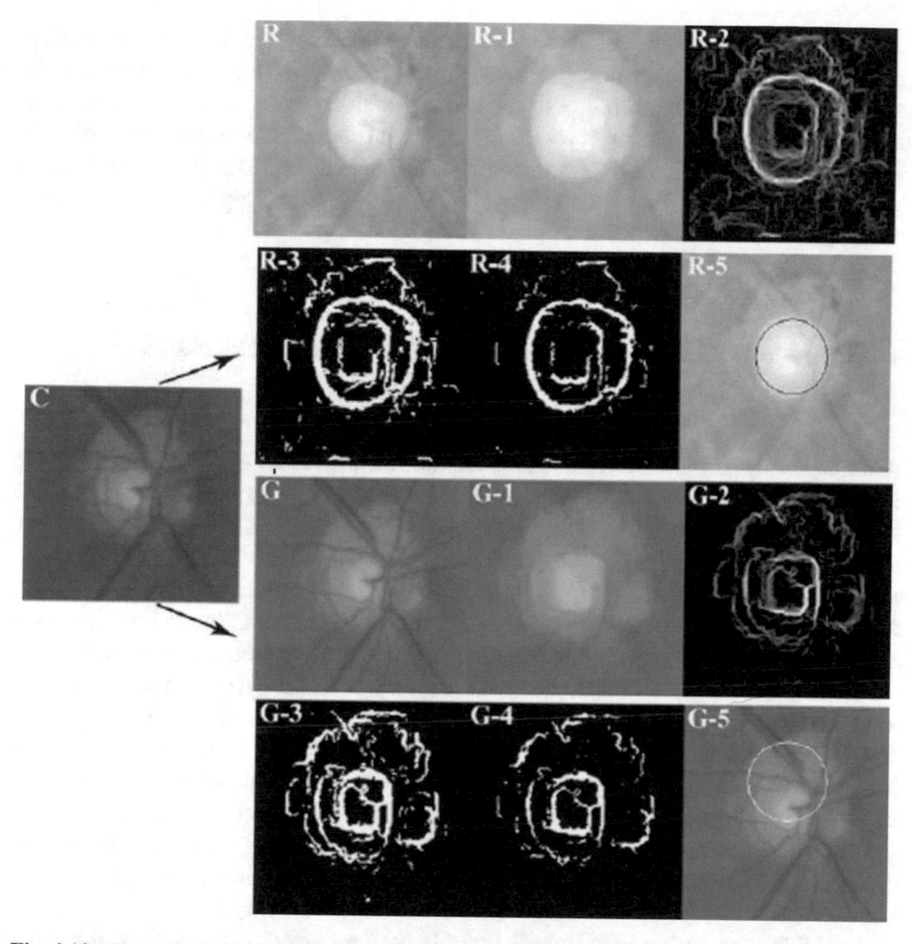

Fig. 4.10 Illustration of the process for the calculation of the circular OD boundary approximation: (*C*) Initial RBG sub-image containing an OD affected by peripapillary atrophy. On the image on the *right*, the *top row* shows the process performed on the *red* channel, whereas the image at the *bottom* depicts the process applied to the green component. (*R*) and (*G*) Subimages extracted from the red and green channels of (*C*), respectively. (*R-1*) and (*G-1*) Vessel elimination. (*R-2*) and (*G-2*) Gradient magnitude image. (*R-3*) and (*G-3*) Binary image. (*R-4*) and (*G-4*) Cleaner version of the binary image. (*R-5*) and (*G-5*) Circular OD boundary approximation. The scores obtained in the Circular Hough Transform algorithm are, 264 for segmentation in (*R-5*) and 130 for segmentation in (*G-5*), so the segmentation selected last would be the one performed on the *red* channel. After [484]

provides an illustration of the process for the calculation of the circular OD boundary approximation.

Most recently, Akyol et al. [359] proposed a method which is comprised of a combination of five main approaches: image processing, key point extraction, texture analysis, visual dictionary, and data mining classifier techniques. In addition, Usman et al. [485] proposed a new model for OD localization which uses template-matching, and is based on vessel-contrast. In this method, first the difference between the average pixel value associated with the inside and the outside region of a red lesion is calculated using a filtering procedure, then a machine leaning method is used to identify haemorrhages using 64 different textural features. The proposed method yielded a sensitivity of 83% and a specificity of 67% when applied to the DRIVE dataset.

4.6.3 Retinal Vessel Classification: Identifying and Sorting Arteries and Veins

Automatic retinal blood vessels classification has also been evolving rapidly over recent years. For the discovery of biomarkers in the retinal vasculature, it is essential to distinguish between arteries and veins [486]. The systems discussed in the current literature are either automatic or semi-automatic. In the work discussed by Saez et al. [487], two approaches (pixel-based or profile-based) are considered for the formation of feature vectors. Pixel-based feature vectors are extracted on the basis of the values of different colour channels of the pixels as well as the mode of the values for the component under study. In the profile-based approach, feature vectors are constructed by taking the mean or median of the colour component in the profile. Vessels are labelled afterwards as veins and arteries using an unsupervised clustering k-means algorithm. The image is divided into overlapping regions so the vessels can be classified multiple times, and feature-vectors are identified after calculating the probabilities of occurrence of the features. Then, the mean of those probabilities is calculated and vessels are labelled as belonging to a particular class according to whether they correspond to a class with the highest probability.

For all images and radii, a sensitivity of 0.7819 for arteries, and 0.8790 for veins was calculated. The mean intensity for the red colour is preferred in [488] for the classification of vessels. The red channel of the image is selected because arteries systematically show a higher intensity than veins in the red channel. The mean intensity of all individual components is then calculated and vessels are classified as arteries on the basis of a higher mean intensity. In their study, the authors examined 15 images to further evaluate the proposed technique, arteries were correctly identified 82% of the time whereas the accuracy in detecting veins was only 50%.

Finally, Estrada et al. [489] proposed a novel, graph-theoretic framework for distinguishing arteries from veins in a fundus image. This group took into consideration the underlying vessel topology to better classify small and midsized vessels. They extended a tree topology estimation framework by incorporating expert, domain-specific features to construct a simple yet powerful global likelihood model. This approach is capable of analysing the entire vasculature, including peripheral vessels, in wide field-of-view fundus photographs. This topology-based method shows significant potential for diagnosing diseases that show retinal vascular changes. Figure 4.11

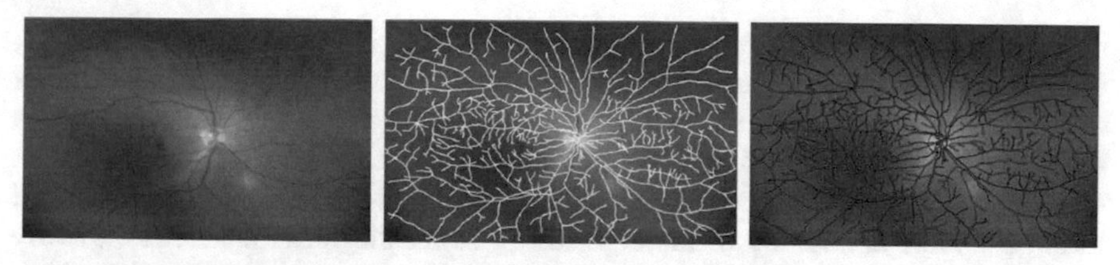

Fig. 4.11 The *left panel* shows retinal arteries and veins as they overlap each other throughout a wide field-of-view color fundus image. The *middle panel* is a constructed planar graph (overlaid in *white*) that captures the projected vascular topology. On the *right panel*, each edge in the graph is identified either as an artery (in *red*) or a vein (in *blue*). After [489]

provides an illustration of arteries and veins as identified using the proposed vascular topology approach.

4.6.4 Automated Image Classification Using Criteria Directly Developed from Clinicians

Currently, most MRI equipment manufacturers are in the process of also developing AI based software for the interpretation of images generated from their scanners. In addition, there are also newly established companies which should soon provide novel AI solutions that will enable complementary interpretation of scans through their own in-house software algorithms. A company at the forefront of such developments that should soon provide automatic interpretation of non-contrast enhanced computed tomography (NCCT) scans (which can have similar database structures as those found in MRI datasets), is Brainomix Ltd. The company is currently developing new software which combines AI based image interpretation with the Alberta Stroke Program Early Computed Tomography Score (ASPECTS), an established 10-point quantitative topographic computed tomography scan score that is currently used by clinicians to assess early ischemic changes in stroke patients. The e-ASPECTS software that Brainomix Ltd developed which is currently undergoing clinical trials across Europe, can provide very quickly an interpretation of the physiological state of regions in the brain in patients, potentially saving valuable clinician time in granting eligibility for endovascular treatment using thrombolytic drugs. As the administration of drugs needs to take place as soon as possible after a stroke episode to minimize damage to the different regions in the brain, the automation of the diagnostic process can have a significant impact on the patient's future quality of life. It is worth noting that, as reported in the work by Herweh et al. (2016), [490] as well as in the work reported by Nagel et al. (2016) [491] that was based on a multicentre trial with 132 patients and 2560 ASPECTS regions, the e-ASPECTS showed a similar performance in terms of ROC sensitivity and specificity, as well as accuracy based on true positive (TP), true negative (TN), false positives (FP), and false negative (FN) scores to that of stroke expert neuroradiologists in the assessment of brain computed tomography of acute ischemic stroke patients. In addition, Bland-Altman plots [492, 493] and associated histograms of score error, showed excellent agreement in terms of the established ground truth in the images. It is also worth noting that Matthews correlation coefficients [494, 495] for e-ASPECTS were higher (0.36 and 0.34) than those of all neuroradiologists (0.32, 0.31, and 0.3 NRAD scores), indicating that through further fine-tuning of the algorithms, better diagnosis than that currently achieved by experts can be potentially achieved. Clearly, the e-ASPECTS methodology is a particularly interesting paradigm of relevance to all imaging modalities discussed in this book as it points towards a direction where a combination of both expert knowledge as well as standardized AI routines can be nicely integrated to provide expert diagnosis with improved consistency, while at the same time providing diagnosis immediately after the patient scans have been concluded.

Chapter 5
Introduction to MRI Time Series Image Analysis Techniques

This chapter discusses opportunities for spatiotemporal enhancement in DCE-MRIs using a tensorial multi-channel framework. Examples from breast tumour reconstruction are provided to showcase the proposed methodology. It is shown that tumour voxels registered in three-dimensional space can be reconstructing better after increasing contrast from background images using the proposed methodology. The algorithm can be used to perform both feature extraction as well as image registration. This chapter also discusses the general structure of supervised learning algorithms for functional MRI datasets. Advances in supervised multivariate learning from fMRI datasets that promise to further elucidate brain disorders are discussed. Finally, the general structure of topological graph kernels in functional connectivity networks is also explained. The prospects for developing machine learning algorithms that would automatically provide spatio-temporal associations of brain activity across different regions using graph theory methodologies are discussed. A more critical view of what may be achieved taking into consideration limitations in the fMRI measurement modality is also provided. Finally, some recent advances from the computer vision community of relevance are also highlighted as possible future research directions.

5.1 Analysis of DCE-MRI Data

Since 1995, MRI has been used extensively for the detection of invasive breast cancer [59, 60, 89, 496]. Because of its high 3D resolution and its ability to acquire kinetic contrast information, it has steadily gained popularity over traditional diagnostic techniques such as X-ray mammography and ultrasound [497]. For breast tumours, lesion diagnostic sensitivities can reach 97% [498]. Moreover, in addition to its wide use in functional neuroscience, the technique has also been extensively used for mapping and identifying brain tumours. In all of these measurement modalities,

X. Yin et al., *Pattern Classification of Medical Images: Computer Aided Diagnosis*, Health Information Science, DOI 10.1007/978-3-319-57027-3_5

multiple images are collected, and one of the problems commonly encountered is how to extract the useful information that simultaneously resides across all the images obtained through separate scans. In the case of DCE-MRI T1-weighted imaging for example, after an intravenous injection of the contrast agent, blood vessels are imaged repeatedly before a tumour or local inflammation can be observed. There can be significant differences in the signal from the contrast agent across the image. This often occurs because the contrast agent is blocked by the regular brain-blood-barrier but is not blocked in the blood vessels generated by the tumour. The concentration of the contrast agent is then measured when it passes from the blood vessels to the extra-cellular space of the tissue and on its path back towards the blood vessels.

However, specificity of breast DCE-MRI is still rather low, with rates of between 30 and 70% [499, 500]. High false positive detection rates on MRI often lead, not only to anxiety for the patient, but may also result in an unnecessary invasive biopsy [497, 499]. This hinders its use as a routine imaging technique in breast cancer patients. Benefits of breast MRI include better cancer detection rates in high-risk women and the provision of additional information regarding the extent of disease in women with known breast cancer.

Computer-aided diagnosis (CAD) approaches for breast MRI are typically employed for automatically identifying tumours from normal tissues when these are at a stage of rapid development [68, 97, 501, 502], whereas the more complex task of classifying a lesion as benign or malignant [63, 104, 501, 503–510] is proving more difficult to address. In order to interpret the patterns resulting from contrast enhancement across a series of MRI volumes, intensity changes per voxel are color-coded by an automated kinetic assessment protocol. However, the technique is not fully automated and requires continuous feedback from experts.

A major challenge in the diagnosis of breast DCE-MRI is the spatiotemporal association of tumour enhancement patterns, a task that humans are not as optimized to perform [63]. With many CAD systems now available commercially, Pan et al. [511] evaluated them to ascertain which system is best in detecting signs of cancer on breast MRIs. The most commonly used CAD systems in the USA are CADstream (CS) (Merge Healthcare Inc., Chicago, IL) and DynaCAD for Breast (DC) (Invivo, Gainesville, FL). Pan et al.'s primary objective (discussed in more detail in the following section) was to compare the CS and DC breast MRI CAD systems for diagnostic accuracy and post processed image quality. The experiments were aimed at evaluating 177 lesions in 175 consecutive patients who underwent second-look ultrasound guided biopsy or MRI-guided biopsy. The results illustrate that the two CAD systems had similar sensitivity and specificity (CS had 70% sensitivity and 32% specificity whereas DC had 81% sensitivity and 34% specificity). Both CS and DC had a high sensitivity for detecting malignant lesions on breast tissue. However, neither system significantly improved specificity for the diagnosis of benign lesions. Assesment was performed on the basis of the Receiver Operating Characteristic curve (or ROC curves). ROC is a plot of the true positive rate against the false positive rate for the different possible cut points of a diagnostic test. The ROC curve plots using both CS and DC systems are illustrated in Fig. 5.1.

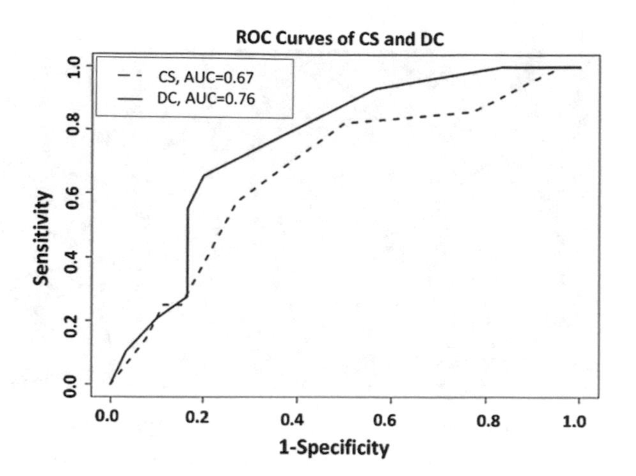

Fig. 5.1 ROC curves of the mean scores for CADstream and DynaCAD for Breast samples. The figure shows the ROC curves based on the two mean diagnostic scores for each software system (CS: CADstream, DC: DynaCAD for Breast, AUC: area under the curve, ROC: receiver operating characteristic). After [511]

5.1.1 *Outlook for Future Tensorial Algebra Based Feature and Image Registration*

In dynamic pattern recognition methods for the analysis of DCE-MRI, the emphasis has been on either high temporal resolution and empirical analysis [159, 512] or high spatial resolution with a stand-alone morphologic feature extraction [512, 513]. Time-series analysis is a time-consuming task due to the often encountered spatiotemporal lesion variability. Changes in spatial intensity of imaged tumours are a further complication as they cause an inherent difficulty in segmentation of an object of interest [377]. In the discussed example, the previously mentioned multi-channel image reconstruction is assumed. Figure 5.2a depicts an imaged ductal carcinoma in situ (DCIS). While the parts depicted by the arrows show the same anatomical structure taken from the same tumour region, the intensity values are different. The intensity indicated by the yellow arrow is higher than the intensity indicated by the red arrows. After conducting intensity based segmentation as illustrated in Fig. 5.2b, the region with low intensity may feature as a gap separating the image into two disconnected parts. The gap forms an area without edge. A multi-channel classification method that considers the associations between spatial and temporal features of high-dimensional images is proposed in order to achieve accurate diagnosis of tumour tissues. Generally, the detection of anomalies in spatiotemporal data is an emergent interdisciplinary topic that involves innovative computer science methods. Mining spatiotemporal patterns is critical for the correct identification of tumour anomalies in DCE-MRI. This task still remains challenging, however, because of the complexity associated with the sparse features in voxel data when this is associated to consecutive scans obtained at separate points in time.

The need for a multi-channel framework that captures a multitude of features extracted using the signal processing routines discussed earlier, leads to a requirement for developing alternative classifiers capable of accommodating a large num-

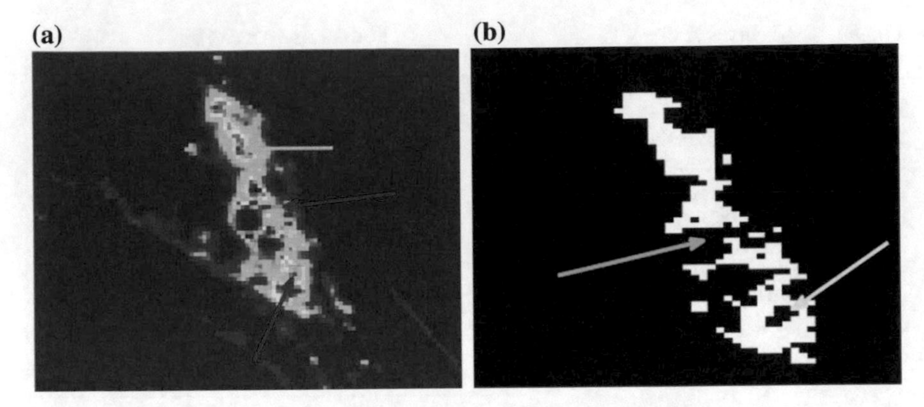

Fig. 5.2 Imaged breast tumours obtained by MRIs. **a** Illustration of intensity inconsistency for breast tumour tissue images. *Yellow arrows* indicate a high intensity and *red arrows* low intensity. **b** Illustration of intensity based segmentation with inhomogeneous boundaries; *yellow arrows* indicate an irregular ring region with a hole inside and the *green arrow* indicates missing areas

ber of input vectors. In addition, recently, tensor decomposition of high-dimensional medical image data, i.e. fMRI, has also gained popularity since it can explore the multi-way structure in the datasets which inherently exists in human organ imaging [514]. Tensors are multimode (multi-way) arrays, where vectors (i.e. one-mode tensors) and matrices (i.e. two-mode tensors) are special cases. The tensor representation captures useful information that is difficult to capture in a conventional vectorial formalism, for example, accounting for specific morphological features such as directional striations in muscle tissue or vessels.

To effectively utilize the additional information contained in tensors, we propose to extend the CELM algorithms for effective tensor classification. Multi-dimensional classifiers do not require a dimensionality reduction of the datasets, thus preserving the information presented at the input stage of the classifier which could otherwise be lost in a conventional dataset fusion framework. Since most standard learning algorithms assume data obtained at separate scans are just vectors composed of different features, it is not straightforward to apply these algorithms on tensorial data. The CELM method (discussed in the previous chapter) enables the identification and learning of inter-mode relations across different features.

As stated earlier, within a THz imaging context, the aim is to preserve the features extracted and ideally present them as separate entities to the classifier. Similarly, within the MRI community, in addition to the components of relevance in a multi-dimensional feature space described earlier, there is a need for observing changes in fMRI signals taking into consideration information obtained at different time stamps so data can also have a tensorial structure. Since an assessment of disease progression is made by cross-correlating images taken from different examinations, again a tensorial framework is often needed. Multi-dimensional classifiers are therefore ideally placed to further explore such cross-correlations.

Currently, there are several approaches for multiclass SVM [515]. The naive approach is constructing and combining several binary classifiers and considering all data as elements within one big optimization problem [516], or by learning interdependent and structured output spaces [517]. Unlike classic SVMs, the complex valued hyper-planes of CELM are calculated using the smallest norm of output weights with the smallest training error in a similar manner as in ELM classification. The technique discards the normal threshold found in SVMs, without calculating support vectors. The extended CELM has significant potential for solving complex valued problems for multiclass classification of tensorial datasets with dramatically reduced computational complexity and significantly improved computational speed. It enables the classification of tensorial data while preserving information associated with adjacent and overlapping data vectors as well as differentially extracted features.

In addition, registration of images is a crucial step in many image processing applications where the final information is obtained by combining multiple input images. In many applications multi-channel images are also available, requiring innovative processing of vector data. Traditional approaches in achieving multichannel image registration can cause inaccuracies by introducing information loss or misinterpretations. An alternative way to perform registration of multichannel images described by associated vectorial datasets is through the use of Geometric Algebras such as Clifford Algebra (discussed in the next chapter). The main advantage of this methods is that it operates on the multichannel signal, instead of scaling the signal down to one dimension (e.g. by averaging) and thereby loosing a lot of information. A further advantage is that it enables the fusion of datasets from heterogeneous sensing modalities, thus allowing for future dataset integration, as will be made possible in the near future through further progress in biomedical sensing.

5.1.2 Performance Measures

Evaluation of diagnostic tests is generally necessary not only for confirming the presence of disease, but also for ruling out the disease in healthy subjects. The diseased subject detection process via DCE-MRI aims to provide a voxel-based classification result. When providing disease diagnosis to patients based on the gold standard, any voxel in MRIs can be classified either as healthy or diseased, and as tumorous or surrounding tissue. Consequently, there are four possibilities; two classifications and two misclassifications. The classifications are the true positive (TP) and the true negative (TN) where the number of tumour voxels and background voxels is correctly detected; the false positive (FP) is the number of pixels not belonging to a vessel, but are mistakenly recognised as one, and the false negative (FN) is the number of pixels belonging to a vessel, but are recognised as background pixels.

One can further derive the probability of a positive test result for patients with disease and the probability of negative test results for patients without disease. Several relevant terms are defined as follows.

Table 5.1 Performance metrics in the diseased tissue detection process via DCE-MRIs

Measure	Description
TPR	TP/deased voxel count
FPR	FP/non-diseased voxel count
Specificity	TN/(TN + FP)
Sensitivity	TP/(TP + FN)
Accuracy (Acc)	(TP +TN)/FOV voxel count

- The true positive rate (TPR) represents the fraction of voxels correctly detected as diseased voxels.
- The false positive rate (FPR) is the fraction of voxels erroneously detected as diseased voxels.
- The accuracy (Acc) is measured by the ratio of the total number of correctly classified voxels (sum of true positives and true negatives) to the number of voxels in the image field of view.
- Sensitivity (SN) reflects the ability of the algorithm to detect the diseased voxels.
- Specificity (SP) is the ability to detect non-diseased voxels. It can be expressed as 1-FPR. The positive predictive value (PPV) gives the proportion of identified diseased voxels which are true diseased voxels.
- The PPV is the probability that an identified diseased voxel is a true positive.

A receiver operating characteristic (ROC) analysis has become a popular method for evaluating the accuracy of medical diagnostic systems. The ROC curve plots the fraction of diseased voxels correctly classified as diseased tissues, namely the TPR, versus the fraction of non-diseased voxels wrongly classified as diseased voxels, namely the FPR. The better the performance of the system is, the closer to the upper left hand corner of the ROC space it registers. The most frequently used performance measure extracted from the ROC curve is the value of the area under the curve (AUC) which is 1 for an optimal system. For MRI images, the TPR and FPR are computed considering only voxels inside the FOV. Table 5.1 summaries the performance metrics used by DCE-MRI image segmentation algorithms. A recently developed algorithm that combines chemometric analystical techniques from spectroscopic datasets with the ROC and AUC metrics is discussed further in [647].

5.2 Tensorial Representations in MRI

Tensorial analysis is directional so interactions of components within the associated matrices provide additional degrees of freedom for data analysis, enabling spatiotemporal data correlations to be made along each co-ordinate direction as shown in Fig. 5.3a. The isolation of such correlations in each co-ordinate plane can provide a clearer picture of disease progression. A third order tensor that may be associated with a DCE-MRI dataset is illustrated in Fig. 5.3b–d. Figure 5.3e illustrates how to flatten the third order tensors along frontal slices.

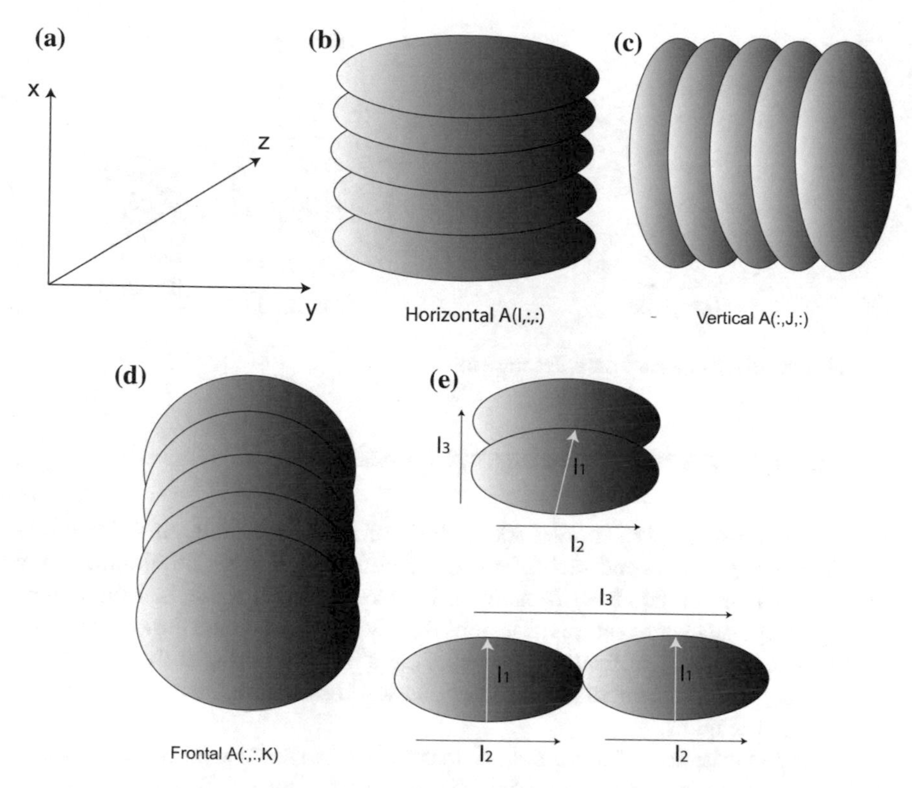

Fig. 5.3 **a** Illustration of the directions associated with the x-, y-, and z-axes. (**b**), (**c**), and (**d**). Illustration of three directional slices of a third order tensor: horizontal, vertical, and frontal, respectively, which are perpendicular to the x-, y-, and z-axes, respectively. **e** Illustration of the way to flatten the third order tensors along the frontal slices. The colon (:) used in the figure indicates all the column elements at a given direction are involved to form an image matrix

Tensor factorisation of a 3D spatial matrix uses multilinear algebra to analyse an ensemble of volume images, to separate and parsimoniously represent high-dimensional spatial datasets into constituent factors [557]. The 3D spatial image datasets are treated as a third order tensor. The image dataset tensor $\mathscr{A}^{(3)} \in \mathbb{R}^{I_1 \times I_2 \times I_3}$ is decomposed [559] or factorised to a core tensor $\mathscr{C} \in \mathbb{R}^{J_1 \times J_2 \times J_3}$ and three different modes of 2D image matrices $\mathbf{X}^{(n)} \in \mathbb{R}^{I_n \times J_n}$, $n = 1, 2, 3$, as illustrated in Fig. 5.4.

In our recent research [385], we explored tensor decomposition for the identification of shape with mirror symmetry. We concluded that if both the first mode matrix (i.e. along the y and the z axes) and second mode matrix (i.e. along the x and the z axes) are symmetric, the frontal plane (along the x and the y axes) is a mirror symmetric plane, and vice versa.

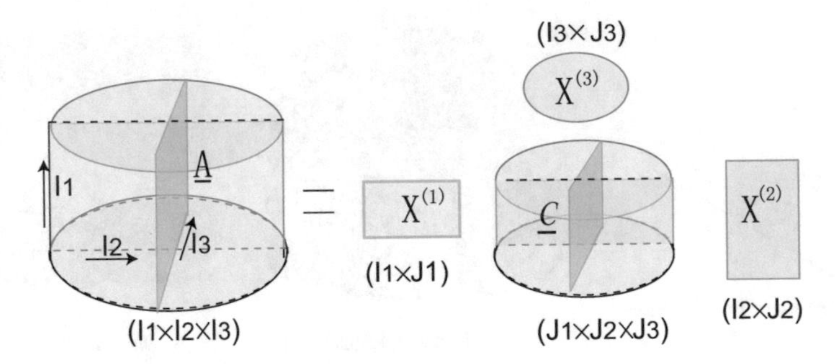

Fig. 5.4 Illustration of a third-order decomposition

5.3 Extensions to Multi-channel Classifiers

By using a tensor algebra framework analysis of spatiotemporally associated features becomes possible, and such advances, therefore, lead to the development of a multidimensional unified MRI framework for processing DCE-MRIs. Mining spatiotemporally associated features of lesions from MRIs can increase the accuracy and efficiency of pattern identification. Current DCE-MRI is not sufficiently accurate for the early detection of tumours because of a lack of association between the spatial and temporal features.

Tensor factorisation of a 3D spatial matrix is a universal methodology that is well suited to the analysis of an ensemble of volume images. In this section, we introduce a novel dynamic tensor reconstruction algorithm after adopting a principal component separation methodology. This is implemented on an offline tensor analysis algorithm (OTA) which results in a combined PCA-OTA algorithm. The algorithm is then implemented on the analysis of dynamic projection matrices for principal component separation of cancerous and healthy tissues.

Before conducting the tensor reconstruction, the intensity-scaled (IS) DCE-MRI datasets are loaded into MatLab (v. R2013b, MathWorks, Natick, MA) and their corresponding enhancement-scaled (ES) datasets are generated. Enhancement of the ES data is defined as the difference per voxel in the intensity of the post-contrast and pre-contrast images. In ES datasets, the reconstruction is performed on the region of interest (ROI) through the use of a pre-processing step according to morphological operations and standard FCM methods. A dynamic tensor data structure is introduced to store the DCE-MR image datasets, as this provides a simple way of extracting data from different dimensions. Another advantage of adopting a tensorial framework in our data structure is that the DCE-MR image data can be easily projected in different directions by using tensor or kronecker products. Tensor factorization is conducted on each three-dimensional (3D) MRI image by decomposing it into three two-dimensional (2D) subspaces (basis images) that are, respectively, associated with each mode (spatial orientations) of observations. These three-modes of dynamic basis images are further aligned to different time frames. For added clarity, we call these aligned basis images with time course, a temporal set of basis images at a different mode.

With the use of HOSVD, the dynamic ES dataset (a dynamic tensor $\mathscr{X}_\tau$) is decomposed into three-mode basis image matrices $\mathscr{A}_\tau^\iota$ and a core tensor C_τ, where $\iota = 1, 2, 3$ is associated with each mode of basis images; $\tau = 1, 2, ..., 6$ corresponds to a single time frame. PCA is applied on a temporal set of basis images. The temporal signal intensity variations $v_i^{\tau\iota}$ for each pixel within the decomposed basis image at each mode are associated with a state vector: $u_i^\iota = u_i^{1\iota}, u_i^{2\iota}, \ldots, u_i^{n\iota}$ ($n = 6$ for ES datasets). The set of all state vectors in one mode of the basis images over a pre-determined time course is defined as $\Upsilon^\iota = \{u_i^\iota\}$, $1 \le i \le \varepsilon$ with ε the number of pixels in the basis image at a different mode ι. The first-order covariance matrix of Υ^ι, Δ^ι, is calculated according to:

$$\Delta^\iota = \frac{1}{\varepsilon} \sum_{u_i^\iota \in \Upsilon^\iota} (u_i^\iota - \bar{u}^\iota)(u_i^\iota - \bar{u}^\iota)^T \text{ and } \bar{u}^\iota = \frac{1}{\varepsilon} \sum_{u_i^\iota \in \Upsilon^\iota} u_i^\iota \tag{5.1}$$

A linear PCA transformation is then applied to obtain the corresponding eigenvectors $E_\varsigma^\iota = \{e_\varsigma^\iota\}$, and eigenvalues $\lambda = \{\lambda_1, \lambda_2, ..., \lambda_6\}$ by solving $\lambda \mathbf{E} = \Delta \mathbf{E}$. A PCA of dynamic basis image datasets at each of the image modes yields 6 eigenvectors. After indexing and sorting according to their eigenvalues, the eigenvector corresponding to the largest eigenvalue is called the first channel eigenvector, the second largest eigenvalue is called second channel eigenvector and so on. As a result, a new mode vector is re-constructed $\mathbf{A}_\varsigma^\iota = \Delta^\iota E_\varsigma^\iota$ for each of the different channels (state points) ($\varsigma = 1, 2, \ldots, 6$). We matricise $\mathbf{A}$ to $\mathscr{A} \in N^\iota \times M^\iota$, to generate ι modes of basis images. To reconstruct a tensor for a 3D MRI approximation, we calculate the tensor product between the averaged core tensor and three modes of filtered basis images. The resultant reconstruction based on the first channel eigenvector nicely retrieves the spatial structure of tumours with uniform enhancement in intensity so subsequent eigenvector values are filtered out. That is $\Gamma_\varsigma = C_{\tau A} \times_1 \mathscr{A}_\varsigma^1 \times_2 \mathscr{A}_\varsigma^2 \times_3 \mathscr{A}_\varsigma^3$, where $C_{\tau_A} = \frac{1}{3}\sum_{\tau=1}^{3} C_\tau$, and $\varsigma = 1$. Finally, we reconstruct the spatio-temporal features in a 3D space. Tensor based multi-channel reconstruction models successfully preserve the intrinsic structures in an image providing a higher contrast per voxel. The generated images, therefore, convey improved diagnostic information. The procedure also allows the simultaneous multi-channel reconstruction of spatial and temporal features simultaneously in relation to DCE-MRIs under a uniform tensor framework. Figure 5.5 illustrates the flow chart of this proposed multi-channel reconstruction algorithm. The pseudo code for multi-channel tensor reconstruction is illustrated in Fig. 5.6. Finally, the multi-channel reconstruction incorporates the FCM technique to segment the tumour region effectively.

Figure 5.7a–c provides an illustration of the differentiation between the fourth post-contrast enhanced images and base line images. Subfigures (d)–(f) show the result of applying the proposed tensor reconstruction algorithm on the subtracted images acquired at different image layers. Subfigures (g)–(i) show the extracted volume image in relation to the tumor region through the application of FCM on

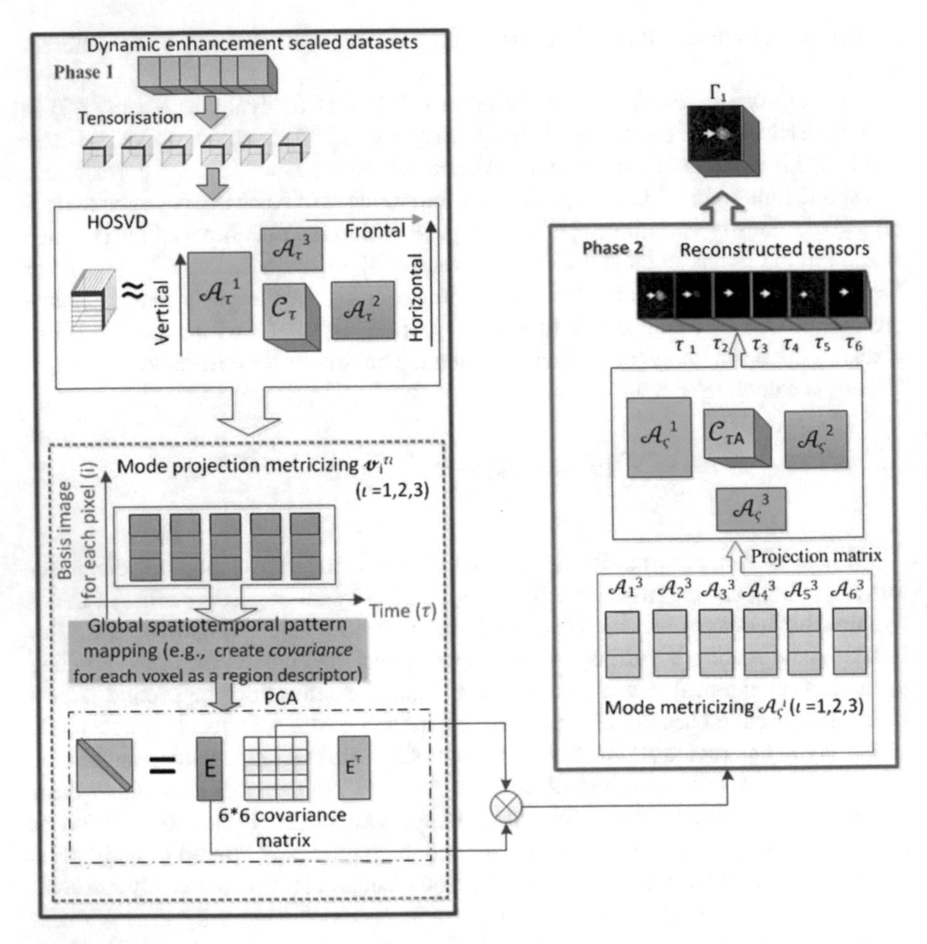

Fig. 5.5 Illustrates the proposed multi-channel tensor reconstruction algorithm

---

Input: The tensors $\mathbf{X}_\tau|_{\tau=1}^{6} \in \mathbb{R}^{N_1 \times N_2 \times N_3}$
Output:
The projection matrix $\tilde{U}_\varsigma^\iota \in \mathbb{R}^{N^\iota \times M^\iota}$ and reconstructed tensor $\Gamma \in \mathbb{R}^{N_1 \times N_2 \times N_3}$, where $\varsigma = \tau$ and $\iota = 1,2,3$
Algorithm:
1. Calculate the three modes of projection matrices U_τ^ι and core tensor $\mathscr{C}$ through the HOSVD algorithm
2. Metricize mode projections by converting each image basis matrix to vector format
3. Compute the 6×6 covariance matrix: $\Delta^\iota(X,Y) = \sum_{i=1}^{\varepsilon} \frac{(x_i-\bar{x})(y_i-\bar{y})}{\varepsilon}$ with $\bar{x} = (\text{mean}(X))$ and $\bar{y} = (\text{mean}(Y))$. The symbol ε is the number of pixels of Δ^ι and X denotes the rows of Δ^ι; and Y denotes the columns of Δ^ι .
4. Calculate the eigenvectors E_ς^ι of the covariance matrix $\Delta^\iota(X,Y)$ and select 6 eigenvectors that correspond to the largest 6 eigenvalues to form the new basis.
5. Project the transformation matrix Δ^ι: $\mathbf{A}_\varsigma^\iota = \Delta^\iota E_\varsigma^\iota$ and matricise $\mathbf{A}_\varsigma^\iota$ for $\mathscr{A}_\varsigma^\iota \in \mathbb{R}^{N^\iota \times M^\iota}$.
6. Calculate the averaged core tensor $\mathscr{C}_{\tau_A}$: $\frac{1}{3}C_{\tau_A} = \sum_{\tau=1}^{3} C_\tau$
7. Reconstruct a tensor Γ_ς through tensor multiplication [560, 31]: $\Gamma_\varsigma = \mathscr{C}_{\tau_A} \times_1 \mathscr{A}_\varsigma^1 \times_2 \mathscr{A}_\varsigma^2 \times_3 \mathscr{A}_\varsigma^3$, where $\varsigma = 1$
8. Generate a reconstructed tensor with tumorous features on the basis of principal component analysis: Γ_1 is the target tensor forfinal output

---

Fig. 5.6 Pseudo code of tensor reconstruction

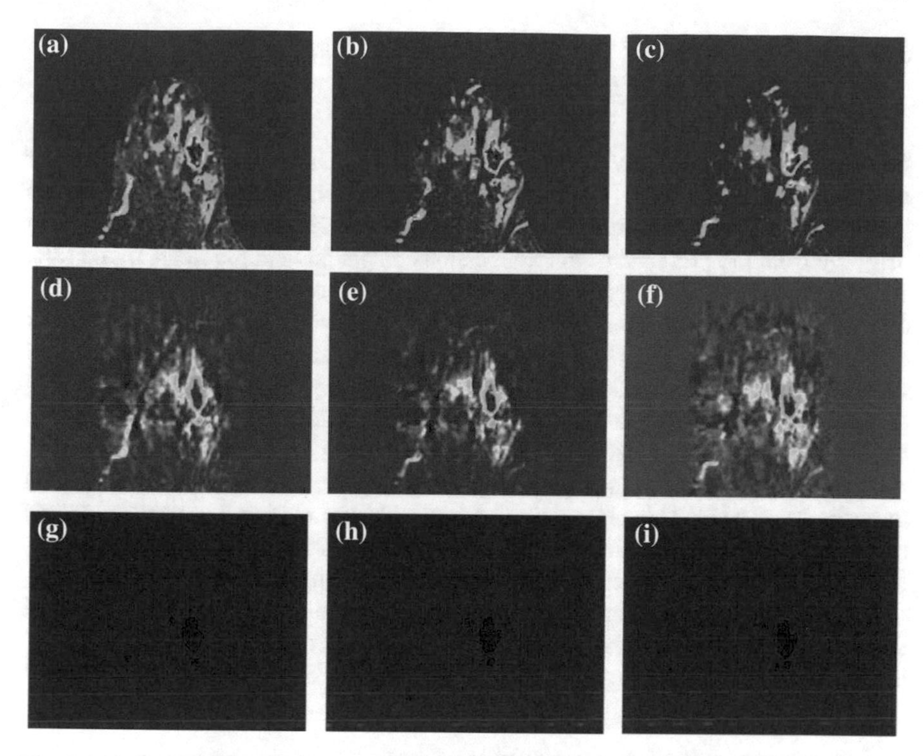

Fig. 5.7 Tensor reconstruction of preprocessed DCE-MRIs. **a–c** Illustration of the differentiation between the fourth post-contrast enhanced images and base line images from three different layers. **d–f** Illustration of the images achieved by applying the proposed tensor reconstruction algorithm. **g–i** Illustration of the extracted volume image in relation to its originally imaged tumor region after applying FCM on the reconstructed images shown in (**d**)–(**f**)

the reconstructed images shown in (d)–(f). The tensorisation of DCE-MRI is reconstructed via multidimensional unified analysis of the MRI data according to tensor factorization. One of the advantages of such reconstruction is the incorporation of the temporal information into spatial voxels. The technique projects four-dimensional time-spatial vectors into a three-dimensional space that shows spatial and temporal information fusion with a decreased number of dimensions. An additional benefit of this methodology is that it makes wide use of the sparsity present in the spatiotemporal matrices which leads to reduced computational cost.

Apart from the properties represented in Fig. 5.2 in Sect. 3.2.3 in relation to the removal of intensity inconsistencies through multi-channel reconstruction, the proposed multi-channel reconstruction has additional advantages, as discussed in the following subsections.

5.3.1 Suppression of Background Voxels Through Multi-channel Reconstruction

Intensity-based classification of MR images has proven to be the Achilles heel of all automated segmentation methods. For example, when differentiating between tumours from healthy breast tissue, the inter-scan or spatial intensity variations often originate from the presence of inhomogeneous magnetic field gradients in the MRI equipment during the image acquisition process. These field variations are often of sufficient magnitude to cause an ambiguity in reconstructed tissue boundaries across different tissue classes to overlap, thereby undermining the fidelity associated with such intensity-based classification. An example of such spatial intensity inhomogeneities is illustrated in Fig. 5.8a. In this figure, the spatial intensities between background and tumour regions are relatively uniform. It is, therefore, difficult to recognize the tumour region from background images on the basis of a variation in intensity [641, 642]. This is investigated further by comparing the results obtained using the proposed hybrid classification and standard FCM classification algorithms. FCM classification is applied on each of the originally dynamic enhanced images.

Figure 5.8a illustrates the original enhanced image associated with a scan at the second time frame. After applying FCM, the red and brown regions (shown in Fig. 5.8b) correspond largely to the tumour region. The blue and green regions

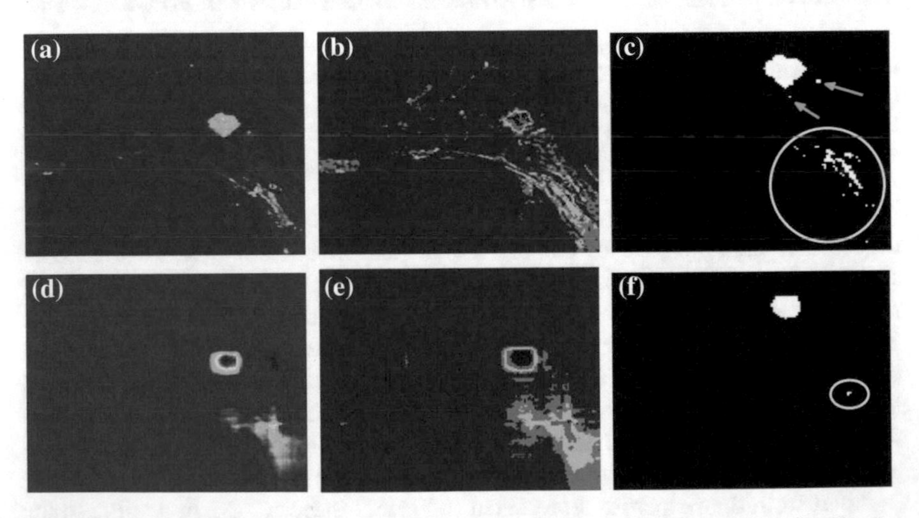

Fig. 5.8 Investigating the effect of spatial intensity inhomogeneities on the proposed classification and FCM. **a** Illustration of the pre-processed images before reconstruction of a granular cell tumour. **b** *Colour coded* images after application of the FCM algorithm on (**a**). **c** Magnification of the extracted tumour region shown in (**b**). The *yellow circle* and *green arrows* indicate a misclassified tumour region. **d** Reconstructed volume image from multiple channels. **e** Illustration of the classified image using the proposed hybrid algorithm. **f** Extracted tumour region according to (**e**). The *yellow circle* indicates that fatty tissue regions that are misclassified as tumour regions and have been shrunk to a very small region depicted as a single dot. This region is small enough to be ignored

in Fig. 5.8b correspond mainly to the background. The extracted tumour regions, as shown in Fig. 5.8c, also include imaged fatty tissues, which are indicated by a yellow circle. The two green arrows denote misclassified tumour regions. The proposed multi-channel reconstruction addresses the problem of removing misclassified tumour voxels well because it consistently produces images showing a consistent depression of the intensity associated with all fatty tissue. Compared to the image in Fig. 5.8a, where there is no obvious variation in intensity between the tumour region and the background, the multi-channel reconstruction shown in Fig. 5.8d, attributes most of the image intensity to the local tumour region and better differentiates tumorous from fatty tissue and background, as indicated by a yellow circle at the bottom right section of the recovered image, shown in Fig. 5.8f. This result can be further visualized based on the proposed hybrid classification assuming five classes, as illustrated in Fig. 5.8e. It can be seen that the tumour region is mainly colour coded in brown, whereas background tissue is colour coded in red, green and blue. The extracted tumour regions including the imaged fatty tissue, are shown in Fig. 5.8f. The FCM classified imaged fatty tissues, indicated by a large yellow circle shown in Fig. 5.8c, have shrunk to a single voxel as indicated by the small yellow circle shown in the recovered image. It should be highlighted that, in Fig. 5.13c, the size of the region associated with the noise pixels is nearly comparable with the size of the region associated with the tumour, leading to difficulty in distinguishing between tumorous and healthy tissues. The proposed hybrid classification shown in Fig. 5.13d makes it easier to identify different tissue types. Reconstruction based on information from the first channel only, recovers tumours voxels from the background well, and this recovery is also correlated with an overall depression in the intensity of the imaged background tissue.

5.3.2 Increased Image Contrast Between Tumours and Background Through Multi-channel Reconstruction

Due to a different intensity distribution associated with different types of tissues, in theory, the background voxels should be more easily separated from tumorous tissue voxels. Frequently, however, interscan intensity inhomogeneities lead to an erroneous depiction of background fatty tissue, and tumour tissue can appear co-located across different parts of the image, as shown in Fig. 5.9a. As a consequence, in certain cases it can become difficult to define clear boundaries. This is further illustrated in Fig. 5.9b, where a single layer associated with the second sequential FCM segment of the enhanced imaged tumour is displayed, and Fig. 5.9c, where sixty layers of identified tumours are superposed after FCM classification. The regions coded in light blue (brighter than background blue) illustrated in Fig. 5.9c correspond to imaged fatty tissue voxels (Fig. 5.9g). This region shows several large fuzzy edges, which implies that many regions of fatty tissue have been misclassified as tumorous tissue. In this case, a clear boundary between tumorous and background tissue needs to be

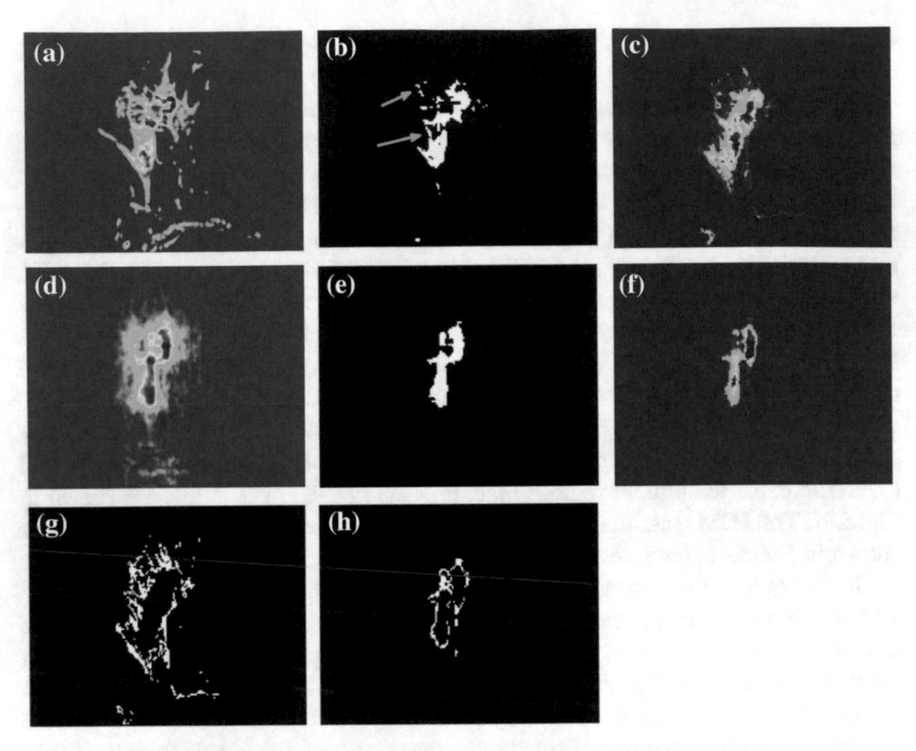

Fig. 5.9 Assessment of an incremental change in intensity contrast between tumours and background through multi-channel reconstruction. **a** Pre-processed images of invasive ductal carcinoma before reconstruction. **b** Illustration of the extracted tumorous regions after the application of FCM classification. The *green arrows* indicate misclassified healthy tissue regions as tumorous regions. **c** Superposition of images after conducting FCM classification for the identified tumour region. **d** Illustration of tumour reconstruction. **e** Resultant classified tumours through the proposed hybrid approach. **f** Superposition images after conducting the proposed hybrid classification. **g** Magnification of the extracted fuzzy edges of the FCM classified tumour segments shown in (**d**). **h** Detail of the smooth reconstructed edge shown in (**f**)

defined. This can be achieved through step-by-step systematic increases in intensity contrast. The first channel reconstruction of imaged tumours, as shown in Fig. 5.9d, addresses this problem well. Compared with Fig. 5.9b, where some joined healthy tissues are clearly visible (as indicated by green arrows), Fig. 5.9e preserves the whole spatial structure of tumours and removes the fatty tissue related background region that has been misclassified as tumorous. Sixty layers of identified tumours in the reconstructed image are superposed and shown in Fig. 5.9f. After classification using the newly proposed hybrid approach, regions denoted by light-blue voxels can be extracted, as illustrated in Fig. 5.9h. The classified voxels form a clear edge region around the tumours, and remove all fuzzy edges as shown in Fig. 5.9g. The proposed multi-channel reconstruction therefore enables us to achieve uniformly enhanced intensity distributions for all image regions associated with the tumours. Furthermore, increased image contrast between tumours and background is also achieved.

5.4 Image Registration of MRIs

In DCE-MRI and fMRI, there are spatial motion artefacts caused by patient movement, respiratory motion, intestinal peristalsis and cardiac pulsations during data collection [526–528]. Especially, for DCE-MRI, signal intensity changes in T1-weighted images when the contrast agent diffuses out from the vascular tissue and accumulates in the interstitial space. These signal intensity variations lead to contrast agent concentration estimation errors which can further amplify errors in pharmacokinetic models of tissue blood volume and vascular permeability, compromising evaluations of therapeutic response [529]. Proper registration of pixels in the chosen co-ordinate frame is a critical step in the data acquisition process as uncorrected voxel displacements from the motion artefacts will corrupt the voxel information.

In DCE-MRI data, there are also further challenges as time progresses after compound injection. Both rigid (alignment using only translation and rotation) and non-rigid algorithms (associated with more complex deformations) have been proposed for image registration, i.e. in DCE-MRIs of kidney [530], breast [531], liver [532], lungs [533, 534] and the heart [535]. Reviews discussing advances in DCE-MRI image registration can be found in [526, 536, 537]. A conceptually straightforward rigid transformation is through manual delineation of the volume images of the target object after aligning the centers of gravity [538]. An automated feature-based algorithm has been presented by Song et al. [539]. In this work, wavelet-based edge detection is followed by the computation of a geometric transformation based on a FT. Zikic et al. proposed a locally rigid registration algorithm with a gradient-based similarity measure to allow for global changes in kidney image feature enhancement [530]. Another approach is to register the images by optimizing the fit of the enhancement curves to a pharmacokinetic model [540, 541]. Nonrigid algorithms include a vertical, deformable transformation minimizing a cost function which suppresses motion and smoothes the enhancement curves [542] while at the same time maximize the mutual information using a cubic B-splines deformation [531, 543]. More recent approaches to registration aim to incorporate additional a priori information based on specific anatomical markers [544], volume preservation of tissue [545] or local rigidity assumptions [546]. Schäfer et al. [547] proposed a regional segmentation approach to study breast tissue lesions taking into consideration whether there was an observed similarity in the tissue perfusion characteristics, thus improving on single voxel-based approaches [548]. This approach has additional advantages from a clinical diagnostics perspective.

Current literature [532] suggests that there are advantages in non-rigid registration when compared to rigid registration. For non-rigid registration, deformable image registration of DCE-MRI time series is accomplished using (normalized) mutual information (MI) [528, 549] approaches. Normally, the images contain edge information between various tissue types. In these studies, a gradient dependent cost function has been proposed to improve image registration. In recent work, it was also shown that normalized gradient fields (NGF) provide a viable alternative to MI for the registration of DCE-MRI images [526].

An alternative approach to non-rigid motion correction uses a Bayesian framework [550] to provide pharmacokinetic parameter estimation in DCE-MRI sequences. In this study, a physiological image formation model was proposed to provide the similarity measure used for motion correction. Hodneland et al. [526] compared a normalized gradients approach with the mutual information approach for motion correction of DCE-MRI datasets, and showed that using cost functions based on normalized gradients can successfully suppress artifacts from moving organs in clinical DCE-MRI records.

An alternative approach, proposed by Lin et al. [551], discusses a respiratory motion-compensated DCE-MRI technique using k-space-weighted image contrast (KWIC) radial filtering. The technique combines the self-gating properties of radial imaging with the reconstruction flexibility provided by the golden-angle view-order strategy. The signal at the k-space center is used to determine the respiratory cycle, and consecutive views during the expiratory phase of each respiratory period are grouped into individual segments. The principle is to divide k-space into concentric rings. The boundary of each circular region is determined by the Nyquist criterion, after assuming that the views within each region have uniform azimuthal spacing.

The feature extraction algorithms mentioned earlier are relevant to both medical image registration as well as motion compensation [552, 553]. An alternative approach to localize anatomical features in DCE-MRI is through the use of level sets, an approach originally proposed in [554, 555]. The method is applicable to post-contrast enhanced MR images to delineate the variable shape of features of interest. Yin et al. [62] proposed such approach to localize anatomical features in breast costal cartilage imaged using DCE-MRI. The contours in each layer are cumulatively added to the first contour to produce the results illustrated in Fig. 5.10a. The shape of the feature of interest clearly varies from layer to layer. The variable shape of contours acquired from a level-set-based segment image actually determines the feature region of interest. This is subsequently used as a guide to specify initial masks for feature extraction. Figure 5.10b shows the superposition of the mask and the level-set based projection of Fig. 5.10a. The motion action of the fourth pair of breast costal cartilages are obtained by re-projecting the resultant segments from transaxial planes to sagittal planes. Rotational motion artefacts in the DCE-MRI are illustrated in Fig. 5.10c.

Pre-processing is necessary in fMRI analysis to clean up artificial noise and prepare images for further processing to establish the network characteristics of the different interconnected brain regions. Motion and slice timing correction, spatial and temporal filter artifacts, as well as intensity normalisation and covariance removal, are common problems when dealing with fMRIs. Motion correction amounts to finding a common orientation for all images within a given imaging session and resampling the original data to this reference orientation. Image alignment is usually

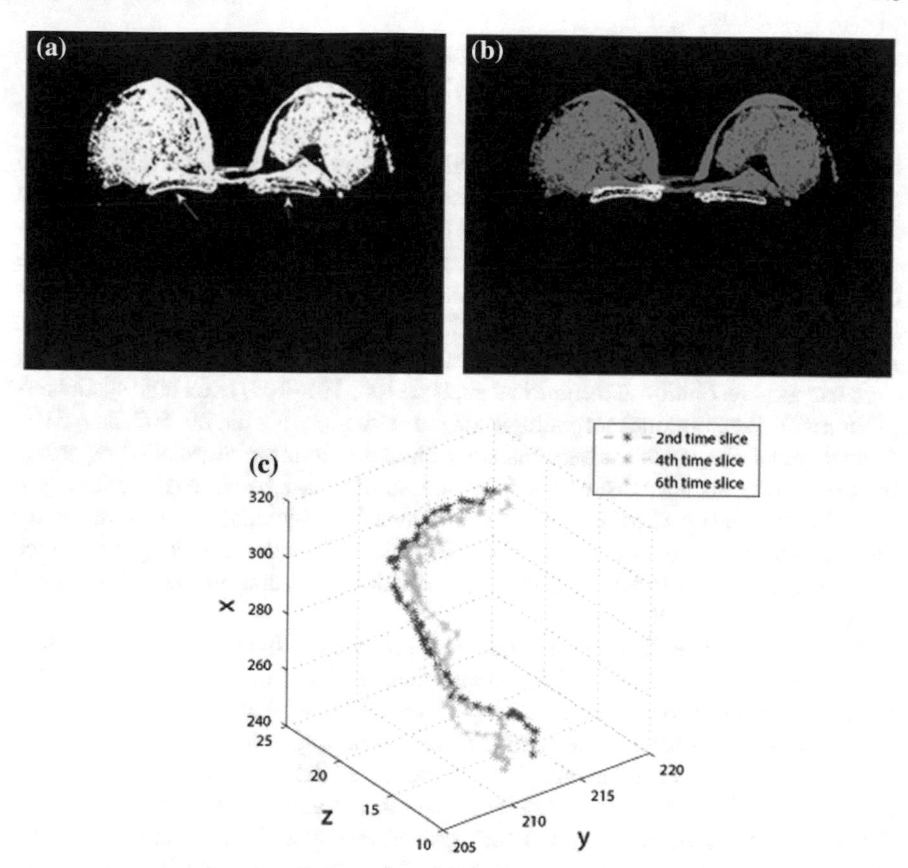

Fig. 5.10 Illustration of magnetic resonance image analysis using tensor algebra. **a** Cumulative contours using the level-set method, with *two white arrows* indicating the positions of features of interest. **b** Illustration of the superposition between the total segment and the level-set based segment. **c** Illustration of the 3D plots of plane centroid produced datasets generated according to the 2nd, 4th, and 6th time slice

achieved by performing a separate 3D image registration of each image in the series with a chosen reference image to remove movement artifacts. To deal with general motion-related intensity variations, it is necessary to remove all trends from the time series that have the same form as that of a the voxel displacement (as measured during the transformation estimation stage in motion correction). This assumes that the artefact will be proportional to the displacement of the voxel from its usual position. However, as there is significant interaction amongst the various artefacts, which also degrade the accuracy of the basic motion correction methods, current research is focusing on simultaneous motion correction and artefact removal methods [556].

5.5 Pattern Identification of Spatiotemporal Association of Features in Tumours from DCE-MRI Data

One of the current challenges in breast DCE-MRI as a screening modality, is reducing false positive detection errors, thereby boosting detection specificity. Computer-aided diagnosis (CAD) approaches for breast MRI are typically employed for automatically identifying tumors from normal tissues when these are at a stage of rapid development [68, 97, 501, 502], whereas the more complex task of classifying a lesion as benign or malignant [63, 104, 501, 503–510] is proving more difficult to address. In dynamic pattern recognation methods, the emphasis has been on either high temporal resolution and empirical analyses [63, 101–104] or on high spatial resolution with a stand-alone morphologic feature extraction [63, 68, 69, 502, 507, 510]. Even though time-series analysis enables radiologists to infer information regarding the tissue state, such assessment is a time-consuming task because of spatiotemporal lesion variability. Currently, most studies consider aggregate measurements for tumour morphological characterization [63, 502, 510] with an initially model-free [502, 510] and data-driven [97, 501] segmentation according to manually marked region-of-interest (ROI).

Common practice in these methods is to process the imaged 3D volumes separately, and then incorporate the temporal information into the spatial databases through a separate processing step. Image reduction based feature extraction enables identification on the basis of the dominant features present in the image. For example, in [98, 99], PCA was applied on enhanced and scaled datasets for a whole 2D object region obtained by DCE-MRIs. This is in contrast to traditional PCA applied in two-dimensional MRI image analysis which ignores any spatial information associated with a time series that records the evolution of disease progression. The analysis of spatiotemporal patterns however, remains a challenging problem [63], and addressing the issues of low specificity and high inter-observer variability found in breast DCE-MRI, requires the development of new software tools.

Representation of multi-dimensional features in a tensor space is a relatively new concept in the computer science and pattern recognition literature. The use of tensor decomposition is motivated by the need to explore multimodal data analysis of the spatiotemporal correlations of sequences existing in DCE-MR images. Recent work [385] shows that there is potential to identify tumour shape by combining non-negative tensor decomposition and directional texture synthesis. The approach uses symmetry information associated with the 3D shapes of the organs under study, and projects this information into the 2D space that is synthesized on the basis of textural features from sparse, decomposed images.

In the following figure (Fig. 5.11), spatial shape datasets with a simple geometry are used for illustration purposes. These images show a three-dimensional mirror symmetry analysis of a spherical object with a radius of 31 pixels. Figure 5.11a illustrates that the flattened basis images are cropped in the middle area after a non-negative tensor decomposition of the sphere. As an example, reconstruction is performed using tensor multiplication of the core tensor, on the basis of first mode

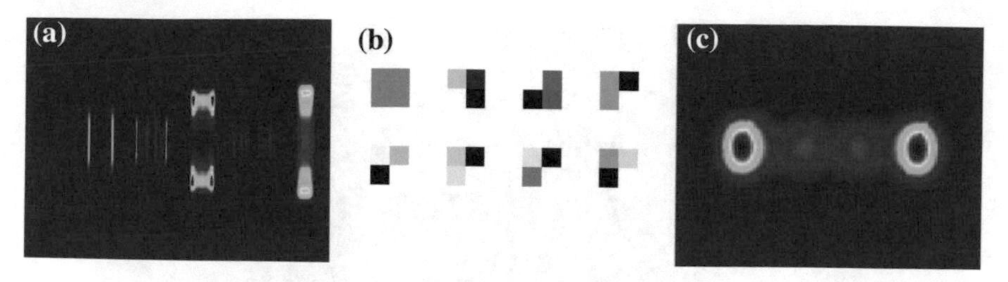

Fig. 5.11 Illustration of three-dimensional mirror symmetry analysis of a spherical object. **a** Non-negative tensor decomposition. **b** Sparse texture extraction. **c** Synthesis of the extracted texture

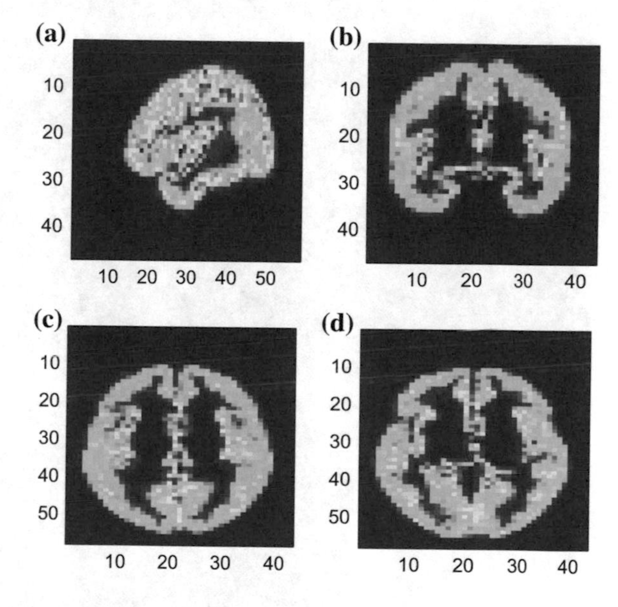

Fig. 5.12 Illustration of the mirror symmetry of brain structural MRI with rough resolution. The brain MRI size is 58 × 47 × 43. **a–c** Illustration of 2D cross-sectional slices along a *horizontal plane*, *vertical plane*, and *frontal plane*. **d** Illustration of a brain slice image with asymmetry along an the x-y plane

and second mode matrices. Figure 5.11b illustrates sparse texture extraction of the spherical object. Figure 5.11c shows the extracted texture on a pixel by pixel basis of the sphere. The resultant synthesised image is symmetric with respect to both vertical and horizontal symmetry axes, implying that the object is symmetric with the frontal plane providing a reflective mirror image.

In the following example, we explore the mirror symmetry of brain structural MRI of white mass as imaged under a rough resolution. The MR image size is 47 × 58 × 43. Figure 5.12a–c illustrate one of the 2D cross-sectional slices along a horizontal plane, vertical plane, and frontal plane. Figure 5.12d illustrates a brain slice image with asymmetry along the x-y plane.

As a first step in the proposed algorithm, the generated 3D images showing either symmetry or asymmetry are assembled and re-mapped into the third order tensors. After this step, non-negative tensor decomposition is applied to factorise the non-negative tensors to factors. The core tensor size is 32 × 32 × 32 and the flatten

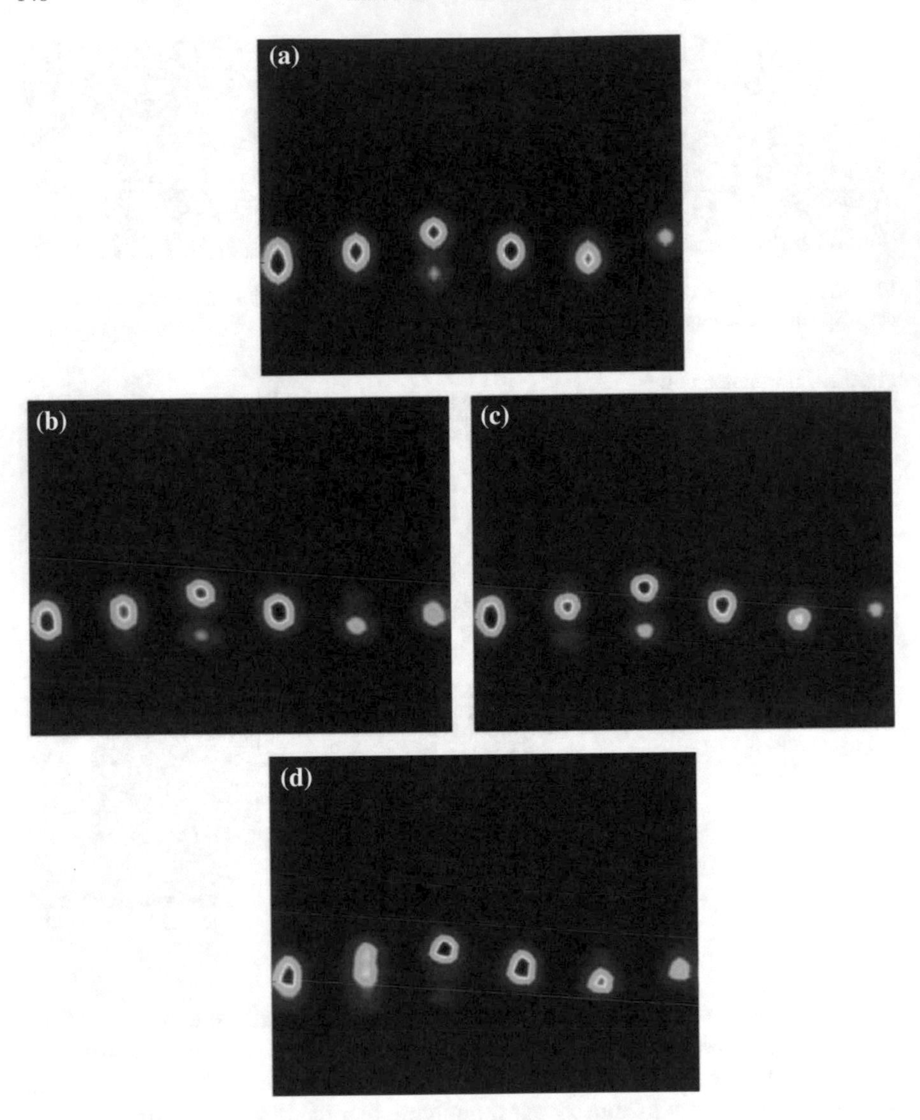

Fig. 5.13 Illustration of the synthesised images related to the generated 3D brain structural MR image with symmetry (refer to Fig. 5.12a–c and asymmetry (refer to Fig. 5.12a, b, and d). **a–d** Illustration of the resultant synthesis for the symmetric brain structural MRI, and the generation of the first (with 15 asymmetric layers), the second (with 25 asymmetric layers), and the third (with 35 asymmetric layers) from asymmetric brain structural MR images, respectively

basis image size is 58×1024. The center region of the basis images is cropped to a size of 58×180. Figure 5.13a–d illustrate the resultant synthesis for the symmetric MRI, and the generation of the first (with 15 asymmetric layers), the second (with 25 asymmetric layers), and the third (with 35 asymmetric layers) from asymmetric MR images.

To ascertain the degree of symmetry (or the lack of it), k means clustering is used to group the synthesis patterns and find the associated 2-dimensional geometric pattern; then histogram images from the synthesis patterns are used to evaluate the degree of intensity symmetry in the image. This way, the analysis of a 3D shape can be mapped into a 2D space, therefore performing the required dimensionality reduction. The above mentioned examples thus propose a way forward towards addressing the challenges associated with tensor decomposition of MRIs for the detection of structural abnormalities in both simulated breast tumours as well as in brain structural MRI.

The proposed methodology is currently most relevant to MRI in clinical practice, but can also benefit the TPI community, especially if such systems are soon to undergo further clinical trials. Such advances are likely to provide improved diagnosis for Alzheimer's Disease and may assist, in the near future, with the early diagnosis of dementia by translating current understanding in cell biology into therapeutic advances [560–562].

5.6 Pattern Classification of Spatiotemporal Association Features in fMRI Data

Over the past several years, through large brain mapping initiatives across the US and Europe, there has been a growing interest in applying pattern classification methods on time series imaging to study the process of brain tissue aging, as well as to diagnose systemic brain disease. FMRI in particular is increasingly used across the clinical and cognitive neuroscience communities, to measure brain activity and reveal brain function. As discussed earlier, this is possible because cerebral blood flow and neuronal activation are coupled. For fMRI, a key challenge is to investigate the associations between spatial and temporal features of fMRIs. Supervised tensor based learning and multivariate classification are two effective supervised classification approaches for the recognition of distributed patterns in relation to fMRI data with consideration of both spatial and temporal futures. For unsupervised learning, the geometric characteristics of a brain network can be discovered from a given neuroimage when extensive datasets regarding both spatial and temporal features are simultaneously recorded.

5.6.1 Supervised Tensor Learning of Brain Disorders in fMRI Datasets

Supervised tensor based learning may be seen as an extension of the methods discussed in the previous sections. Some of the earliest works establishing its formulation were discussed by Tao et al. [563] and Signoretto et al. [564]. These works formulate the learning problem as an optimization task of support tensor machines (STMs); essentially a generalization of the standard support vector machines (SVMs) from vector spaces to tensor spaces. The objective of such learning algorithms is to generate a hyperplane by which the samples with different labels are divided at distances as far away as possible on a Cartesian co-ordinate hyperplane. A problem often encountered however, is that tensor data may not be linearly separable in the input space. This problem may be addressed by considering nonlinear transformation of the original tensorial data, after taking into consideration the interrelationships of the dataset within the tensor itself. He et al. studied the problem of supervised tensor learning with nonlinear kernels which can preserve the structure of tensor data [565]. The proposed solution is an extension of kernels from vector spaces to tensor spaces, thus taking the multidimensional tensorial structure into account. This is achieved by representing each tensor object as a sum of rank-one tensors in the original space and mapping them into the tensor product feature space for kernel learning. The tensor kernel mapping on a rank-one tensor can be represented as follows:

$$\phi : \prod_{n=1}^{N} \otimes x^{(n)} \rightarrow \prod_{n=1}^{N} \otimes \phi\left(x^{(n)}\right) \in \mathbb{R} I_1 \times I_2 \times \ldots \times I_N \tag{5.2}$$

Two image tensors of $\mathscr{X}$, $\mathscr{Y}$ can be decomposed via candecomp/parafac (CP) tensor factorization as $\mathscr{X} = \sum_{r=1}^{R} \prod_{n=1} x_r^{(n)}$ and $\mathscr{Y} = \sum_{r=1}^{R} \prod_{n=1} y_r^{(n)}$, respectively. By using the concept of the kernel function, we can directly derive the naive tensor product kernels with $R = 1$ as

$$\kappa(\mathscr{X}, \mathscr{Y}) = \prod_{n=1}^{N} \prod_{n=1}^{N} \kappa\left(x^{(n)} y^{(n)}\right). \tag{5.3}$$

To achieve a compact and informative presentation of the original tensorial dataset using a simple rank-one tensor, the challenge is how to design a feature mapping function when the value of R is more than one. Based on the definition of the kernel function, if the feature space is a high-dimensional space of the original space, the tensor data can be directly factorised in the feature space in the same way as if it was in the original space by performing the following mapping:

$$\phi : \sum_{r=1}^{R} \prod_{n=1}^{N} \otimes x_r^{(n)} \rightarrow \sum_{r=1}^{R} \prod_{n=1}^{N} \otimes \phi\left(x^{(n)}\right) \tag{5.4}$$

This transformation enables the mapping of the raw data tensors into new high-dimensional tensors which also retain the original structure and inter-relations in the data. The process can be regarded as a mapping of the original data into a tensor feature space followed by a CP factorization in the feature space. This transformation is known as the dual-tensorial mapping function, and is illustrated in Fig. 5.14.

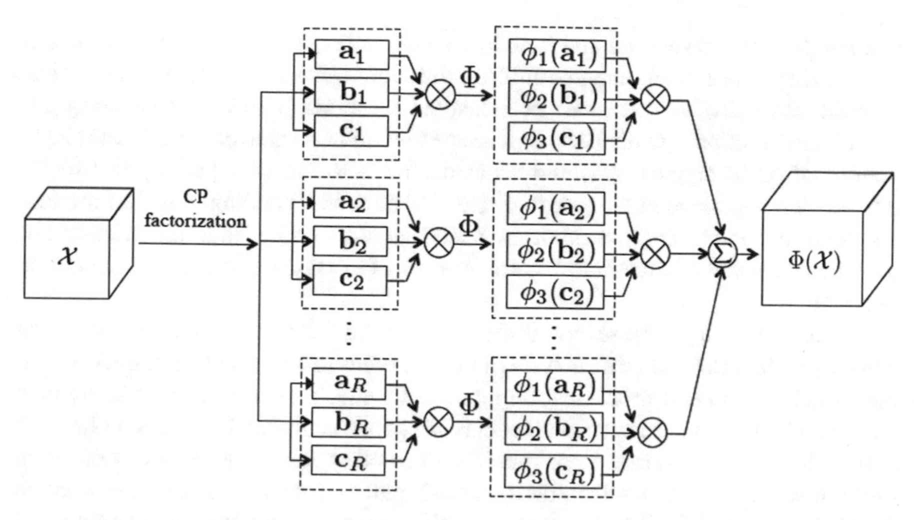

Fig. 5.14 Conceptual diagram for illustration of dual-tensor mapping. The symbols a, b, and c are the basis factors obtained by projecting the data tensor onto the feature subspace after conducting the CP facorization. After [565]

After mapping the CP factorization of the data into the tensor product feature space, the kernel itself is just the standard inner product of tensors in that feature space:

$$\kappa\Big(\sum_{r=1}^{R}\prod_{n=1}^{N}\otimes x_r^{(n)}, \sum_{r=1}^{R}\prod_{n=1}^{N}\otimes x_r^{(n)}\Big) = \sum_{i=1}^{R}\sum_{j=1}^{R}\prod_{(n=1)}^{N}\kappa\left(x_i^{(n)}, y_j^{(n)}\right) \tag{5.5}$$

However, the dual-tensorial mapping function cannot automatically consider the spatio-temporally complex information that can be found in most neuroimaging datasets in an integral manner. Han et al., applied a deep learning algorithm, known as hierarchical convolutional sparse auto-encoder, to extract robust features and conserve the detailed information associated with the neuroimaging process to perform classification [566]. This seems to be a particularly interesting research direction so the use of deep learning networks is further discussed in the following chapter.

5.6.2 Supervised Multivariate Learning of Brain Disorders from fMRI Data

Traditionally, univariate or voxel based analysis approaches have been used to analyse neuroimaging data (for example, General Liner Model and Voxel Based Morphometry) [567]. These are significantly less powerful than tensorial learning techniques and only appropriate in cases where the group differences are spatially distributed and subtle [356]. Structural and functional MRI data are inherently multivariate in nature, since each scan contains information about, for example, tissue structure or brain activation, at thousands of measured locations (voxels). Considering that most brain functions are distributed processes involving a network of different interconnected brain regions, it would seem desirable to use the spatially distributed information contained in the data to obtain a better understanding of brain functions under normal and diseased conditions. Such spatially distributed information can be investigated using Multivariate Pattern Analysis (MVPA) using Machine Learning in fMRI.

As discussed in [357], several different machine learning techniques have been used for multivariate pattern analysis in fMRI studies in order to gain an understanding of different neural processes. Support vector machines and linear discriminant analysis were applied to successfully classify patterns of fMRI activation observed due to the visual presentation of pictorial cues of various categories of objects in [568]. It was demonstrated that, fMRI activity patterns in early visual areas, contain detailed orientation information that can reliably predict subjective perception using linear SVM in [569]. The basic MVPA method is a straightforward application of pattern classification techniques, where the patterns to be classified are (typically) vectors of voxel activity values.

Figure 5.15 illustrates the four basic steps in an MVPA analysis. The first step, feature selection, involves deciding which voxels will be included in the classification analysis, as shown in Fig. 5.15a; Box 1 describes the feature selection process in more detail. The second step, pattern assembly, involves sorting the data into discrete 'brain patterns' corresponding to the pattern of activity across the selected voxels at a particular time in the experiment, as shown in Fig. 5.15b. Brain patterns are labeled according to which experimental condition generated the pattern; this labeling procedure needs to account for the fact that the hemodynamic response measured by the scanner is delayed and smeared out in time, relative to the instigating neural event. The third step, classifier training, involves feeding a subset of these labeled patterns into a multivariate pattern classification algorithm. Based on these patterns, the classification algorithm learns a function that maps the voxel activity patterns to the experimental conditions, as shown in Fig. 5.15c. The fourth step is generalization testing: Given a new pattern of brain activity (not previously presented to the classifier), the trained classifier should be validated on the basis of how correctly it can determine the experimental condition associated with that pattern, as shown in Fig. 5.15d.

Multivariate pattern analysis (MVPA) has been gaining popularity within the neuroimaging community, and has been used in studies of both adult healthy and clinical populations. These studies have shown that information present in neuroimaging data can be used to decode intentions and perceptual states, as well as discriminate between healthy and diseased regions in the brain [570]. Depression is characterized by a mood change that typically includes sadness and anhedonia or an impaired ability to experience pleasure [571]. Neuroimaging studies in major depression disorder have identified neurophysiologic abnormalities in multiple areas of the orbital and medial prefrontal cortex, the amygdala, and related parts of the striatum and

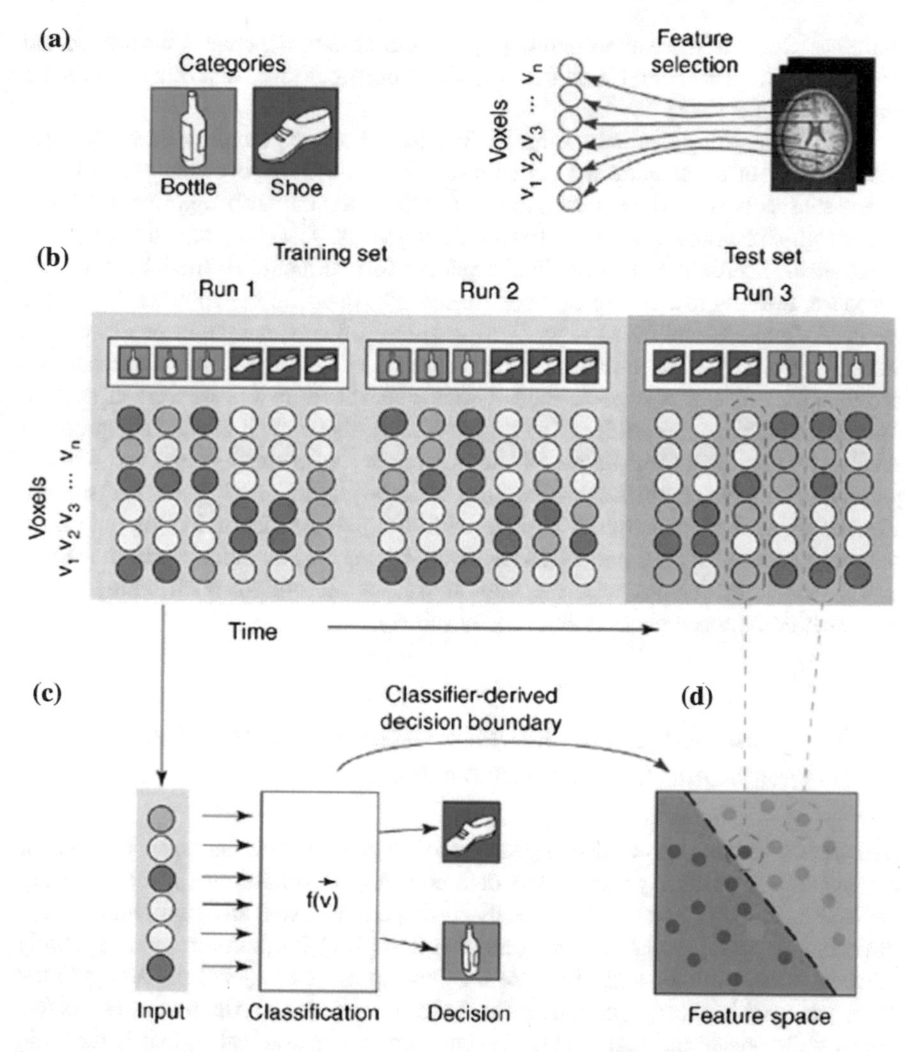

Fig. 5.15 Illustration of a hypothetical experiment and how it could be analyzed using MVPA. **a** Subjects view stimuli from two object categories (*bottles and shoes*). A 'feature selection' procedure is used to determine which voxels will be included in the classification analysis. **b** The fMRI time series is decomposed into discrete brain patterns that correspond to the pattern of activity across the selected voxels at a particular point in time. Each brain pattern is labeled according to the corresponding experimental condition (*bottle vs. shoe*). The patterns are divided into a training set and a testing set. **c** Patterns from the training set are used to train a classifier function that maps between brain patterns and experimental conditions. **d** The trained classifier function defines a decision boundary (*red dashed line, right*) in the high-dimensional space of voxel patterns. Each dot corresponds to a pattern and the *color* of the *dot indicates* its category. The *background color* of the figure corresponds to the predicted classes that the region belongs to. The trained classifier aims to asign a label to the patterns from the test set. The figure shows one example of the classifier correctly identifying a bottle pattern (*green dot*) as a bottle, and one example of the classifier misidentifying a shoe pattern (*blue dot*) as a bottle. After [357]

thalamus. Some of these abnormalities appear mood state-dependent and are located in regions where cerebral blood flow increases during normal and other pathologic emotional states [572].

Machine learning methods using MVPA, have been explored by Fu et al. [573] who used them to examine the patterns of cerebral activity over the whole brain. These studies have also been used to identify and predict neurocognitive states and to distinguish healthy individuals from patient groups. The study aimed to diagnose psychiatric disorders and to predict responses to treatment. To model the BOLD response, training/test examples were created by averaging the volumes within the event. A linear kernel SVM algorithm provided a direct extraction of the weight vector as an image. To validate the performance of the classifier, a leave-one-out cross-validation test was performed. Group classification was performed at each intensity of facial expression and a combined analysis from all the facial expression levels was conducted for diagnosis and comparison of acutely depressed unipolar patients and healthy control subjects, along with the predictors of treatment response. Figure 5.16 shows the cerebral regions with the greatest discriminating activation pattern. Because this is a result of a multivariate process, it encompasses the whole brain, where the regions with the highest weight vectors are contributing to the demarcation between patients and control subjects.

5.6.3 Topological Graph Kernel on Multiply Thresholded Functional Connectivity Networks

Although a tensor can be decomposed into several factors, unconstrained tensor decomposition resulting from fMRI data may not be suitable for node discovery because each factor does not necessarily correspond to a spatially contiguous region nor does it necessarily match an anatomical region [574]. Furthermore, many spatially adjacent voxels in the same structure may not appear as they are not active in the same factor which is anatomically impossible. Therefore, in order to discover active nodes while preserving anatomical adjacency, known anatomical regions in the brain are used as masks and constraints are added to enforce the close matching of the discovered factors and these masks [575].

A structural representation is an alternative approach to addressing the above problem. In brain connectivity studies, graphs have been shown to be suitable for representing the location of activity in the brain and account for the movement of the information. Usually, topological descriptors such as modularity, centrality and node-degree distribution, are computed to characterize these networks. Despite the analysis of these topological properties of a graph, which may be useful in elucidating the correlations between functionality and localization of brain activity, the application of classifiers on graph data would be a more robust approach [576].

Graph kernels are one of the most recent methods that can be used in pattern recognition studies [577]. They are particularly useful in the analysis of the more

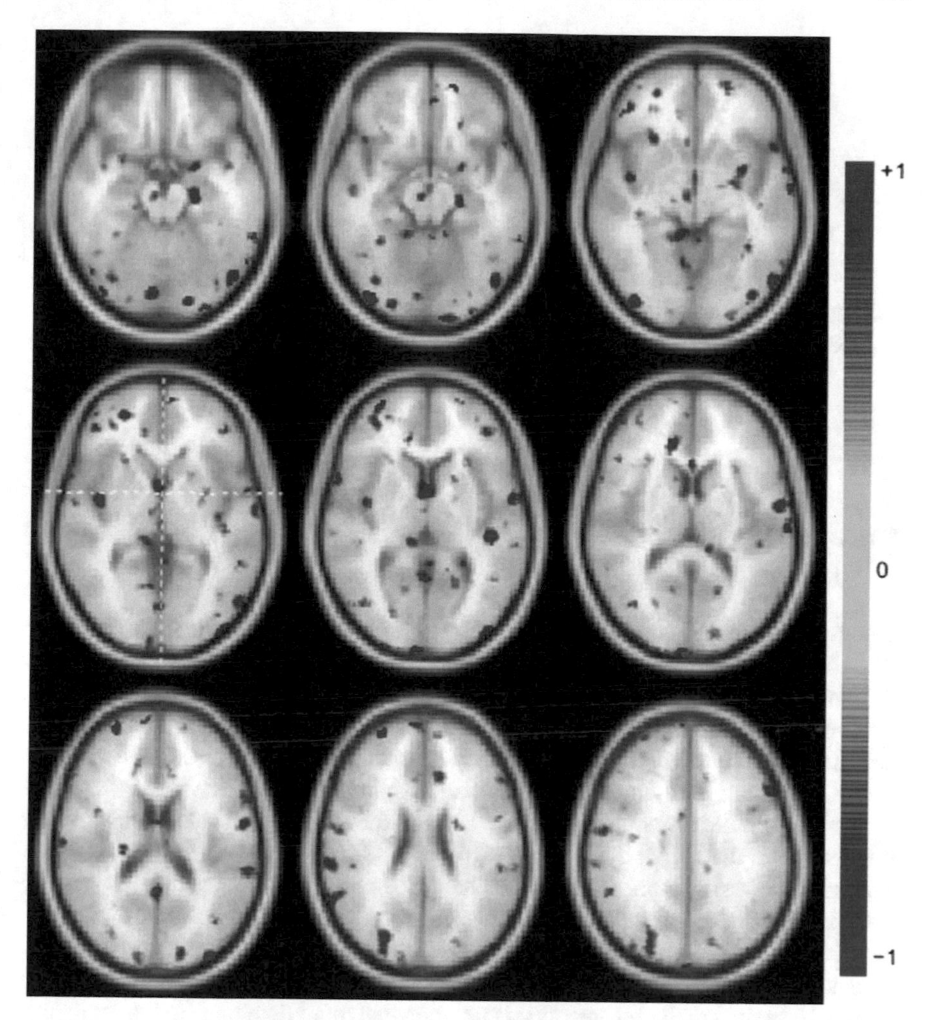

Fig. 5.16 Cerebral regions that showed the greatest discrimination between patients and healthy control subjects during presentation of the highest intensity of sad faces based on single events modeling. A linear kernel SVM algorithm allows the direct extraction of the weight vector from analysed fMRIs. Regions with the largest weight vectors provide a stronger contribution to the classification decision. Increasingly positive weight vector values indicate the subjects are patients (*red*) whereas negative values are associated with healthy control subjects (*blue*). Transverse brain images are presented with z-coordinates ranging from −18 to +30 and the section where z = 0 is indicated by crosshairs (*left hand side* second row). After [573]

complex graph data types, capturing the semantics inherent in the graph structure [578, 579]. After a graph kernel is defined, many learning algorithms such as SVM, can be implemented. A number of methods have been proposed to construct a graph kernel. Graph kernels can mainly be divided into the following three classes: (1) kernels based on common random walks and paths between two graphs [580–582],

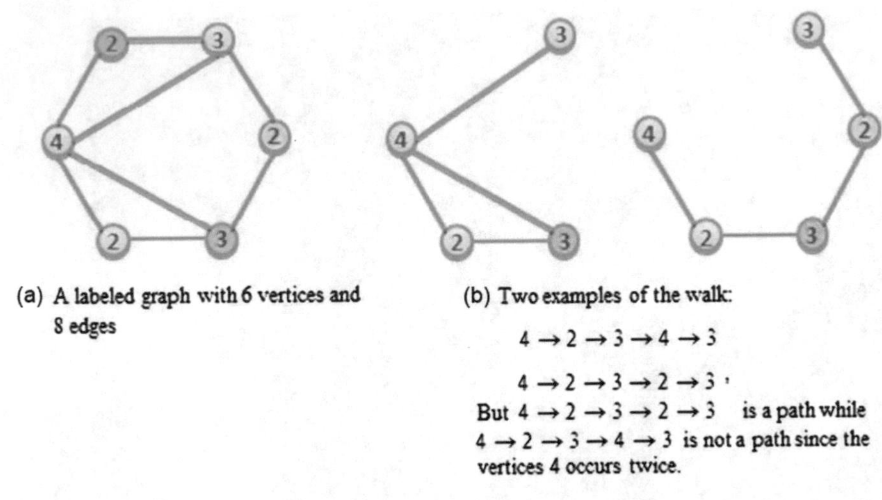

Fig. 5.17 Illustration of relevant annotations and typical walk found in labeled graphs. After [577]

(2) kernels based on common limited-size subgraphs between two graphs [583], and (3) kernels based on common subtree patterns between two graphs [584]. All of the above kernels have been successfully applied to a variety of problems such as image classification [585] and protein function prediction [580] etc. More recently, there have also been studies applying graph kernel methodologies to neuroimaging studies. For example, they may be used to discriminate between healthy controls from patients with schizophrenia on the basis of the derived functional connectivity of individual networks in the brain [586].

In graph classification, labelled graphs are analysed after nodes and edges are labeled with numerical values, as shown in Fig. 5.17a. The shortest-path kernel is one of the kernels that can be applied to such graphs. A path in a graph relates to a sequence of nodes in such way that consecutive nodes in the sequence are connected by an edge in the graph and any node is not repeated more than once in the sequence. Path length relates to the number of edges along the path that must be traversed to reach from one node to another. In a weighted graph, the definition of path length changes according to the sum of the weights of the traversed edges. The shortest path again corresponds to the path with the minimum length.

For a graph $G(V, E)$ in which V and E are the sets of nodes and edges respectively, the shortest-path kernel transforms each graph $G(V, E_G)$ into a shortest-path graph $S(V, E_S)$. The shortest-paths graph S includes the same set of nodes as the original graph G, and there is an edge between the nodes in S which are connected by a path in G. Every edge in S between nodes v_i and v_j is labeled by the length of shortest path between these two nodes in G. The Floyd algorithm provides a way of incorporating the shortest path information into the kernel functions and uses a similar strategy. The shortest path kernel between two graphs is converted into a simple comparison between corresponding shortest-paths graphs [587]. In this transform, a shortest-paths graph S contains the same set of nodes as the input graph I. Unlike in the input graph, there exists an edge between all nodes in S which are connected by a walk in I. Every edge in S between nodes v_i and v_j is labeled by the shortest distance between these two nodes. Floyd's algorithm is used to solve the all-pairs-shortest-paths problem that can be applied to determine all the shortest distance edge labels in S.

To clarify the above description, a mathematical expression of the shortest-path kernel is provided below, after assuming in the following example that there are two graphs $G(V, E_G)$ and $\hat{G}(\hat{V}, \hat{E}_G)$ which are transformed into the corresponding shortest-paths graphs $S(V, E_S)$ and $\hat{S}(\hat{V}, \hat{E}_S)$, respectively. Then the shortest-path kernel can be defined over $S(V, E_S)$ and $\hat{S}(\hat{V}, \hat{E}_S)$ as

$$\kappa_{\text{shortlest-path}}(S, \hat{S}) = \sum_{e \in E_S} \sum_{\hat{e} \in \hat{E}_S} \kappa^1_{\text{walk}}(e, \hat{e}) \tag{5.6}$$

where κ^1_{walk} is a positive definite kernel of walks length 1 or a kernel on edges.

Therefore the shortest-path kernel [587] is converted to a walk kernel on the Floyd-transformed graphs after considering walks of length 1 only. The symbol κ^1_{walk} is defined based on the approach of Kashima et al. (2003) which chooses a positive definite kernel on nodes and a positive definite kernel on edges. A kernel on pairs of walks of length 1, κ^1_{walk}, is then defined as the product of kernels on nodes and edges encountered along the walk. An elegant approach to determine all pairs of matching walks is based on the methodology discussed by Gartner et al. [581]. Assuming that there are two input graphs $G = (V, E)$ and $\hat{G} = (\hat{V}, \hat{E})$ related through a direct product graph $G_\times$:

$$\kappa_\times(G, \hat{G}) = \sum_{i,j=1}^{|V_\times|} \left[\sum_{n=0}^{\infty} \lambda_n A_\times^n \right]_{ij} \tag{5.7}$$

where $A_\times$ is the adjacency matrix of $G_\times$. The adjacency matrix A of G is defined as

$$[A]_{ij} = \begin{cases} 1, & \text{if}(v_i, v_j) \in E \\ 0, & \text{otherwise} \end{cases} \tag{5.8}$$

Here, $G_\times = (V_\times, E_\times)$, is defined through the following mapping:

$$V_\times(G, \hat{G}) = \{(v_1, \omega_1) \in V \times \hat{V} : \text{label}(\text{v}_1) = \text{label}(\omega_1)\} \tag{5.9}$$

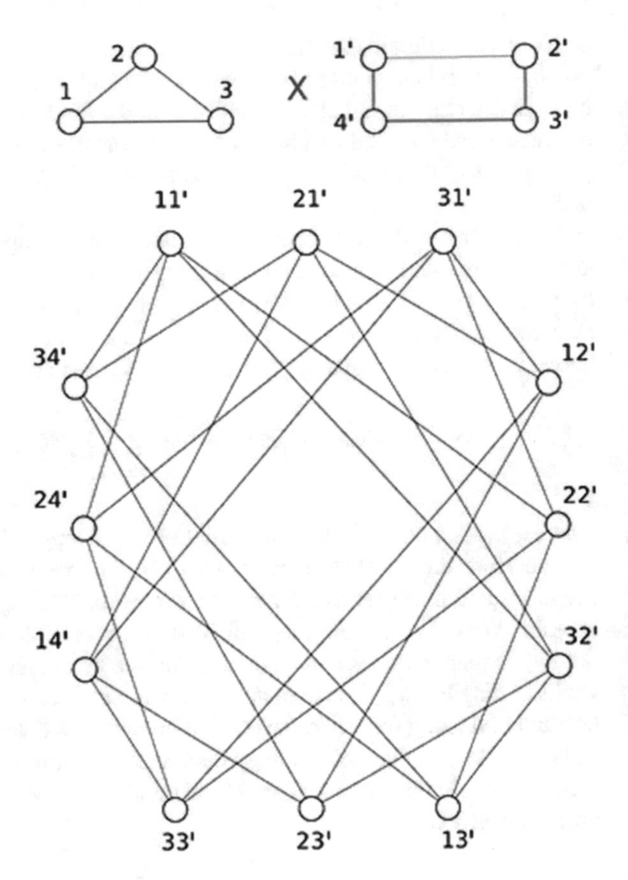

Fig. 5.18 Two graphs (*top left* and *right*) and their direct product (*bottom*). Each node of the direct product graph is labeled with a pair of nodes; an edge exists in the direct product if and only if the corresponding nodes are adjacent in both original graphs. For instance, nodes 11' and 32' are adjacent because there is an edge between nodes 1 and 3 in the first graph, and 1'and 2' in the second graph. After [579]

$$E_{\times}(G, \hat{G}) = \{(v_1, \omega_1), (v_2, \omega_2) \in V^2(G_1 \times G_2 : \\ (v_1, v_2) \in E \wedge (\omega_1, \omega_2) \in \hat{E} \\ \wedge \text{label}(\text{v}_1, \text{v}_2) = \text{label}(\omega_1, \omega_2)\} \tag{5.10}$$

where λ_n must be chosen appropriately for $k_\times$ to converge. A graph kernel may thus be seen as a measure of similarity between walks that are not identically labeled [580]. Node and edge labels along the walks are compared via kernel functions. The direct product of two graphs $G(V, E)$ and $\hat{G}(\hat{V}, \hat{E})$ can be illustrated in Fig. 5.18.

Generally, an undirected graph is one where the edges do not have a particular orientation, whereas a directed graph is characterized by edges that have a defined orientation. A graph is called a labeled graph if its vertices are assigned labels from the vertex label alphabet. At this point it is worth distinguishing between a walk and a path. A walk is a finite sequence of neighboring vertices, whereas a path is a walk such that all its vertices are distinctive. Tracing a walk in the product graph corresponds to simultaneously tracing common walks in the two original graphs. Common labeled walks of length k can now be computed from the adjacency matrix

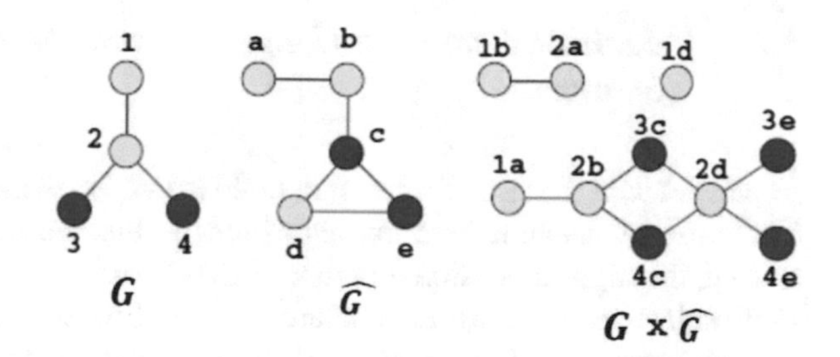

Fig. 5.19 Product graph consisting of pairs of identically labeled nodes and edges from G and $\hat{G}$

of the product graph A_x^k, noting that the structure of the product graph ensures that only walks with matching labels are counted.

Another example of a product graph that consists of pairs of identically labeled nodes and edges is shown in Fig. 5.19. In this figure, for the yellow lablled nodes from the two graphs G and $\hat{G}$, the joint nodes exist between 1a and 2b and 2a and 1b as there is an edge between 1 and 2 in the graph of G and a and b in the graph $\hat{G}$. The blue labelled nodes in the product graph are labelled 3c, 4c and 3e, 4e respectively. Nodes 3c and 2b are adjacent, considering edges exist between nodes 2 and 3. The same applies for the nodes between 4c and 2b. The yellow labled nodes 1d and 2d are the nodes in the product graph. The node 2d is connected with nodes 3d, 4d and 3e, 4e in the product graph as edges exist between each of the two nodes in both original graphs. Node 1d is isolated as no edge exist in the other nodes that correspond to the original graphs.

Graph kernels are based on limited-size subgraphs. A subtree is a subgraph of a graph which has no cycles (i.e. any two vertices are connected by exactly one simple path). A subtree pattern extends the notion of a subtree by allowing repetitions of nodes and edges. However, these same nodes (edges) are treated as distinct nodes (edges). A subtree pattern of height 2 from the directed graph is illustrated in Fig. 5.20. The repetitions of nodes in the unfolded subtree pattern on the right are also shown.

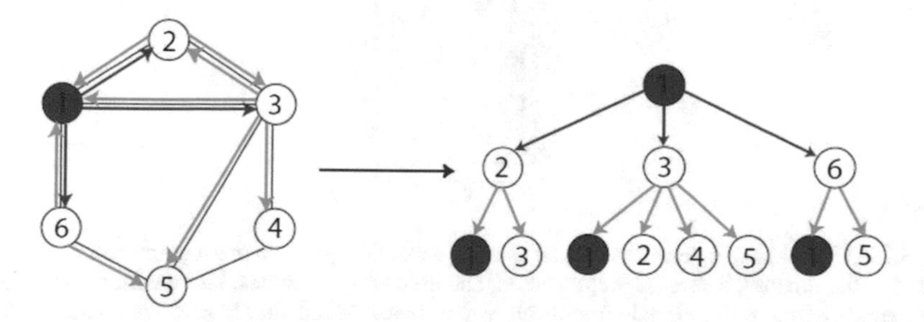

Fig. 5.20 A subtree pattern of height 2 rooted at the node 1 from the directed graph. After [579]

5.6.4 Machine Learning Using Information from Brain Graphs

In parallel with the rise of interest in brain networks, there has also been an increase in the use of machine-learning algorithms in the neuroscience community [588]. Indeed, the high-dimensional nature of fMRI data hinders the application of many multivariate methods using standard statistical techniques. This has prompted an increasing number of researchers to rely on regularization methods commonly found in machine learning and signal processing in addition to well-established univariate analysis techniques. Predictive modeling using machine-learning techniques has been suggested by Richiardi et al. [589], and is now commonly applied to various subdisciplines such as cognitive, clinical, affective, and social neuroscience. Figure 5.21 illustrates an emerging approach that applies machine-learning techniques to brain connectivity data.

Finally, it is worth noting that regression techniques have also been proposed in [590] for support vector regression (SVR). They showed that it is possible to

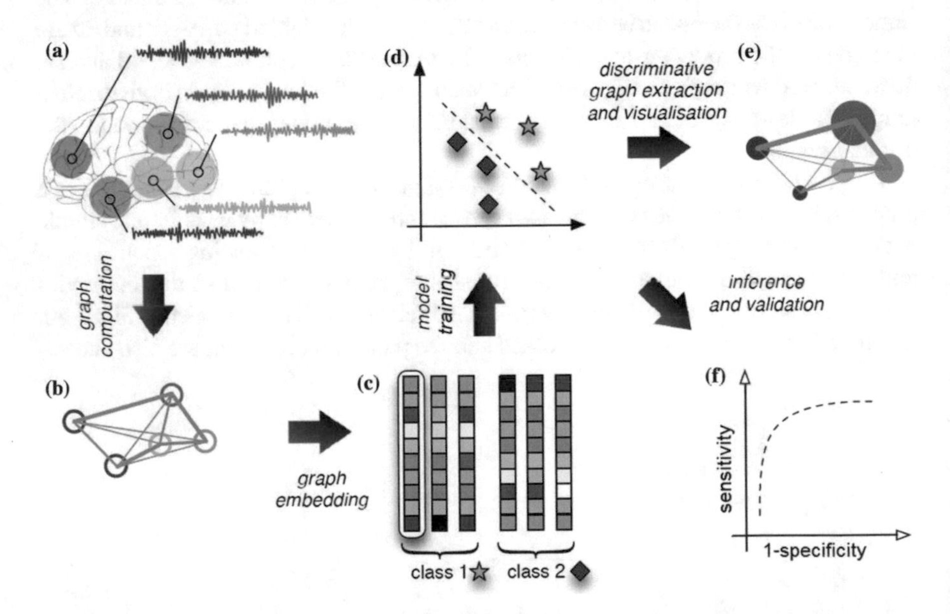

Fig. 5.21 Overview of a generic machine learning scheme to perform brain graph mining. **a** In the first step, the imaging dataset is preprocessed, and divided into regions, along with the associated representative time series signals from each region. **b** A labelled simple graph is computed from the correlations in the regional time series, where edge labels correspond to statistical dependency between brain regions, and brain regions are mapped to graph vertices. **c** The graph is converted into a vector space, for further statistical machine learning which is shown in the plot in (**d**). An interpretation of the classified pattern for brain-space visualisation is generated in (**e**). Finally, there is a step for the validation of the graph classification techniques as shown in (**f**) e.g. to elicit imaging markers in clinical applications. After [589]

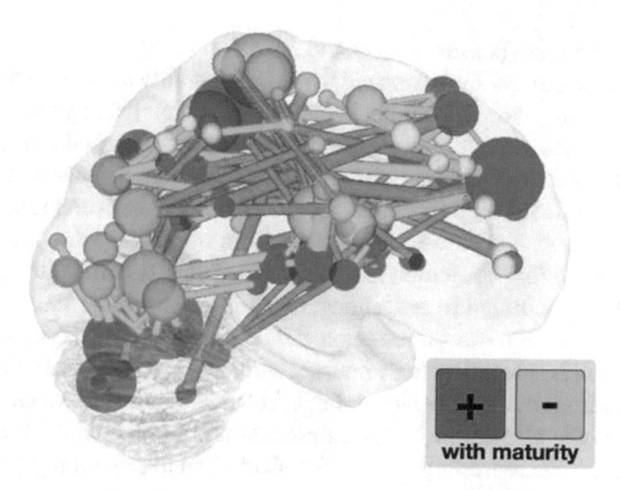

Fig. 5.22 Illustration of mapping showing different levels of importance in edges associated with the networks associated with distinct locations in the brain. The average SVR weight of 156 edges that were selected in all cross-validation folds is shown in a sagittal projection. The width of edges is proportional to their weight according to the regression coefficients vector value. Edges that are red indicates increased label value with age, whereas green labelling indicates a decreased label value. The importance of individual vertices is indicated by the size of the associated spheres, and sphere color indicates the functional subnetwork to which the vertex is part. After [589, 590]

perform age prediction from resting-state brain fMRIs scans. In their work, meta-analyses were used to define 160 regions of interest, yielding graphs with 12,270 different edge labels. Univariate filter feature selection was then performed, with the use of correlation operations between edge label with age. The approach aimed to reduce dimensionality to 200 edges on a separate data set. Following this step, a radial basis function kernel was used with an SVM solver to predict age from these 200 edges. Figure 5.22 illustrates a brain-space map of the more predictive edges.

5.6.5 Additional Considerations Regarding MRI Feature Extraction Methodologies

As discussed by Logothetis and Pfeuffer (2004), [593] a comparison of local field potentials (LFPs), single- and multi-unit spiking activity with highly spatio-temporally resolved BOLD fMRI responses from the visual cortex of monkeys showed that the largest magnitude changes were observed in LFPs, furthermore, the impulse response of the neurovascular system is both animal- and site-specific, and that LFPs yield a better estimate of BOLD responses than the multi-unit responses. These findings suggest that the BOLD contrast mechanism reflects the input and intracortical processing of a given area rather than its spiking output [591–593, 595].

Further to the above studies in a critical review by N. K. Logothetis in Nature [594] he suggested that the current limitations of the fMRI modality are not related to physics or poor engineering, and are unlikely to be resolved by increasing the sophistication and power of the scanners; they are instead due to the circuitry and functional organization of the brain, as well as to inappropriate experimental protocols that ignore this organization. The fMRI signal cannot easily differentiate between function-specific processing and neuromodulation, between bottom-up and top-down signals, and it may potentially confuse excitation and inhibition [596]. The magnitude of the fMRI signal cannot be quantified to reflect accurately differences between brain regions, or between tasks within the same region [597]. The origin of the latter problem is not due to our current inability to estimate accurately cerebral metabolic rate of oxygen ($CMRO_2$) from the BOLD signal, but to the fact that haemodynamic responses are sensitive to the size of the activated population of cells, which may change as the sparsity of neural representations varies spatially and temporally [598]. In cortical regions in which stimulus- or task-related perceptual or cognitive capacities are sparsely represented (for example, instantiated in the activity of a very small number of neurons), volume transmission which probably underlies the altered states of motivation, attention, learning and memory may dominate haemodynamic responses and make it impossible to deduce the exact role of the area in the task at hand. Neuromodulation is also likely to affect the ultimate spatiotemporal resolution of the signal. In addition, electrical measurements of brain activity, including invasive techniques with single or multiple electrodes, also fall short of providing real answers about network activity. It is thus widely accepted that single-unit recordings and firing rates are better suited to the study of cellular properties than of neuronal assemblies; furthermore, field potentials share much of the ambiguity discussed in the context of the fMRI signal [599]. From the above discussion, it follows that our future understanding of perception or cognition will ultimately depend on the development and application of integrative approaches. Single cell recordings, large electrode or tetrode-array recordings, monitoring of action potentials and slow waves must be employed in combination with neuroimaging using calibrated BOLD signals, cerebral blood flow (CBF), volume (CBV) and MR spectroscopy (MRS) of cerebral metabolites and neurotransmitters to obtain the information required for studying the brain's capacity to generate various behaviors. The recent development of high-field MRI and functional CBF imaging as well as MR spectroscopic imaging [chemical shift imaging (CSI)] point to the direction that such integrative approaches can and must be applied in systems neuroscience. Integrative approaches, however, require the interdisciplinary education of researchers and a thorough understanding of, at least, the basics of closely associated research fields. A multimodal approach using multichannel heterogeneous measurement modalities with appropriate sensor fusion techniques as discussed in the following chapters may thus provide new opportunities for further interpreting brain function and disorders.

5.6.6 *Recent Relevant Advances from the Computer Vision Community*

The idea of using multiple kernels in SVM classification where each kernel captures a different feature in the channel (e.g. the distribution of edges in an image) is not new and there is considerable work performed in this direction by the computer vision community [600]. In addition, nonlinear SVMs can be efficiently approximated by several linear ones [601] to simplify the computational aspects as well as provide a more systematic evaluation of algorithms used in biomedical classification problems. The computer vision community has also been making important advances in object localization which can provide better class segmentation which are also of relevance to the biomedical community [605]. Convex optimization routines may be adopted in the process of learning local feature descriptors [602] and deep matching [603] as well as recent advances in convolutional neural networks [604] are particularly promising emerging methodologies. To this effect, improved description of textural features that can be adopted by both the clinicians as well as the computer vision community would also be an important development that will facilitate the better tuning and evaluation of future algorithms [606].

Chapter 6
Outlook for Clifford Algebra Based Feature and Deep Learning AI Architectures

As stated in previous chapters, the interpretation of medical images requires advances in image segmentation and analysis, shape approximation, three-dimensional (3D) modelling, and registration of volumetric data. In the last few years, Clifford Algebra has emerged as a generic methodology for image processing and pattern recognition. Its attractiveness stems from the fact that it uses a more generic class of operators for the representation and solution of complex geometric problems. One of the main goals in this chapter is to discuss the new opportunities that Clifford algebras can provide to solve problems encountered in multichannel image processing and pattern recognition. In addition, we place into context recent advances in deep learning, as a new very promising classification modality which despite its success in other fields, is yet to be fully explored and applied to medical image analysis. The incorporation of geometric (Clifford) neurons to a deep learning framework seems to be a particularly exciting future research direction.

6.1 Prospects for Medical Image Analysis Under a Clifford Algebra Framework

The necessity for a multi-channel framework [89] that captures a multitude of features extracted using the signal processing routines discussed earlier, leads to a need for developing alternative classifiers capable of accommodating a large number of input vectors. Multi-dimensional classifiers do not require a dimensionality reduction of the datasets, thus preserving the information presented at the input stage of the classifier which could otherwise be lost in a conventional dataset fusion framework. Within a THz imaging context, the aim is to preserve the features extracted and ideally present them as separate entities to the classifier. Similarly, within the MRI community, in addition to the components of relevance in a multi-dimensional feature space described earlier, there is a need for observing changes in fMRI signals taking into consideration information obtained at different time stamps so data structures can have a tensorial structure. In addition, since an assessment of disease progres-

X. Yin et al., *Pattern Classification of Medical Images: Computer Aided Diagnosis*, Health Information Science, DOI 10.1007/978-3-319-57027-3_6

sion is made by cross-correlating images taken from different examinations, again a tensorial framework is often needed. Multi-dimensional classifiers are, therefore, ideally placed to further explore such cross-correlations.

Currently, there are several approaches to multiclass SVM [17, 59, 60, 350, 515]. The most promising way forward however, is through a Clifford algebra framework [518]. This framework allows us to express in a compact way several geometric entities in a multiclass context. Real and complex-valued support multi-vectors can be accommodated using the multi-vector Gramm matrix formalism. Through the Clifford product, one obtains the direct sum of linear spaces to achieve multiple outputs. A single kernel involving the Clifford product is used to provide nonlinear multi-vector input-output mappings reducing the complexity of the computation.

In a Clifford algebra framework, the geometric product of two vectors $\boldsymbol{a}$ and $\boldsymbol{b}$ is defined as a sum of their inner product (symmetric part) and their wedge product (antisymmetric part)

$$\mathbf{ab} = \mathbf{a} \cdot \mathbf{b} + \mathbf{a} \wedge \mathbf{b} \tag{6.1}$$

where the inner product $\mathbf{a} \cdot \mathbf{b}$ and the outer product $\mathbf{a} \wedge \mathbf{b}$ are defined as

$$\mathbf{a} \cdot \mathbf{b} = \frac{1}{2}(\mathbf{ab} + \mathbf{ba}) \tag{6.2}$$

$$\mathbf{a} \wedge \mathbf{b} = \frac{1}{2}(\mathbf{ab} - \mathbf{ba}) \tag{6.3}$$

The inner product of two vectors is the standard scalar or dot product and produces a scalar. The outer or wedge product of two vectors is called a bivector, an oriented area in the plane containing $\boldsymbol{a}$ and $\boldsymbol{b}$, formed by sweeping $\boldsymbol{a}$ along $\boldsymbol{b}$. The outer product is immediately generalizable to higher dimensions, so a trivector $\mathbf{a} \wedge \mathbf{b} \wedge \mathbf{c}$ is interpreted as the oriented volume formed by sweeping the area $\mathbf{a} \wedge \mathbf{b}$ along vector $\boldsymbol{c}$. The outer product of $\boldsymbol{k}$ vectors is a $\boldsymbol{k}$-vector or $\boldsymbol{k}$-blade, and such a quantity is said to have grade $\boldsymbol{k}$ and a multivector $\mathbf{A} \in \mathfrak{g}_n$ is the sum of $\boldsymbol{k}$-blades of different or equal grade. For an n-dimensinal space $\mathbf{V}^n$, orthonormal basis vectors are introduced $\{\mathbf{e}_i\}$, $i = 1, ..., n$ such that $e_i \cdot e_j = \delta_{ij}$, so that a basis that spans 1, $\{\mathbf{e}_i\}$, $\{\mathbf{e}_i \wedge \mathbf{e}_j\}$, $\{\mathbf{e}_i \wedge \mathbf{e}_j \wedge \mathbf{e}_k\}$, $\ldots$, $\mathbf{e}_1 \wedge \mathbf{e}_2 \wedge \ldots \wedge \mathbf{e}_n = \mathbf{I}$ is generated, where $\boldsymbol{I}$ corresponds to the hypervolume associated with the dataset. The set of all $\boldsymbol{k}$-vectors is a vector space $\bigwedge^{k} \mathbf{V}^n$ spanned by vectors

$$\binom{\mathbf{n}}{\mathbf{k}} := \frac{n!}{(n-k)!k!} \tag{6.4}$$

and the geometric algebra $\mathfrak{g}_n$ is spanned by a number of

$$\sum_{k=0}^{n} \binom{\mathbf{n}}{\mathbf{k}} = 2^n \tag{6.5}$$

elements where $\mathfrak{g}_n = \overset{0}{\bigwedge} \mathbf{V}^n \oplus \overset{1}{\bigwedge} \mathbf{V}^n \oplus \overset{2}{\bigwedge} \mathbf{V}^n \oplus \ldots \oplus \overset{n}{\bigwedge} \mathbf{V}^n$ corresponds to the linear n dimensional vector space. Any multivector of $\mathfrak{g}_n$ is expressed in terms of the basis of these subspaces. In the case of a three-dimensional space, this has $2^3 = 8$ elements:

$$\{1 \text{ (scalar)}, \ \{\mathbf{e}_1, \ \mathbf{e}_2, \ \mathbf{e}_3\} \text{ (vectors)}, \ \{\mathbf{e}_1\mathbf{e}_2, \ \mathbf{e}_2\mathbf{e}_3, \mathbf{e}_3\mathbf{e}_1\}$$
$$\text{(bivectors)}, \ \{\mathbf{e}_1\mathbf{e}_2\mathbf{e}_3\} \text{ (trivectors)} \equiv \mathbf{I}\}$$

In $\mathfrak{g}_{3,0,0}$ a typical multivector $\mathbf{v}$ will be of the form $\mathbf{v} = \boldsymbol{\alpha}_0 + \boldsymbol{\alpha}_1\mathbf{e}_1 + \boldsymbol{\alpha}_2\mathbf{e}_2 + \boldsymbol{\alpha}_3\mathbf{e}_3 + \boldsymbol{\alpha}_4\mathbf{e}_2\mathbf{e}_3 + \boldsymbol{\alpha}_5\mathbf{e}_3\mathbf{e}_1 + \boldsymbol{\alpha}_6\mathbf{e}_1\mathbf{e}_2 + \boldsymbol{\alpha}_7\mathbf{I}_3 = \langle\mathbf{v}\rangle_0 + \langle\mathbf{v}\rangle_1 + \langle\mathbf{v}\rangle_2 + \langle\mathbf{v}\rangle_3$, where the $\boldsymbol{\alpha}_i$'s are real numbers and $\langle\mathbf{v}\rangle_0 = \boldsymbol{\alpha}_0 \in \overset{0}{\bigwedge} \mathbf{V}^n$, $\langle\mathbf{v}\rangle_1 = \boldsymbol{\alpha}_1\mathbf{e}_1 + \boldsymbol{\alpha}_2\mathbf{e}_2 + \boldsymbol{\alpha}_3\mathbf{e}_3 \in \overset{1}{\bigwedge} \mathbf{V}^n$, $\langle\mathbf{v}\rangle_2 = \boldsymbol{\alpha}_4\mathbf{e}_2\mathbf{e}_3 + \boldsymbol{\alpha}_5\mathbf{e}_3\mathbf{e}_1 + \boldsymbol{\alpha}_6\mathbf{e}_1\mathbf{e}_2 \in \overset{2}{\bigwedge} \mathbf{V}^n$, $\langle\mathbf{v}\rangle_3 = \boldsymbol{\alpha}_7\mathbf{I}_3 \in \overset{3}{\bigwedge} \mathbf{V}^n$.

As discussed in more detail in [518] in Clifford algebra, rotations are performed by rotors $\mathbf{R}$, which are even-grade elements of the algebra that satisfy $\boldsymbol{R}\widetilde{\boldsymbol{R}} = 1$, where $\widetilde{\boldsymbol{R}}$ stands for the conjugate of $\mathbf{R}$. Rotors may be combined in a straightforward manner. For an input comprising of D multivectors and one multivector output, i.e., each data ith-vector has D multivector entries $\mathbf{x}_i = [x_{i1}, \ x_{i2} \ , \ldots, x_{iD}]^T$, where $x_{ij} \in \mathfrak{g}_n$ and D is its dimension. Thus, the ith-vector dimension is $D \times 2^n$, then each data ith-vector $\mathbf{x}_i \in \mathfrak{g}_n^D$. This ith-vector will be associated with one output of the total of all 2^n possibilities given by the following multivector output:

$$\begin{aligned} \boldsymbol{y}_i &= \boldsymbol{y}_{i_s} + \boldsymbol{y}_{i_{e1}} + \boldsymbol{y}_{i_{e2}} \\ &\quad + \cdots + \boldsymbol{y}_{i_I} \in \{\pm 1 \pm \boldsymbol{e}_1 \pm \boldsymbol{e}_2 \cdots \pm \boldsymbol{I}\} \end{aligned} \tag{6.6}$$

where the first subindex s stands for the scalar part outputs. For the classification, Clifford-SVM separates these multivector-valued samples into 2^n groups by selecting a good enough function from the set of functions:

$$\begin{aligned} f(\boldsymbol{x}) &= \omega^{\dagger^T} \boldsymbol{x} + \boldsymbol{b} \qquad (6.7) \\ &= [\boldsymbol{\omega}_1^\dagger, \boldsymbol{\omega}_2^\dagger, \ldots, \boldsymbol{\omega}_D^\dagger]^T [\boldsymbol{x}_1, \boldsymbol{x}_2, \ldots, \boldsymbol{x}_D] + \boldsymbol{b} \\ &= \sum_{i=1}^{D} \boldsymbol{\omega}_i^\dagger \boldsymbol{x}_i + \boldsymbol{b} \qquad (6.8) \end{aligned}$$

where $\boldsymbol{\omega}_i^\dagger \boldsymbol{x}_i$ corresponds to the Clifford product of two multi-vectors, $\boldsymbol{\omega}_i^\dagger$ is the reversion of the multivector $\boldsymbol{\omega}_i$, $\boldsymbol{x}$, $\boldsymbol{\omega} \in \mathfrak{g}_n^D$ and $f(\boldsymbol{x}), \boldsymbol{b} \in \mathfrak{g}_n$. An entry of the normal of the optimal hyperplane $\boldsymbol{\omega} = [\boldsymbol{\omega}_1, \ \boldsymbol{\omega}_2, \ldots, \ \boldsymbol{\omega}_D]^T$ is given by $\boldsymbol{\omega}_k = \boldsymbol{\omega}_{ks} + \ldots + \boldsymbol{\omega}_{ke1e2}\boldsymbol{e}1\boldsymbol{e}2 + \ldots + \boldsymbol{\omega}_{kI}\boldsymbol{I}$.

This problem is solved by considering a loss function ε using linear constraint quadratic programming:

$$\min L(\boldsymbol{\omega}, \boldsymbol{b}, \varepsilon) = \frac{1}{2}\boldsymbol{\omega}^{\dagger^{\mathrm{T}}}\boldsymbol{\omega} + \boldsymbol{C}\sum_{\mathrm{i,j}} \varepsilon_{\mathrm{ij}} \tag{6.9}$$

subject to

$$y_{ij}(f(\boldsymbol{x}_i))_j = y_{ij}(\boldsymbol{\omega}^{\dagger^T}\boldsymbol{x}_i + \boldsymbol{b})_j >= 1 - \varepsilon_{ij} \tag{6.10}$$

$$\varepsilon_{ij} >= 0 \qquad \text{for all } i,\ j \tag{6.11}$$

where ε_{ij} stands for the slack variables, i indicates the data ith-vector and j indexes the multivector component, i.e., $j = 1$ for the coefficent of the scalar part, $j = 2$ for the coefficient of $\boldsymbol{e}1$, ..., $j = 2^n$ for the coefficient of $\boldsymbol{I}$.

An entry ω_k of the optimal hyperplane $\boldsymbol{\omega}$ is computed using l multivector samples using the following expressions:

$$\omega_{ks} = \sum_{j=1}^{l}\Big((\boldsymbol{\alpha}_s)_j(\boldsymbol{y}_s)_j\Big)(\boldsymbol{x}_{ks})_j \tag{6.12}$$

$$\omega_{ke1} = \sum_{j=1}^{l}\Big((\boldsymbol{\alpha}_{e1})_j(\boldsymbol{y}_{e1})_j\Big)(\boldsymbol{x}_{ke1})_j \tag{6.13}$$

…

$$\omega_{kI} = \sum_{j=1}^{l}\Big((\boldsymbol{\alpha}_I)_j(\boldsymbol{y}_I)_j\Big)(\boldsymbol{x}_{iI})_j \tag{6.14}$$

where $(\boldsymbol{\alpha}_s)_j,\ (\boldsymbol{\alpha}_{e1})_j, \ldots,\ (\boldsymbol{\alpha}_I)_j,\ j = 1, \ldots,\ l$, are the Lagrange multipliers. Further details as well as an extension of this approach to non-linear Clifford-SVM using a Clifford algebra kernel $K(\boldsymbol{x},\ \boldsymbol{y})$ that performs the mapping component-wise are discussed in [518]. Concise introductions to geometric algebras can be found in [519] and in [520–523]. The representation of rigid body motions within a Clifford algebra framework, as would be needed to account for movement of patients during MRI scans, can be addressed using the analysis discussed in [524]. Furthermore, a Matlab implementation of the Clifford framework can be found in [525]. As will be discussed in the following section, the above analysis places geometric algebras at the center of a future deep learning framework suitable for both MRI as well as THz imaging datasets.

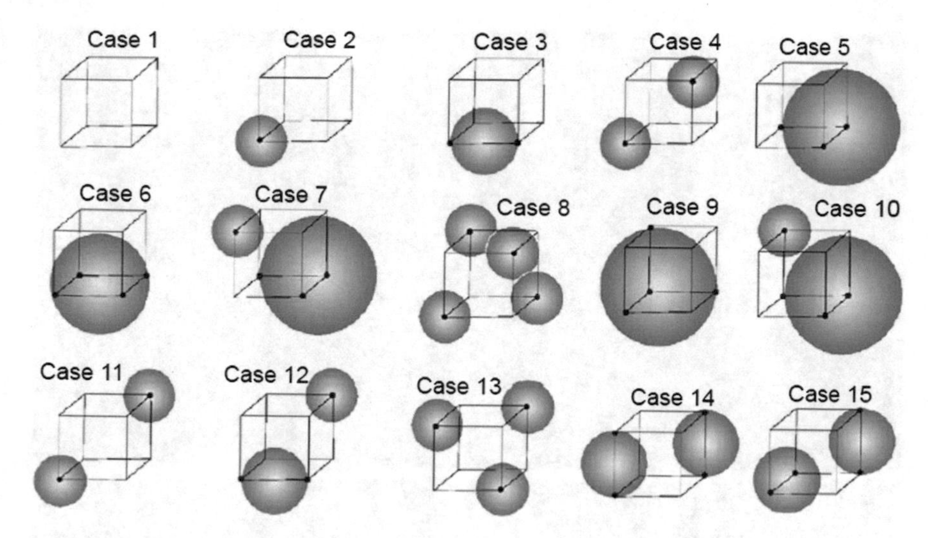

Fig. 6.1 The basic 15 cases of surface intersecting cubes. The spheres are numbered starting at left-superior corner, from 1 to 15. After [607]

An illustration of the use of geometric/Clifford algebra for medical image volume representation is provided in the work discussed by Jorge and Eduardo [607]. In their work, the marching cubes concept is introduced. This concept uses spheres to account for 15 basic cases of surface intersecting cubes, as illustrated in Fig. 6.1. Figure 6.2 shows a CT image of the skull with balloons (only one slide), for the case of a patient with a tumour. The segmentation results as well as approximation of the surface obtained by using circles, are based on a 2D version implementation of the marching cubes.

6.2 Outlook for Developing a Geometric Neuron Deep Learning of Time Series Datasets in Medical Images

Within the context of approximation theory, any given continuous function $g(x)$ representing MRI or THz-TPI/OCT datasets can be seen as a superposition of weighted functions [60]:

$$y(\boldsymbol{x}) = \sum_{j=1}^{N} \boldsymbol{\omega}_j \boldsymbol{\sigma}_j(\boldsymbol{w}_j^T \boldsymbol{x} + \boldsymbol{\theta}_j) \tag{6.15}$$

where $\sigma(.)$ is a continuous discriminatory function which can have the shape of a sigmoid, $\boldsymbol{\omega}_j \in \mathbf{R}$ and $\boldsymbol{x}, \ \boldsymbol{\theta}_j, \ \boldsymbol{w} \in \Re^n$. The finite sums of the form of Eq. 6.15 are dense if $|g(\boldsymbol{x}) - y(\boldsymbol{x})| < \varepsilon$ for a given $\varepsilon > 0$ and for all $\boldsymbol{x} \in [0, 1]^n$. This is known

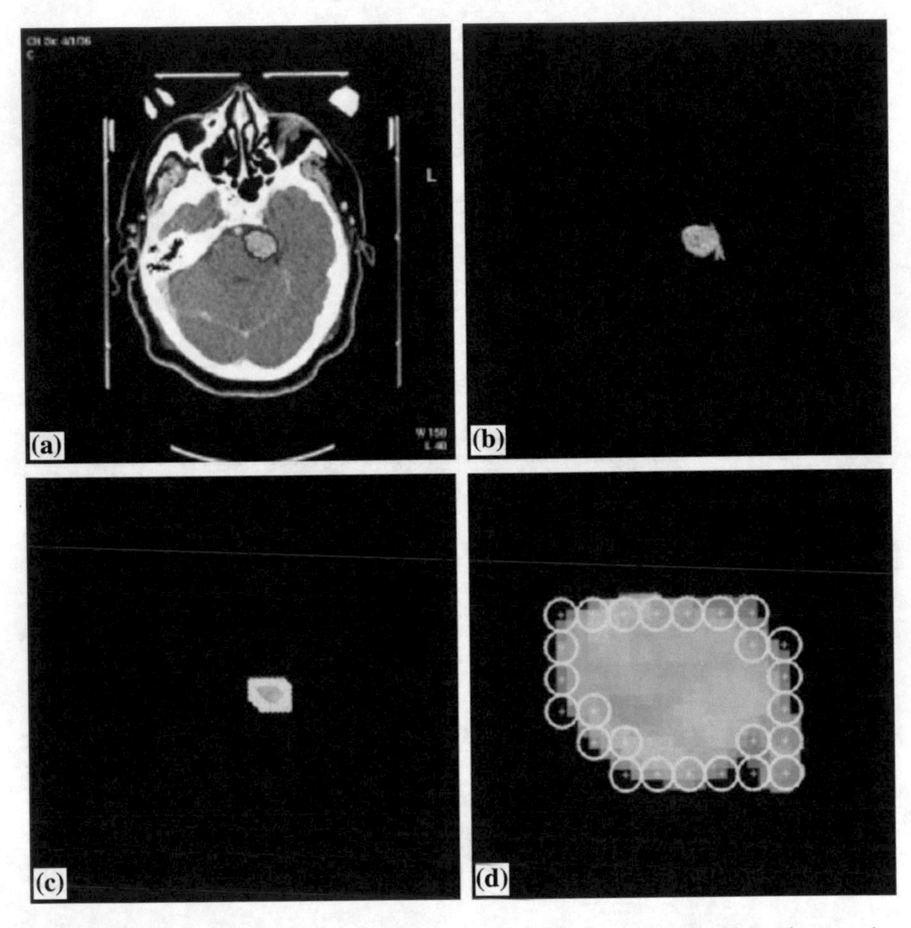

Fig. 6.2 Patient cranial image: **a** original of one CT slide; **b** segmented object (the tumor); **c** approximation by circles, 2D version of marching cube idea; **d** zoom of (**c**) for better visualization. After [607]

as the a density theorem and is a fundamental concept in approximation theory and nonlinear system modelling [608–610]. Multilayer feed-forward networks are known to be good universal approximators and can thus be used in the estimation process of the above function. As discussed in [611], the above expression depicting a scalar product can be conveniently extended to the case of a Clifford or geometric product, as illustrated in Fig. 6.3.

The function $f(\boldsymbol{m})$ for an n-dimensional multivector $\boldsymbol{m}$ is given from:

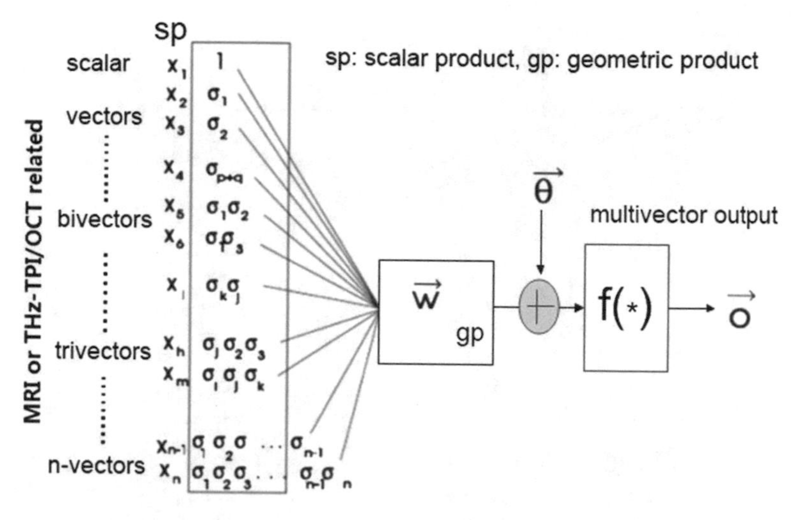

Fig. 6.3 Geometric neuron based on the McCulloch-Pitts neuron for MRI or THz-TPI/OCT datasets based on the generic framework discussed in [611]. The symbol *sp* denotes scalar product and *gp* denotes geometric product

$$\begin{aligned} f(\boldsymbol{m}) &= f(\boldsymbol{m}_0 + \boldsymbol{m}_i\boldsymbol{\sigma}_i + \boldsymbol{m}_j\boldsymbol{\sigma}_j + \boldsymbol{m}_k\boldsymbol{\sigma}_k + \ldots + \boldsymbol{m}_{ij}\boldsymbol{\sigma}_i \wedge \boldsymbol{\sigma}_j \\ &\quad + \ldots + \boldsymbol{m}_{ijk}\boldsymbol{\sigma}_i \wedge \boldsymbol{\sigma}_j \wedge \boldsymbol{\sigma}_k + \ldots + \boldsymbol{m}_n \wedge \boldsymbol{\sigma}_1 \wedge \boldsymbol{\sigma}_2 \wedge \ldots \wedge \boldsymbol{\sigma}_n) \\ &= f(\boldsymbol{m}_0) + f(\boldsymbol{m}_i)\boldsymbol{\sigma}_i + f(\boldsymbol{m}_j)\boldsymbol{\sigma}_j + f(\boldsymbol{m}_k)\boldsymbol{\sigma}_k + \ldots \\ &\quad + f(\boldsymbol{m}_{ij})\boldsymbol{\sigma}_i \wedge \boldsymbol{\sigma}_j + \ldots + f(\boldsymbol{m}_{ijk})\boldsymbol{\sigma}_i \wedge \boldsymbol{\sigma}_j \wedge \boldsymbol{\sigma}_k + \ldots \\ &\quad + f(\boldsymbol{m}_n) \wedge \boldsymbol{\sigma}_1 \wedge \boldsymbol{\sigma}_2 \wedge \ldots \wedge \boldsymbol{\sigma}_n. \end{aligned} \tag{6.16}$$

The standard scalar product in the neuron is replaced by the Clifford product

$$\boldsymbol{\omega x} + \boldsymbol{\theta} = \boldsymbol{\omega} \cdot \boldsymbol{x} + \boldsymbol{\omega} \wedge \boldsymbol{x} + \boldsymbol{\theta} \tag{6.17}$$

so the output is

$$\boldsymbol{o} = f(\boldsymbol{\omega x} + \boldsymbol{\theta}) = f(\boldsymbol{\omega} \cdot \boldsymbol{x} + \boldsymbol{\omega} \wedge \boldsymbol{x} + \boldsymbol{\theta}) \tag{6.18}$$

which is composed of the scalar product expression

$$f(\boldsymbol{\omega} \cdot \boldsymbol{x} + \boldsymbol{\theta}) = f(s_0) \equiv f(\sum_{i=1}^{N} \boldsymbol{\omega}_i \boldsymbol{x}_i + \boldsymbol{\theta}) \tag{6.19}$$

and an additional expression:

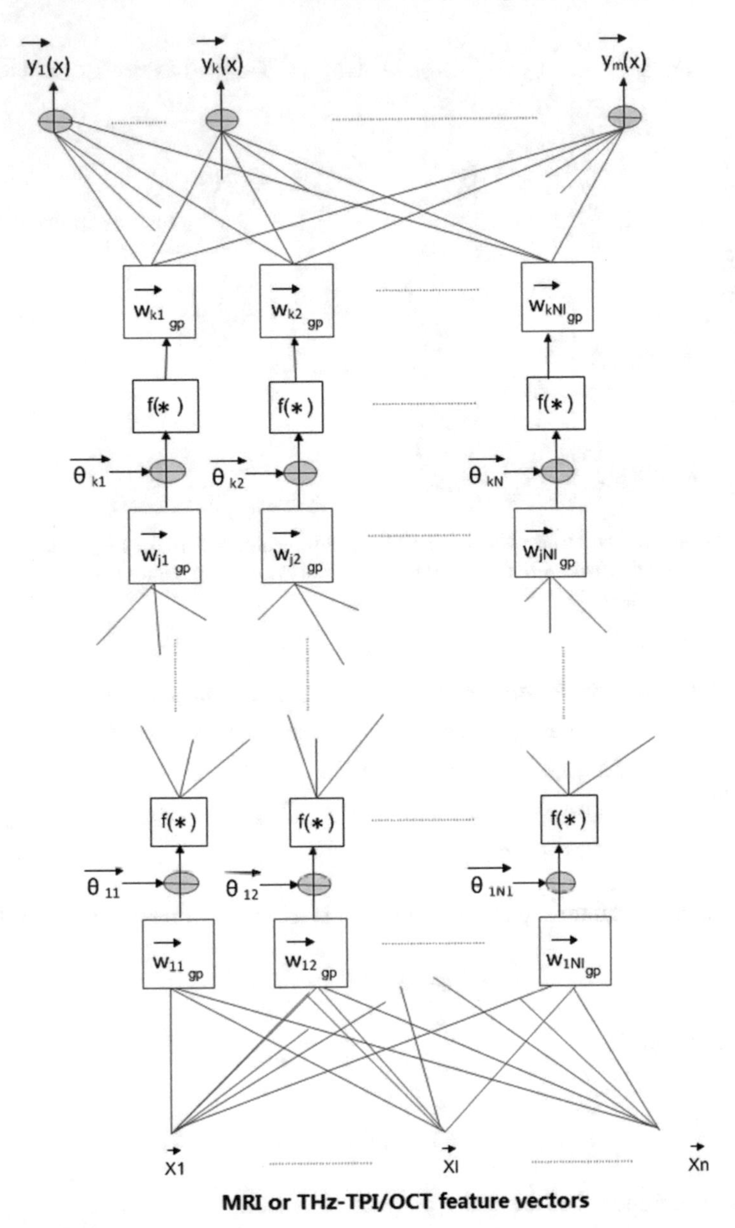

Fig. 6.4 Illustration of a multilayered geometric neuron that enables simplification of the learning rule as discussed in [611]. In the training of geometric feed forward networks, the weights of the output layer could be real values (the output weight multivectors could be scalars of k-grade)

$$f(\boldsymbol{\omega x} + \boldsymbol{\theta} - \boldsymbol{\theta}) = f(\boldsymbol{s}_1)\boldsymbol{\sigma}_1 + f(s_2)\boldsymbol{\sigma}_2 + f(s_3)\boldsymbol{\sigma}_3 + f(s_4)\boldsymbol{\sigma}_1\boldsymbol{\sigma}_2 \\ +... + f(s_5)\boldsymbol{\sigma}_1\boldsymbol{\sigma}_3 + f(s_6)\boldsymbol{\sigma}_2\boldsymbol{\sigma}_3 + f(\boldsymbol{s}_7)\boldsymbol{\sigma}_1\boldsymbol{\sigma}_2\boldsymbol{\sigma}_3. \tag{6.20}$$

A general representation of the geometric multilayered perception is shown in Fig. 6.4 below. The general expressions incorporating the geometric product of the outputs of hidden and output layers are:

$$\boldsymbol{o}_j = f_j(\sum_{i=1}^{N_i} \boldsymbol{\omega}_{ji} \cdot \boldsymbol{x}_{ji} + \boldsymbol{\omega}_{ji} \wedge \boldsymbol{x}_{ji} + \boldsymbol{\theta}_j) \tag{6.21}$$

$$\boldsymbol{y}_k = f_k(\sum_{j=1}^{N_j} \boldsymbol{\omega}_{kj} \cdot \boldsymbol{o}_{kj} + \boldsymbol{\omega}_{kj} \wedge \boldsymbol{o}_{kj} + \boldsymbol{\theta}_k) \tag{6.22}$$

The updating equation for the multivector weights of any hidden layer j is given from

$$\boldsymbol{\omega}_{ij}(t+1) = \eta[(\sum_{k}^{N_k} \delta_{kj} \otimes \overline{\boldsymbol{\omega}_{kj}}) \odot \boldsymbol{F}'(\mathbf{net}_{ij})] \\ \otimes \overline{\boldsymbol{o}_i} + \alpha \boldsymbol{\omega}_{ij}(t), \tag{6.23}$$

and for any k-output with a linear activation function:

$$\boldsymbol{\omega}_{jk}(t+1) = \eta[(\boldsymbol{y}_{k_t} - \boldsymbol{y}_{k_\alpha}) \odot \boldsymbol{F}'(\mathbf{net}_{jk})] \\ \otimes \overline{\boldsymbol{o}_j} + \alpha \boldsymbol{\omega}_{jk}(t), \tag{6.24}$$

$\Downarrow$

$$\boldsymbol{\omega}_{jk}(t+1) = \eta(\boldsymbol{y}_{k_t} - \boldsymbol{y}_{k_\alpha}) \otimes \overline{o_j} + \alpha \boldsymbol{\omega}_{jk}(t),$$

where $\boldsymbol{F}$ is the activation function, t is the update step, η and α are the learning rate and the momentum respectively, $\otimes$ is the Clifford or geometric product, $\odot$ is a scalar component by component product and $\overline{(\cdot)}$ is a multivector anti-involution operator (reversion or conjugation).

So far, the discussion has focused on methods for developing hyper-complex kernel based algorithms preserving and potentially fusing the information found in the extracted features of MRI or THz-TPI/OCT datasets. One further problem encountered, especially within an imaging context is that some of the mathematical functions describing malignant or benign tissue can be highly non-linear displaying a very large number of variations across the domain of interest. In the case of large voxel variations across an image for example, direction of excitatory signal and its intensity, as well as tissue texture can vary significantly and independently. An analytical understanding of these factors contributing to the overall observed variation may often be too complex to be captured in a single machine learning framework (as already discussed). An intuitive strategy, as discussed in [612], is first extracting low-level features that are invariant to small geometric variations such as edge detectors from Gabor filters, and then transforms them gradually to make them invariant to contrast changes and contrast inversion. This should be followed by focusing on the presence of edges, the detection of more complex but local shapes, up to the identification of more abstract categories associated with sub-objects and objects which are parts of the image, until these can be integrated. The above process is based on multiple stages of transformation and representation similar to cognition. Therefore, future AI based expert systems are likely to need to mimic such architectures in order to perform automated diagnosis.

Artificial neurons, performing an affine transformation followed by a non-linearity, form the basis of multi-layer neural networks which may be used to perform a learning task. In most of the neural networks encountered in the literature, 'shallow architectures' of up to 3 layers are discussed, the reason being that a 3-layered architecture can successfully approximate any function. Shallow architectures, however, have limitations, as some functions cannot be efficiently represented in terms of the number of tunable elements. It is not uncommon for them to fail to efficiently represent and, hence, learn a task of interest.

In contrast, 'deep architectures' (where depth of architecture refers to the depth of that graph, i.e., the longest path from an input node to an output node) are often associated with up to ten levels of representation at different levels of abstraction and have shown improved ability in learning. The development of Deep Belief Networks (DBNs) [613] is paving the way for a new class of unsupervised learning algorithms that greedily train one layer at a time. In essence, these architectures guide the training of intermediate levels of representation, this is a task performed locally at each level. As discussed in [612], once a good representation has been found at each level, it can be used to initialize and successfully train a deep neural network by supervised gradient-based optimization. DBNs can therefore be successfully applied in dimensionality reduction [614], classification tasks [615–619], regression [620], texture analysis [621, 622], segmentation [623] as well as motion [626] and it is only a matter of time before they are systematically used by the biomedical community in the processing of MRI and THz-TPI as well as OCT datasets.

Other aspects of the human brain that a biomedical AI system would have to emulate to provide human-like responses include a distributed and sparse representation [625, 627] as not all neurons are simultaneously used in a decision making process. Another aspect closely associated with human cognition is that of locality of representation, which is intimately connected with the notion of local generalization. Many existing machine learning methods are local in input space: to obtain a learned function that behaves differently in different regions of data-space, they require the fragmentation of that space and the use of different tunable parameters for each of these regions. This, of course, can be addressed partly with the Clifford algebra framework (discussed earlier) by adjusting the number of components used in the

Clifford product. Furthermore, there is the problem of making a choice for presenting local or distributed representations of data structures for learning to a classifier. In contrast to learning methods based on local generalization, the total number of patterns that can be distinguished using a distributed representation scales, possibly exponentially, with the dimension of the representation (i.e., the number of learned features). This is a common problem in the AI literature known as multi-task learning [628–630]. Deep learning algorithms address this issue by learning intermediate representations which can be shared across tasks. Hence, they can use data from similar tasks in the training process [631] to boost classification performance. This approach also provides a solution in instances where data is poorly labelled [632]. It may be argued that the simultaneous learning of a broad set of interrelated concepts enables the kind of broad generalizations that human experts appear to do well.

Unfortunately, from a computational perspective, the task of training deep architectures with many layers is not a trivial one. Very often the first problem encountered is that of initializing the network. Some work in this direction has been performed by Hinton [613] who introduced unsupervised learning algorithms that could be exploited to initialize deep neural networks. The auto-encoder is a simple unsupervised algorithm for learning a one-layer model that computes a distributed representation for its input [633], and stacked auto-encoders [616, 634] can provide greedy layer-wise training of deep networks. This is an important step, as within the AI community, there is a belief that part of the success of current learning strategies for deep architectures is connected to the optimization of lower layers.

It is also not uncommon that in order to improve the learning ability of a neural network, boosting is performed. Boosting adds one more layer level to its base learners so that a vote or linear combination of the outputs of the base learners can be used in the learning process [635]. Stacking [636] is another meta-learning algorithm that adds one layer in order to improve the generalization ability of the network. As discussed in [612], theoretical results suggest that it is not the absolute number of levels that matters, but the number of levels relative to how many are required to efficiently represent the target function (the more complex the function, the larger the number of levels needed). Furthermore, when a function needs a very large shallow architecture for successful representation, an alternative is to consider a compactly represented deep architecture.

Another important class of classifiers worth exploring with MRI, THz-TPI and OCT datasets, is that of decision trees [624]. A review of decision tree classifiers can be found in [638]. Decision trees need at least as many training examples as there are variations of interest in the target function, and they cannot generalize to new variations not covered in the training set. To improve on their generalization ability, one may consider soft decision tree algorithms [643]. These define an important class of hierarchical structures composed of internal decision nodes and terminal leaves. In the hard decision tree, a single path from the root to one of the leaves is traversed, whereas in the case of soft decision trees, all children are selected but selection is probabilistic, after allocating different weights with probabilities given by a sigmoid gating function. An alternative decision tree model [644], where a node can be a leaf and an internal node at the same time is also very promising and is worth considering in classification problems of MRI and THz-TPI datasets. Unlike traditional trees which solve incremental sub-problems greedily, budding trees solve the optimization problem taking all the parameters into account one tree at a time. During training, as new nodes are added, the existing node parameters are not fixed but the whole tree is continuously updated so as to better take account of the changes in the model. Budding trees have a soft architecture and provide a continuous and differentiable response in terms of their parameters and hence can be trained using a continuous optimization method like gradient-descent. With the utilization of the chain rule, the parameters in all the layers and nodes can be trained together, each proportional to its responsibility.

Other general aspects that may have to be taken into consideration when aiming to improve the learning process is that the number of samples necessary to achieve a particular error rate with a Gaussian kernel machine is exponential in the input dimension. Therefore, there are diminishing returns from a strategy of developing extensive libraries of MRI or THz/OCT images to train the classifier. The geometric algebra framework seems more appropriate in this respect, as the kernel is multidimensional with its value being optimized in each dimension. Furthermore, a larger number of inputs in the classifier imply better similarity between the inputs, which also ensures smoothness in the learning function facilitating the learning process. Finally, it is worth noting that the modeling of temporal dependencies as associated with disease progression is also an area open for further development as changes in the data structure would have to be captured by the dynamics of a network, and a dynamically reconfigured network has more degrees of freedom to perform such tasks than a static one.

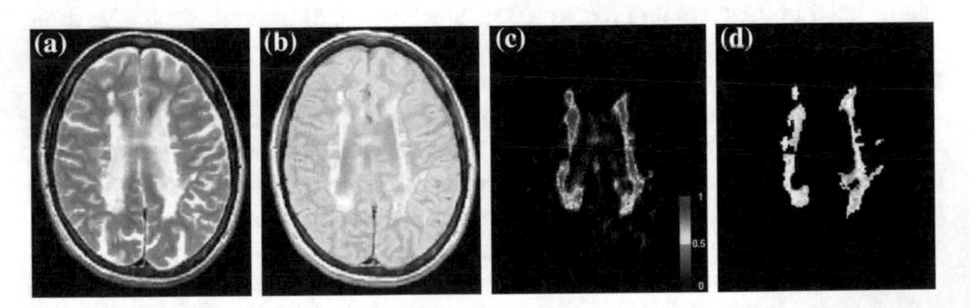

Fig. 6.5 Illustration of a probabilistic segmentation example based entirely on unlabelled data. **a** T2 input image, **b** PD input image, **c** probabilistic segmentation result, **d** ground truth. DSC = 73.15% After [645]

6.3 Prospects for Alternative Classifiers in Deep Learning of Unlabelled Medical Image Data

Recently, an automatic method for multiple sclerosis (MS) lesion segmentation of multi-channel 3D MR images was proposed in [645]. The novelty of the method lies in the fact that it can learn the spatial image features needed for training a supervised classifier entirely from unlabelled data. This is in contrast to the previously discussed supervised methods, which typically require the user to preselect or design the features to be used. The method can learn an extensive set of image features with minimal user effort and bias. In addition, by separating the feature learning process from the classifier training process that uses labelled (pre-segmented data), feature learning can take advantage of the much more widely available unlabelled data. The method uses deep learning and a random forest for supervised classification. In their reported work, the authors carried out quantitative validation using 1450 T2-weighted and proton density (PD) weighted pairs of MRIs of MS patients, where 1400 pairs were used for feature learning (100 of those for labelled training), and 50 pairs were used for testing. The results demonstrate that the learned features are very similar to those features isolated and identified by experts in terms of segmentation accuracy. They also showed that segmentation performance increased with the amount of unlabelled data used, even when the number of labelled images was fixed. An example of a segmentation result with a larger lesion load is shown in Fig. 6.5.

Chapter 7
Concluding Remarks

This book considers four different imaging modalities THz-TPI, MRI, fundus imaging and OCT. It is shown that, because of the complementarity between THz-TPI and MRI datasets along with OCT techniques, there is potential for developing a unified biomedical signal processing framework. THz-TPI is currently being explored as a viable alternative imaging modality to assess disease progression in a non-invasive manner. DCE-MRI is well established and is regularly used in clinical environments. In contrast, TPI has yet to gain popularity although there is a general recognition of its potential to provide complementary information to clinicians.

TPI scans provide information from individual pixels that show wavelength dependent attenuation, dispersion and phase delay according to the state of hydration of the tissue and the wavelength-dependent extinction coefficient of the sample. Specific vibrational signatures may also be identified in the frequency domain after Fourier transformation of the time-domain data. Hyper-spectral imaging can provide additional information for de-noising or classification. Similarly, MRI datasets are based on observations of de-excitation lifetimes so there are common grounds for a unified approach in processing these signals. In both cases, specific signatures may be identified as biomarkers, thereby assisting the molecular identification of compounds. Alternative imaging modalities such as fluorescence lifetime imaging, 2-photon microscopy, electron spin resonance spectrometry and dynamic neutron polarization techniques have also been mentioned as there are potential synergies with existing TPI, MRI or OCT modalities. These modalities may also benefit from the unified signal processing framework discussed.

Signal de-noising assuming Gaussian noise is probably more advanced in the THz community, whereas routines for Rician noise suppression are more advanced in the MRI community. Techniques that have been developed by the THz community such as adaptive apodization, adaptive wavelet decomposition and fractional order system identification are likely to benefit the MRI as well as the OCT community. The fitting of ARX, ARMAX subspace or fractional order identification models or the approximation of time domain signatures or spectral features with wavelet coefficients in both datasets, can provide a more parsimonious signal representation. This enables the extraction of lifetimes in a very parsimonious manner so classification can be

X. Yin et al., *Pattern Classification of Medical Images: Computer Aided Diagnosis*, Health Information Science, DOI 10.1007/978-3-319-57027-3_7

improved. Modelling using fractional order routines is an emerging modality of particular interest for all imaging systems. In all of the three modalities where pulses are used as excitation modalities, there is scope for selective sample excitation by pulse shaping methodologies.

In contrast to the above well-established signal processing approaches, pixel feature classification of retinal blood vessels can be performed using machine learning techniques that assign one or more classes to the individual pixels in a retinal image. Pixel feature classification is typically performed using a supervised approach. Originally, pixel intensity was used as the only feature in most studies. More recently, however, n-dimensional multi-feature vectors have been utilized. These incorporate information regarding pixel contrast with the surrounding region, their proximity to an edge, and similarity measures. Other multi-feature vectors utilizing local convolutions with multiple Gaussian derivative, Gabor, or other wavelet kernels [119], may also be used. Furthermore, alternative de-noising algorithms based on entropic principles have been developed by the fundus photography community, but have yet to be tested with MRI or THz-TPI or OCT datasets. Current 3-D imaging modalities are focusing on volume segmentation along with 3-D rendering and visualization. Some interferometric techniques are very well developed by the OCT community and these topologies may be further adopted and implemented by the THz community. Similarly, the null-balance polarizing techniques developed by the continuous wave THz community are equivalent to normal incidence ellipsometry and may thus be implemented with optical fibres for the OCT community. Retinal image segmentation from OCT measurements can benefit from advances in fundus imaging segmentation modalities, but, segmentation in THz-TPI is not sufficiently well developed. Advances in de-embedding different layers of tissue developed by the OCT community are also particularly useful to the THz-TPI community. Processing time in OCT can also be an issue as discussed in [646], and can also benefit from methods developed by the MRI community.

In contrast to fundus imaging and OCT, both MRI and THz-TPI systems are characterized by slow image acquisition rates. This can be distressing to patients in a clinical environment and leads to movement artefacts which need to be corrected. Compressed sensing techniques and techniques based on sparser data acquisition with k-space under-sampling are more developed in the MRI community and can benefit THz imaging systems when these are operated as a tomographic modality as opposed to imaging in a single plane. Correction algorithms using image registration can account for the movement of organs in DCE-MRI, but have yet to be used by the TPI community.

To achieve accurate detection and diagnosis of tumours, emphasis should be placed on the analysis of spatiotemporal features using a unified perspective. Automatic classification of both THz and MRI data sets is feasible using either SVM or ELM classifiers. In the case of SVM and ELM algorithms, their complex extensions are more useful because features in amplitude and phase or time and frequency respectively, may be simultaneously presented to the classifier as different entities. For both THz TPI as well as MRI datasets, treating the real and complex components in the datasets as separate entities from the de-noising step all the way to the classification step by adopting the complex extensions of the preferred classifier, is advantageous from a de-noising perspective as filtering can be optimized in each domain. This is also advantageous from a classification perspective because separately tuned kernels can improve classification accuracy. Textural information as well as PCA or ICA extracted features are associated with non-local features in an image or spectrum so will probably need to be processed within a distributed learning AI context. Some of these methodologies also have the potential to benefit the analysis of fundus images, leading to better segmentation.

Functional MRIs can record BOLD responses related to neural activity and are important in the analysis of neuronal diseases in the brain. Furthermore they can elucidate the functional aspects of the brain as a result of network alteration following disease or trauma. Two generic types of pattern mining methods based on neuronal connectivity information were discussed: the first is based on multivariable pattern classification, whereas the second makes use of the spatio-temporal correlations of the data structures across different regions in the brain. Multivariate pattern analysis has been used extensively in neuroimaging studies over the last few years because it also provides an assessment of the subject's mental state. Network analysis of regions in the brain using graph theoretical approaches provides a powerful means for quantifying functional connectivity. In addition, it is considered to be efficient in identifying functional changes due to psychiatric and neurological disorders [639]. THz-TPI has not been used systematically in brain imaging studies because of the thickness of the associated tissue but if further developed, it could in principle complement the current fMRI and OCT modalities for regions in the periphery of the skull.

Tensorial image registration enables the simultaneous consideration of additional measurement parameters such as polarization, hyperspectral components, morphological or textural features such as tissue folds and striations, and enable this type of information to be incorporated into the input space of the classifiers. This leads to a need for developing multi-channel kernels based on quaternion or other division 2 algebras. An alternative more versatile approach is to assume a Clifford algebra framework. In principle, such an approach should lead to improved classification accuracy. Multi-channel classifiers also enable fusion of information from other alternative complementary sensing modalities. Furthermore, they enable the integration of information acquired at different time stamps before being presented to the classifier. This can be important from a disease progression diagnostics perspective.

The work also makes a case for the further development of deep learning architectures. As discussed extensively in [612], the open problems that deep AI is trying to address require an ability of the networks to perform generalization at higher levels of abstraction, an ability to learn complex, highly-varying functions with a number of variations much greater than the number of training examples, an ability to perform unsupervised learning and learning from mostly unlabelled data in a semi-supervised setting, as well as demonstrate capability to exploit the synergies present in multi-task learning. These are generic problems which will have to be addressed eventually by the biomedical community through systematic investigations on the basis of sensitivity specificity and accuracy performance metrics.

What is clear, however, is that the variety of features that can be extracted using both MRI and THz TPI and OCT sensing modalities require novel and more elaborate classifier architectures to be developed. Synergies from adopting multilayer networks in conjunction with formulations using geometric algebras and geometric neurons are likely to play a central role in future classifier developments for biomedical applications. In addition, there is the potential for developing unlabelled data classifiers, which will make further use of very large datasets. This is an alternative methodology that becomes more relevant as existing databases become larger and more comprehensive.

The current open problems encountered from an AI perspective are making a case for researchers to develop more generic transferable skills which will pave the way for a unified data analysis and visualization framework that can be used across many sensing modalities. The further development and integration of the algorithms discussed, has the potential to advance biomedical AI by providing an improved and eventually fully automated quantitative assessment of disease proliferation.

Finally, it is worth noting that throughout this book a case was made for adopting a unified approach to the further processing of the various datasets generated through different imaging systems. A case was thus made of the possible benefits from convergent evolution of algorithms. It is anticipated however, that most of the future solutions that will eventually prevail as the most successful for each of the above imaging modalities, will go through several evolutionary steps, taking into consideration the extensive testing that is needed in clinical environments. As a result, it is expected that research will lead to solutions showing divergent evolutional characteristics.

References

1. S. Bow, *Pattern Recognition and Image Preprocessing*, Signal Processing and Communications Series (Marcel Dekker Inc, NY, USA, 2002)
2. S. Mickan, D. Abbott, J. Munch, X.-C. Zhang, T. van Doorn, Analysis of system trade-offs for terahertz imaging. Microelectron. J. **31**(7), 503–514 (2000)
3. E. Pickwell, V.P. Wallace, Biomedical applications of terahertz technology. J. Phys. D Appl. Phys. **39**(17), R301–R310 (2006)
4. W. Withayachumnankul, G.M. Png, X. Yin, S. Atakaramians, I. Jones, H. Lin et al., T-ray sensing and imaging. Proc. IEEE **95**(8), 1528–1558 (2007)
5. P. Siegel, Terahertz technology in biology and medicine. IEEE Trans. Microw. Theory Tech. **52**(10), 2438–2447 (2004)
6. S. Hadjiloucas, L. Karatzas, J.W. Bowen, Measurements of leaf water content using terahertz radiation. IEEE Trans. Microw. Theory Tech. **47**(2), 142–149 (1999)
7. S. Hadjiloucas, J.W. Bowen, Precision of quasioptical null-balanced bridge techniques for transmission and reflection coefficient measurements. Rev. Sci. Instrum. **70**(1), 213–219 (1999)
8. D. Mittleman, R. Neelamani, R.B.J. Rudd, M. Koch, Recent advances in terahertz imaging. Appl. Phys. B Lasers Opt. **68**(6), 1085–1094 (1999)
9. R.M. Woodward, V.P. Wallace, R.J. Pye, B.E. Cole, D. Arnone, E.H. Linfield- et al., Terahertz pulse imaging of ex vivo basal cell carcinoma. J. Investig. Dermatol. **120**(1), 72–78 (2003)
10. V.P. Wallace, A.J. Fitzgerald, S. Shankar, N. Flanagan, R. Pye, J. Cluff- et al., Terahertz pulsed imaging of basal cell carcinoma ex vivo and in vivo. J. Investig. Dermatol. **151**(2), 424–432 (2004)
11. X.-X. Yin, B.W.-H. Ng, D. Abbott, B. Ferguson, S. Hadjiloucas, Application of auto regressive models of wavelet sub-bands for classifying terahertz pulse measurements. J. Biol. Syst. **15**(4), 551–571 (2007)
12. X.X. Yin, B.W.H. Ng, B. Ferguson, S.P. Mickan, D. Abbott, Statistical model for the classification of the wavelet transforms of T-ray pulses, in *Proceeding of 18th International Conference on Pattern Recognition* (2006), pp. 236–239
13. T. Lahtinen, J. Nuutinen, E. Alanen, M. Turunen, L. Nuortio, T. Usenius- et al., Quantitative assessment of protein content in irradiated human skin. Int. J. Radiat. Oncol. Biol. Phys. **43**(3), 635–638 (1999)
14. H. Frölich, The biological effects of microwaves and related questions. Adv. Electron. Electron Phys. **53**, 85–152 (1980)
15. W. Grundler, F. Kaiser, Experimental evidence for coherent excitations correlated with cell growth. Nanobiology **1**, 163–176 (1992)
16. D.M. Mittleman, R. Jacobsen, M. Nuss, T-Ray imaging. IEEE J. Sel. Top. Quantum Electron. **2**(679), 679–692 (1996)
17. X.-X. Yin, B.W.-H. Ng, B.M. Fischer, B. Ferguson, D. Abbott, Support vector machine applications in terahertz pulsed signals feature sets. IEEE Sens. J. **7**(12), 1597–1608 (2007)

X. Yin et al., *Pattern Classification of Medical Images: Computer Aided Diagnosis*, Health Information Science, DOI 10.1007/978-3-319-57027-3

18. X.-X. Yin, K.M. Kong, J.W. Lim, B.W.H. Ng, B. Ferguson, S.P. Mickan, D. Abbott, Enhanced T-ray signal classification using wavelet preprocessing. Med. Biol. Eng. Comput. **45**(6), 611–616 (2007)
19. B. Fischer, M. Hoffmann, H. Helm, P.U. Jepsen, Chemical recognition in terahertz time-domain spectroscopy and imaging, semiconductor science and technology. Semicond. Sci. Technol. **20**(7), S246–S253 (2005)
20. D. Martin, E. Puplett, Polarised interferometric spectrometry for the millimetre and submillimetre spectrum. Infrared Phys. **10**, 105–109 (1970)
21. D.H. Martin, J.W. Bowen, Long-wave optics. IEEE Trans. Microw. Theory Tech. **41**(10), 1676–1690 (1993)
22. S. Smye, J. Chamberlain, A. Fitzgerald, E. Berry, The interaction between terahertz radiation and biological tissue. Phys. Med. Biol. **46**(9), R101–R112 (2001)
23. P.F. Taday, I.V. Bradley, D.D. Arnone, M. Pepper, Using terahertz pulse spectroscopy to study the crystalline structure of a drug: A case study of the polymorphs of ranitidine hydrochloride. J. Pharm. Sci. **92**(4), 831–838 (2003)
24. X. Yin, B.W.H. Ng, J.A. Zeitler, K.L. Nguyen, L.F. Gladden, D. Abbott, Local computed tomography using a THz quantum cascade laser. IEEE Sens. J. **10**(11), 1718–1731 (2010)
25. S. Hadjiloucas, J. Bowen, Precision of quasi-optical null-balanced bridge techniques for transmission and reflection coefficient measurements. Rev. Sci. Instrum. **70**, 213–219 (1999)
26. R. Donnan, B. Yang, Enhanced rapid and accurate sub-THz magneto-optical characterization of hexaferrite ceramics. J. Magn. Magn. Mater. **323**(15), 1992–1997 (2011)
27. B. Yang, R. Wylde, D. Martin, P. Goy, R. Donnan, S. Caroopen, The determination of the gyrotropic characteristics of hexaferrite ceramics from 75 to 600 GHz using an ultra-wideband vector-network-analyser. IEEE Trans. Microw. Theory Tech. **58**(12), 3587–3597 (2010)
28. W. Sun, B. Yang, X. Wang, Y. Zhang, R. Donnan, Accurate determination of terahertz optical constants by vector network analyzer of fabry-perot response. Opt. Lett. **38**(24), 5438–5441 (2013)
29. R.M. Woodward, B. Cole, V.P. Walace, D.D. Arnone, R. Pye, E.H. Linfield et al., Terahertz pulse imaging in reflection geometry of human skin cancer and skin tissue. J. Investig. Dermatol. **47**(21), 3853–3863 (2002)
30. B. Ferguson, S. Wang, D. Gray, D. Abbott, X.C. Zhang, Identification of biological tissue using chirped probe THz imaging. Microelectron. J. **33**(12), 1043–1051 (2002)
31. X.X. Yin, B.W.H. Ng, D. Abbott, *Terahertz Imaging for Biomedical Applications: Pattern Recognition and Tomographic Reconstruction* (Springer Science & Business Media, Berlin, Germany, 2012)
32. C. Rønne, P. Åstrand, S.R. Keiding, THz spectroscopy of liquid H2O and D2O. Phys. Rev. Lett. **82**(14), 2888–2891 (1999)
33. X.-X. Yin, B.W.H. Ng, B. Ferguson, D. Abbott, Wavelet based local tomographic image using terahertz techniques. Digit. Signal Proc. **19**(4), 750–763 (2009)
34. B. Ferguson, S. Wang, H. Zhong, D. Abbott, and X.-C. Zhang, Powder retection with T-ray imaging, in *Proceeding of SPIE Terahertz for Military and Security Applications*,vol. 5070, eds. by R.J. Hwu and D.L. Woolard (SPIE, USA, 2003), pp. 7–16
35. B.S.-Y. Ung, J. Li, H. Lin, B.M. Fischer, W. Withayachumankul, D. Abbott, Dual-mode terahertz time-domain spectroscopy system. IEEE Trans. Terahertz Sci. Technol. **3**(2), 216–220 (2013)
36. A. Pashkin, M. Kempa, H. Nemec, F. Kadlec, P. Kuzel, Phasesensitive time-domain terahertz reflection spectroscopy. Rev. Sci. Instrum. **74**(11), 4711–4717 (2003)
37. C.M. Watts, D. Shrekenhamer, J. Montoya, G. Lipworth, J. Hunt, T. Sleasman, S. Krishna, D.R. Smith, W.J. Padilla, Terahertz compressive imaging with metamaterial spatial light modulators. Nat. Photonics **8**, 605–609 (2014)
38. A. Horestani, J. Naqui, D. Abbott, C. Fumeaux, F. Martén, Two-dimensional displacement and alignment sensor based on reflection coefficients of open microstrip lines loaded with split ring resonators. Electron. Lett. **50**(8), 620–622 (2014)

39. M. Herrmann, M. Tani, K. Sakai, Display modes in time-resolved terahertz imaging. Jpn. J. Appl. Phys. Part 1 Regul. Pap. Short Notes Rev. Pap. **39**(11), 6254–6258 (2000)
40. X.X. Yin, B.W.H. Ng, B. Ferguson, S.P. Mickan, D. Abbott, 2-D wavelet segmentation in 3-D T-ray tomography. IEEE Sens. J. **7**(3), 342–343 (2007)
41. O. Sushko, R. Dubrovka, R. Donnan, Sub-terahertz spectroscopy reveals that proteins influence the properties of water at greater distances than previously detected. J. Chem. Phys. **142**(5), Art Number: 055101 (2015)
42. O. Sushko, R. Dubrovka, R. Donnan, Terahertz spectral domain computational analysis of hydration shell of proteins with increasingly complex tertiary structure. J. Phys. Chem. B **117**(51), 16486–16492 (2013)
43. M. Naftaly, *Terahertz Metrol.* (Artech House, Boston London, 2015)
44. S. Hadjiloucas, G.C. Walker, J.W. Bowen, One-port de-embedding technique for the quasi-optical characterization of integrated components. IEEE Sens. J. **13**(1), 111–123 (2013)
45. S. Hadjiloucas, R. Galvão, J. Bowen, R. Martini, M. Brucherseifer, H.P. Pellemans et al., Measurement of propagation constant in waveguides using wideband coherent THz spectroscopy. J. Opt. Soc. Am. B **20**(2), 391–401 (2003)
46. R. Galvão, S. Hadjiloucas, V. Becerra, J. Bowen, Subspace system identification framework for the analysis of multimoded propagation of THz-transient signals. Meas. Sci. Technol. **16**(5), 1037–1053 (2005)
47. S. Qian, *Time-Frequency and Wavelet Transforms* (Prentice Hall Inc, New Jersey, USA, 2002)
48. T. Froese, S. Hadjiloucas, R. Galvão, V. Becerra, C. Coelho, Comparison of extrasystolic ECG signal classifiers using discrete wavelet transforms. Pattern Recogn. Lett. **27**(5), 393–407 (2006)
49. E. Berry, R.D. Boyle, A.J. Fitzgerald, J.W. Handley, Time frequency analysis in terahertz pulsed imaging, in *Proceeding of Computer Vision Beyond the Visible Spectrum (Advances in Pattern Recognition)*, ed. by B. Bhanu, I. Pavlidis (Springer Verlag, London, UK, 2005), pp. 290–329
50. A. Meyer-Base, *Pattern Recognition for Medical Imaging* (Elsevier, California, USA, 2003)
51. S. Hadjiloucas, R. Galvão, J. Bowen, Analysis of spectroscopic measurements of leaf water content at thz frequencies using linear transforms. J. Opt. Soc. Am. A **19**(12), 2495–2509 (2002)
52. R. Galvão, S. Hadjiloucas, J. Bowen, C. Coelho, Optimal discrimination and classification of THz spectra in the wavelet domain. Opt. Express **11**(12), 1462–1473 (2003)
53. J.W. Handley, A. Fitzgerald, E. Berry, R. Boyle, Wavelet compression in medical terahertz pulsed imaging. Phys. Med. Biol. **47**(21), 3885–3892 (2002)
54. R.K.H. Galvão, S. Hadjiloucas, K.H. Kienitz, H. Paiva, R. Afonso, Fractional order modeling of large three-dimensional RC networks. IEEE Trans. Circuits Syst. I **60**(3), 624–637 (2013)
55. R.K.H. Galvão, K.H. Kienitz, S. Hadjiloucas, G. Walker, J. Bowen, S.F.C. Soares- et al., Multivariate analysis of random three-dimensional RC networks in the time and frequency domains. IEEE Trans. Dielectr. Electr. Insul. **20**(3), 995–1008 (2013)
56. L.A. Jacyntho, M.C.M. Teixeira, E. Assunção, R. Cardim, R.K.H. Galvão, S. Hadjiloucas, Identification of fractional-order transfer functions using a step excitation. IEEE Trans. Circuits Syst. II Express Briefs **62**(9), 896–900 (2015)
57. J.Y. Park, H.J. Choi, G.-E. Nam, K.-S. Cho, J.-H. Son, In vivo dual-modality terahertz/magnetic resonance imaging using superparamagnetic iron oxide nanoparticles as a dual contrast agent. IEEE Trans. Terahertz Sci. Technol. **2**(1), 93–98 (2012)
58. G. Chavhan, P. Babyn, B. Thomas, M. Shroff, E. Haacke, Principles, techniques, and applications of T2*-based MR imaging and its special applications. Radiographics **29**(5), 1433–1449 (2009)
59. X.-X. Yin, S. Hadjiloucas, Y. Zhang, M.Y. Su, Y. Miao, D. Abbott, Pattern identification of biomedical images with time series: Contrasting THz pulse imaging with DCE-MRIs. Artif. Intell. Med. **67**, 1–3 (2016)
60. X.X. Yin, Y. Zhang, J. Cao, J.L. Wu, S. Hadjiloucas, Exploring the complementarity of THz pulse imaging and DCE-MRIs: Toward a unified multi-channel classification and a deep learning framework. Comput. Methods Programs Biomed. **137**, 87–114 (2016)

61. A. Karahaliou, K. Vassiou, N.S. Arikidis, S. Skiadopoulos, T. Kanavou, L. Costaridou, Assessing heterogeneity of lesion enhancement kinetics in dynamic contrast enhanced MRI for breast cancer diagnosis. Br. J. Radiol. **83**(988), 296–309 (2010)
62. X.X. Yin, B.W.-H. Ng, Q. Yang, A. Pitman, K. Ramamohanarao, D. Abbott, Anatomical landmark localization in breast dynamic contrast-enhanced MR imaging. Med. Biol. Eng. Comput. **50**(1), 91–101 (2012)
63. S.H. Lee, J.H. Kim, N. Cho, J.S. Park, Z. Yang, Y.S. Jung et al., Multilevel analysis of spatiotemporal association features for differentiation of tumor enhancement patterns in breast DCE-MRI. Med. Phys. **37**(8), 3940–3956 (2010)
64. N. Bhooshan, M.L. Giger, S.A. Jansen, H. Li, L. Lan, G.M. Newstead, Cancerous breast lesions on dynamic contrast-enhanced MR images: computerized characterization for image-based prognostic markers. Radiology **254**(3), 680–690 (2010)
65. X.-X. Yin, B.W.-H. Ng, K. Ramamohanarao, A. Baghai-Wadji, D. Abbott, Exploiting sparsity and low-rank structure for the recovery of multi-slice breast MRIs with reduced sampling error. Med. Biol. Eng. Comput. **50**(9), 991–1000 (2012)
66. C.F. Beckmann, S.M. Smith, Tensorial extensions of independent component analysis for multisubject FMRI analysis. Neuroimage **25**(1), 294–311 (2005)
67. W. Chen, M.L. Giger, L. Lan, U. Bick, Computerized interpretation of breast MRI: investigation of enhancement-variance dynamics. Med. Phys. **31**(5), 1076–1082 (2004)
68. Y. Zheng, S. Englander, S. Baloch, E. Zacharaki, Y. Fan, M.D. Schnall- et al., STEP: spatiotemporal enhancement pattern for MR-based breast tumor diagnosis. Med. Phys. **37**(7), 3192–3204 (2009)
69. S. Agner, S. Soman, E. Libfeld, M. McDonald, K. Thomas, S. Englander- et al., Textural kinetics: a novel dynamic contrast enhanced (DCE)-MRI feature for breast lesion classification. J. Digit. Imaging **24**(3), 446–463 (2011)
70. M. Mahrooghy, A.B. Ashraf, D. Daye, C. Mies, M. Feldman, M. Rosen-et al., Heterogeneity wavelet kinetics from DCE-MRI for classifying gene expression based breast cancer recurrence risk, in *Proceeding of Medical Image Computing and Computer-Assisted Intervention—MICCAI 2013*, eds. by K. Mori, I. Sakuma, Y. Sato, C. Barillot, N. Navab. LNCS16(Part II), (Springer-Verlag, Berlin, Heidelberg, 2013), pp. 295–302
71. F. Bloch, Nuclear induction. Phys. Rev. **70**(7–8), 460–474 (1946)
72. H. Torrey, Bloch equations with diffusion terms. Phys. Rev. **104**(3), 563–565 (1956)
73. C. Neuman, Spin echo of spins diffusing in a bounded medium. J. Chem. Phys. **60**, 4508–4511 (1974)
74. E. Stejskal, J. Tanner, Spin diffusion measurements: spin echoes in the presence of time-dependent field gradient. J. Chem. Phys. **42**(1), 288–292 (1965)
75. M. Neeman, J. Freyer, L. Sillerud, Pulsed-gradient spin-echo studies in nmr imaging. effects of the imaging gradients on the determination of diffusion coefficients. J. Magn. Reson. **90**(2), 303–312 (1990)
76. G. Cleveland, D. Chang, C. Hazlewood, H. Rorschach, Nuclear magnetic resonance measurement of skeletal muscle: anisotropy of the diffusion coefficient of the intracellular water. Biophys. J. **16**(9), 1043–1053 (1976)
77. L. Garrido, V. Wedeen, K. Kwong, U. Spencer, H. Kantor, Anisotropy of water diffusion in the myocardium of the rat. Circ. Res. **74**(5), 789–793 (1994)
78. J. Tanner, Self diffusion of water in frog muscle. Circ. Res. **28**(1), 107–116 (1979)
79. R. Henkelman, G. Stanisz, J. Kim, M. Bronskill, Anisotropy of NMR properties of tissues. Magn. Reson. Med. **32**(5), 592–601 (1994)
80. M. Moseley, Y. Cohen, J. Kucharczyk, J. Mintorovitch, H. Asgari, M. Wendland, J. Tsuruda, D. Norman, Diffusion-weighted MR imaging of anisotropic water diffusion in cat central nervous system. Radiology **176**(2), 439–445 (1990)
81. M. Moseley, J. Kucharczyk, H. Asgari, D. Norman, Anisotropy in diffusion-weighted MRI. Magn. Reson. Med. **19**(2), 321–326 (1991)
82. P. Basser, J. Mattiello, D. Le Bihan, Estimation of the effective self-diffusion tensor from the NMR spin echo. J. Magn. Reson. Ser. B **103**(3), 247–254 (1994)

83. P. Basser, J. Mattiello, D. Le Bihan, Estimation of the effective self-diffusion tensor from the NMR spin echo. Biophys. J. **66**(1), 259–267 (1994)
84. J. Mattiello, P. Basser, D. Le Bihan, Analytical expression for the b matrix in NMR diffusion imaging and spectroscopy. J. Magn. Reson. Ser. A **108**(2), 131–141 (1994)
85. J. Mattiello, P. Basser, D. Le Bihan, The b matrix in diffusion tensor echo-planar imaging. Magn. Reson. Med. **37**(2), 292–300 (1997)
86. P. Basser, S. Pajevic, C. Pierpaoli, J. Duda, A. Aldroubi, In vivo fiber-tractography in human brain using diffusion tensor MRI (DT-MRI) data. Magn. Reson. Med. **44**(4), 625–632 (2000)
87. D. Jones, A. Simmons, S. Williams, M. Horsfield, Noninvasive assessment of axonal fiber connectivity in the human brain via diffusion tensor MRI. Magn. Reson. Med. **42**(1), 37–41 (1999)
88. S. Mori, B. Crain, V. Chacko, P. van Zijl, Three-dimensional tracking of axonal projections in the brain by magnetic resonance imaging. Ann. Neurol. **45**(2), 265–269 (1999)
89. X.-X. Yin, S. Hadjiloucas, J.-H. Chen, Y. Zhang , J.-L. Wu , M.-Y. Su, Tensor based multichannel reconstruction for breast tumours identification from DCE-MRIs. PLoS One **12**(3), Article Number: e0172111 (2017)
90. T. Conturo, N. Lori, T. Cull, E. Akbudak, A. Snyder, J. Shimony, R. McKinstry, H. Burton, M. Raichle, Tracking neuronal fiber pathways in the living human brain. Proc. Natl. Acad. Sci. **96**(18), 10422–10427 (1999)
91. P.J. Basser, D.K. Jones, Diffusion-tensor MRI: Theory, experimental design and data analysis. NMR Biomed. **15**(7–8), 456–467 (2002)
92. J. Simpson, H. Carr, Diffusion and nuclear spin relaxation in water. Phys. Rev. **111**(5), 1201–1202 (1958)
93. R. Mills, Self-diffusion in normal and heavy water in the range 1–45 degree. J. Phys. Chem. **77**(5), 685–688 (1973)
94. D. Le Bihan, J. Delannoy, R. Levin, Temperature mapping with MR imaging of molecular diffusion: application to hyperthermia. Radiology **171**(3), 853–857 (1989)
95. U. Castellani, M. Cristani, C. Combi, V. Murino, A. Sbarbati, P. Marzola, Visual MRI: Merging information visualization and non-parametric clustering techniques for MRI dataset analysis. Artif. Intell. Med. **44**(3), 171–282 (2008)
96. C. Lavinia, M. de Jongea, M. Van de Sandeb, P. Takb, A.J. Nederveena, M. Maas, Pixel-by-pixel analysis of DCE MRI curve patterns and an illustration of its application to the imaging of the musculoskeletal system. Magn. Reson. Imaging **25**(5), 604–612 (2007)
97. M.J. Stoutjesdijk, J. Veltman, M. Huisman, N. Karssemeijer, J. Barents, H. Huisman, Automatic analysis of contrast enhancent in breast MRI lesions using mean shift clustering for roi selection. J. Magn. Reson. Imaging **26**(3), 606–614 (2007)
98. E. Eyal, H. Degani, Model-based and model-free parametric analysis of breast dynamic-contrast-enhanced MRI. NMR Biomed. **22**(1), 40–53 (2009)
99. J.E. Levman, P.M.A.L. Warner, E. Causer, A vector machine formulation with application to the computer-aided diagnosis of breast cancer from DCE-MRI screeening examinations. J. Digit. Imaging **27**(1), 145–151 (2014)
100. M. Rakoczy, D. McGaughey, M.J. Korenberg, J. Levman, A.L. Martel, Feature selection in computer-aided breast cancer diagnosis via dynamic contrast-enhanced magnetic resonance images. J. Digit. Imaging **26**(2), 198–208 (2013)
101. H. Hawighorst, M. Libicher, M.V. Knopp, T. Moehler, G.W. Kaufmann, G.V. Kaick, Evaluation of angiogenesis and perfusion of bone marrow lesions: role of semiquantitative and quantitative dynamic MRI. J. Magn. Reson. Imaging **10**(3), 286–294 (1999)
102. C.S.P. van Rijswijk, M.J.A. Geirnaerdt, A.H.M. Taminiau, F. van Coevorden, A.H. Zwinderman, T.Pope et al., Soft-tissue tumours: value of static and dynamic gadopentate dimeglumine-enhanced MR imaging in prediction of malignancy. Radiology **233**(2), 493–502 (2004)
103. K.L. Verstraete, P. Lang, Bone and soft tissue tumors: the role of contrast agents for MR imaging. Eur. J. Radiol. **34**(3), 229–246 (2000)
104. J. Levman, T. Leung, P. Causer, D. Plewes, A.L. Martel, Classification of dynamic contast-enhanced magnetic resonance breast lesions by support vector mechines. IEEE Trans. Med. Imaging **27**(5), 688–696 (2008)

105. J. Yao, Breast tumor analysis in dynamic contrast enhanced MRI using texture features and wavelet transform. IEEE J. Sel. Top. Signal Process. **3**(1), 94–100 (2009)
106. C. Tanner, D.J. Hawkes, M. Khazen, P. Kessar, M.O. Leach, Does registration improve the performance of a computer aided diagnosis system for dynamic contrast-enhanced MR mammography?, in *IEEE International Symposium on Biomedical Imaging*, (2006), pp. 466–469
107. S. Marrone, G. Piantadosi, R. Fusco, A. Petrillo, M. Sansone, C. Sansone, Automatic lesion detection in breast DCE-MRI, in *Proceeding of The 17th International Conference on Image Analysis and Processing (ICIAP2013)*, ed. by A. Petrosino. LNCS8157 (Part II), (Springer-Verlag, Berlin, Heidelberg, 2013), pp. 359–368
108. M. Lustig, D. Donoho, J.M. Pauly, Sparse MRI: the application of compressed sensing for rapid MR imaging. Magn. Reson. Imaging **58**(6), 1182–1195 (2007)
109. L. Duvillaret, F. Garet, L. Coutaz, De-noising techniques for terahertz responses of biological samples. IEEE J. Sel. Top. Quantum Electron. **2**(3), 739–746 (1996)
110. L. Duvillaret, F. Garet, J.-L. Coutaz, Highly precise determination of optical constants and sample thickness in terahertz time-domain spectroscopy. Appl. Opt. **38**(2), 409–415 (1999)
111. T.D. Dorney, R.G. Baraniuk, D.M. Mittleman, Material parameter estimation with terahertz time-domain spectroscopy. J. Opt. Soc. Am. A **18**(7), 1562–1571 (2001)
112. I. Pupeza, R. Wilk, M. Koch, Highly accurate optical material parameter determination with thz time-domain spectroscopy. Opt. Express **15**(7), 4335–4350 (2007)
113. M. Scheller, C. Jansen, M. Koch, Analyzing sub-100 nm samples with transmission terahertz time domain spectroscopy. Opt. Commun. **282**(7), 1304–1306 (2009)
114. R. Wilk, I. Pupeza, R. Cernat, M. Kochh, Highly accurate thz time-domain spectroscopy of multilayer structures. IEEE J. Sel. Top. Quantum Electron. **14**(2), 392–398 (2008)
115. G.P. Kniffin, L.M. Zurk, Model-based material parameter estimation for terahertz reflection spectroscopy. IEEE Trans. Terahertz Sci. Technol. **2**(2), 231–241 (2012)
116. G.K. Aguirre, J.A. Detre, J. Wang, Perfusion fmri for functional neuroimaging. Int. Rev. Neurobiol. Neuroimaging Part A **66**, 213–236 (2005)
117. E. Özarslan, P.J. Basser, MR diffusion-"diffraction" phenomenon in multi-pulse-field-gradient experiments. J. Magn. Reson. **188**(2), 285–294 (2007)
118. J.M. Papy, L. De Lathauwer, S. Van Huffel, Exponential data fitting using multilinear algebra: The single-channel and multi-channel case. Numer. Linear Algebr. Appl. **12**, 809–826 (2005)
119. M. Abramoff, M. Garvin, M. Sonka, Retinal imaging and image analysis. IEEE Rev. Biomed. Eng. **3**, 169–208 (2010)
120. J.D. Lewis, G. Destito, A. Zijlstra, M.J. Gonzalez, J.P. Quigley, M. Manchester, H. Stuhlmann", Nat. Med. **12**, 354–360 (2006)
121. D. Huang, E.A. Swanson, C.P. Lin, J.S. Schuman, W.G. Stinson, W. Chang, M.R. Hee, T. Flotte, K. Gregory, C.A. Puliafito, J.G. Fujimoto, Optical Coherence Tomography. Science **254**, 1178–1181 (1991)
122. R.J. Cooper, E. Magee, N. Everdell, S. Magazov, M. Varela, D. Airantzis, A.P. Gibson, J.C. Hebden, MONSTIR II: a 32-channel, multispectral, time-resolved optical tomography system for neonatal brain imaging. Rev. Sci. Instrum. **85**(5). Article Number 053105 (2016)
123. L.A. Dempsey, R.J. Cooper, S. Powell, A. Edwards, C.-W. Lee, S. Brigadoi et al., Whole-head functional brain imaging of neonates at cot-side using time-resolved diffuse optical tomography, in *SPIE Proceedings on Diffuse Optical Imaging V*, Article Number 953818 (2015)
124. L.A. Dempsey, R.J. Cooper, T. Roque, T. Correia, E. Magee, S. Powell et al., Data-driven approach to optimum wavelength selection for diffuse optical imaging. J. Biomed. Opt. **20**(1). Article Number 016003 (2015)
125. S. Powell, L. Dempsey, R.J. Cooper, A. Gibson, J.C. Hebden, S. Arridge, Real-time dynamic image reconstruction in time-domain diffuse optical tomography, in *Biomedical Optics 2016 OSA Technical Digest (online)*, Article Number: OM4C.5 (2016)
126. Y. Pan, H. Xie, G.K. Fedder, Endoscopic optical coherence tomography based on a micro-electromechanical mirror. Opt. Lett. **26**(24), 1966–1968 (2001)

127. H. Xie, Y. Pan, G.K. Fedder, Endoscopic optical coherence tomographic imaging with a CMOS-MEMS micromirror. Sens. Actuators A **103**(1–2), 237–241 (2003)
128. L. Xi, C. Duan, H. Xie, H. Jiang, Miniature probe combining optical-resolution photoacoustic microscopy and optical coherence tomography for in vivo microcirculation study. Appl. Opt. **52**(9), 1928–1931 (2013)
129. X. Dai, L. Xi, C. Duan, H. Yang, H. Xie, H. Jiang, Miniature probe integrating optical-resolution photoacoustic microscopy, optical coherence tomography, and ultrasound imaging: proof-of-concept. Opt. Lett. **40**(12), 2921–2924 (2015)
130. M.S. Mahmud, D.W. Cadotte, B. Vuong, C. Sun, T.W. Luk, A. Mariampillai, V.X. Yang, Review of speckle and phase variance optical coherence tomography to visualize microvascular networks. J. Biomed. Opt. **18**(5). Aritcle Number 050901 (2013)
131. A.G. Markelz, A. Roiberg, E.J. Heilweil, Pulsed terahertz spectroscopy of DNA, bovine serum albumin and collagen between 0.1 and 2.0 THz. Chem. Phys. Lett. **320**(1–2), 42–48 (2000)
132. P. Martel, P. Calmettes, B. Hennion, Vibrational modes of hemoglobin in red blood cells. Biophys. J. **59**(2), 363–377 (1991)
133. P. Siegel, Terahertz technology. IEEE Trans. Microw. Theory Tech. **50**(3), 910–928 (2002)
134. P.U. Jepsen, J.K. Jensen, U. Møller, Characterization of aqueous alcohol solutions in bottles with thz reflection spectroscopy. Opt. Express **16**(13), 9318–9331 (2008)
135. A.G. Markelz, Terahertz dielectric sensitivity to biomolecular structure and function. Spectrochim. Acta Part A Mol. Biomol. Spectrosc. **14**(1), 180–190 (2008)
136. M. Brucherseifer, M. Nagel, P.H. Bolivar, H. Kurz, A. Bosserhoff, R. Büttner, Label-free probing of the binding state of DNA by time-domain terahertz sensing. Appl. Phys. Lett. **77**(24), 4049–4051 (2000)
137. A. Mazhorova, A. Markov, A. Ng, R. Chinnappan, O. Skorobogata, M. Zourob- et al., Label-free bacteria detection using evanescent mode of a suspended core terahertz fiber. Opt. Express **20**(5), 5344–5355 (2012)
138. T. Chen, Z. Li, W. Mo, Identification of biomolecules by terahertz spectroscopy and fuzzy pattern recognition. Spectrochim. Acta Part A Mol. Biomol. Spectrosc. **106**, 48–53 (2013)
139. A. Menikh, S.P. Mickan, H. Liu, R. MacColl, X.-C. Zhang, Label-free amplified bioaffinity detection using terahertz wave technology. Biosens. Bioelectron. **20**(3), 658–662 (2004)
140. A. Menikh, R. MacColl, C. Mannella, X. Zhang, Terahertz biosensing technology: Frontiers and progress. ChemPhysChem **3**(8), 655–658 (2002)
141. B. Fischer, M. Hoffmann, H. Helm, R. Wilk, F. Rutz, T. Kleine-Ostmann- et al., Terahertz time-domain spectroscopy and imaging of artificial RNA. Opt. Express **13**(14), 5205–5215 (2005)
142. M.K. Choi, K. Taylor, A. Bettermann, D.W. van der Weide, Broadband 10–300 GHz stimulus-response sensing for chemical and biological entities. Phys. Med. Biol. **47**(21), 3777–3789 (2002)
143. M. Herrmann, R. Fukasawa, O. Morikawa, Terahertz imaging. Terahertz Optoelectronics **97**, 331–381 (2005)
144. J. Nishizawa, T. Sasaki, K. Suto, T. Tanabe, K. Saito, T. Yamada- et al., THz transmittance measurements of nucleobases and related molecules in the 0.4- to 5.8-THz region using a GaP THz wave generator. Opt. Commun. **246**(1–3), 229–239 (2005)
145. M. Walther, B. Fischer, M. Schall, H. Helm, P.U. Jepsen, Far-infrared vibrational spectra of all-trans, 9-cis and 13-cis retinal measured by THz time-domain spectroscopy. Chem. Phys. Lett. **332**(3–4), 389–395 (2000)
146. I. Jones, T.J. Rainsford, B. Fischer, D. Abbott, Towards T-ray spectroscopy of retinal isomers: a review of methods and modelling. Vib. Spectrosc. **41**(2), 144–154 (2006)
147. C.J. Strachan, P.F. Taday, D. Newnham, K.C. Gordon, J.A. Zeitler, M. Pepper- et al., Using terahertz pulsed spectroscopy to study crystallinity of pharmaceutical materials. Chem. Phys. Lett. **390**(1–3), 20–24 (2004)
148. C.J. Strachan, P.F. Taday, D. Newnham, K.C. Gordon, J.A. Zeitler, M. Pepper- et al., Using terahertz pulsed spectroscopy to quantify pharmaceutical polymorphism and crystallinity. J. Pharm. Sci. **94**(4), 837–846 (2005)

149. C.J. Strachan, P.F. Taday, D.A. Newnham, K.C. Gordon, J.A. Zeitler, M. Pepper- et al., Terahertz pulsed spectroscopy and imaging in the pharmaceutical setting—a review. J. Pharm. Pharmacol. **59**(2), 209–223 (2005)
150. A.I. McIntosh, B. Yanga, S.M. Goldupb, M. Watkinsonb, R.S. Donnana, Crystallization of amorphous lactose at high humidity studied by terahertz time domain spectroscopy. Chem. Phys. Lett. **558**, 104–108 (2013)
151. C. Hayes, A. Padhani, M. Leach, Assessing changes in tumour vascular function using dynamic contrast enhanced magnetic resonance imaging. NMR Biomed. **15**, 154–163 (2002)
152. A. Jackson, D.L. Buckley, G.J.M. Parker, M. Ah-See, *Dynamic Contrast-Enhanced Magnetic Resonance Imaging in Oncology* (Springer-Verlag, Heidelberg, Germany, 2005)
153. P.D. Friedman, S.V. Swaminathan, R. Smith, SENSE imaging of the breast. Am. J. Roentgenol. **184**(2), 448–451 (2005)
154. S. Ljunggren, A simple graphical representation of fourier-based imaging methods. J. Magn. Reson. **54**(2), 338–343 (1983)
155. D. Twieg, The k-trajectory formulation of the NMR imaging process with applications in analysis and synthesis of imaging methods. Med. Phys. **10**(5), 610–621 (1983)
156. T. Parrish, X. Hu, Continuous update with random encoding (CURE): a new strategy for dynamic imaging. Magn. Reson. Med. **33**(3), 326–336 (1995)
157. R.C. Semelka, N.L. Kelekis, D. Thomasson, M.A. Brown, G.A. Laub, HASTE MR imaging: description of technique and preliminary results in the abdomen. J. Magn. Reson. Imaging **6**(4), 698–699 (1996)
158. D.S. Smith, E.B. Welch, X. Li, L.R. Arlinghaus, M.E. Loveless, T. Koyama- et al., Quantitative effects of using compressed sensing in dynamic contrast enhanced MRI. Phys. Med. Biol. **56**(15), 4933–4946 (2011)
159. H. Wang, Y. Miao, K. Zhou, Y. Yu, S. Bao, Q. He- et al., Feasibility of high temporal resolution breast DCE-MRI using compressed sensing theory. Med. Phys. **37**(9), 4971–4981 (2010)
160. L. Chen, M.C. Schabel, E.V.R. DiBella, Reconstruction of dynamic contrast enhanced magnetic resonance imaging of the breast with temporal constraints. Magn. Reson. Imaging **28**(5), 637–645 (2010)
161. J.F. Cai, E.J. Candès, Z. Shen, A singular value thresholding algorithm for matrix completion. SIAM J. Optim. **20**(4), 1956–1982 (2010)
162. L. Astolfi, F. Cincotti, D. Mattia, S. Salinari, C. Babiloni, A. Basilisco, P. Rossini, L. Ding, Y. Ni, B. He, M. Marciani, F. Babiloni, Estimation of the effective and functional human cortical connectivity with structural equation modeling and directed transfer function applied to high-resolution EEG. Magn. Reson. Imaging **22**(10), 1457–1470 (2004)
163. A. Luna, J.C. Vilanova, L.C. Hygino Da Cruz Jr., S.E. Rossi, in *Functional Imaging in Oncology, Biophysical Aspects and Technical Approaches*, (Springer Verlag Berlin, Heidelberg, 2014)
164. X.-C. Zhang, Terahertz wave imaging: horizons and hurdles. Phys. Med. Biol. **47**(21), 3667–3677 (2002)
165. D.L. Woolard, T.R. Globus, B.L. Gelmont, M. Bykhovskaia, A.C. Samuels, D. Cookmeyer, J.L. Hesler, T.W. Crowe, J.O. Jensen, J.L. Jensen, W.R. Loerop, Submillimeter-wave phonon modes in DNA macromolecules. Phys. Rev. E **65**, Article Number 051903 (2002)
166. A.J. Fitzgerald, S. Pinder, A.D. Purushotham, P. O'Kelly, P.C. Ashworth, V.P. Wallace, Classification of terahertz-pulsed imaging data from excised breast tissue. J. Biomed. Opt. **17**(1), Article Number 016005 (2012)
167. A.J. Fitzgerald, V.P. Wallace, M. Jimenez-Linan, L. Bobrow, R.J. Pye, A.D. Purushotham- et al., Terahertz pulsed imaging of human breast tumors. Radiology **239**(2), 533–540 (2006)
168. E. Pickwell, B.E. Cole, A.J. Fitzgerald, V.P. Wallace, M. Pepper, Simulation of terahertz pulse propagation in biological systems. Appl. Phys. Lett. **84**(12), 2190–2192 (2004)
169. C. Yu, S. Fan, Y. Sun, E. Pickwell-MacPherson, The potential of terahertz imaging for cancer diagnosis: a review of investigations to date. Quant. Imaging Med. Surg. **2**(1), 33–45 (2012)
170. G.-B. Huang, Q.-Y. Zhu, C.-K. Siew, Extreme learning machine: theory and applications. Neurocomputing **70**(1–3), 489–501 (2006)

171. V.P. Wallace, A.J. Fitzgerald, E. Pickwell, R.J. Pye, P.F. Taday, N. Flanagan, T. Ha, Terahertz pulsed spectroscopy of human Basal Cell Carcinoma. Appl. Spectrosc. **60**, 1127–1133 (2006)
172. P. Knobloch, C. Schildknecht, T. Kleine-Ostmann, M. Koch, S. Hoffmann, M. Hofmann, E. Rehberg, M. Sperling, K. Donhuijsen, G. Hein, K. Pierz, Medical THz imaging: an investigation of histo-pathological samples. Phys. Med. Biol. **47**, 3875–3884 (2002)
173. G.M. Png, J.-W. Choi, B.W.-H. Ng, S.P. Mickan, D. Abbott, X.-C. Zhang, The impact of hydration changes in fresh bio-tissue on THz spectroscopic measurements. Phys. Med. Biol. **53**, 3501–3517 (2008)
174. J. OConnor, P. Tofts, K. Miles, L. Parkes, G. Thompson, A. Jackson, Dynamic contrast-enhanced imaging techniques: CT and MRI. Br. J. Radiol. **84**(2), S112–S120 (2011)
175. M.A. Lindquist, The statistical analysis of fMRI data. Stat. Sci. **23**(4), 439–464 (2008)
176. M. Tonouchi, Cutting-edge terahertz technology. Nat. Photonics **1**, 97–105 (2007)
177. W. Shi, Y.J. Ding, Continuously tunable and coherent terahertz radiation by means of phase-matched difference-frequency generation in zinc germanium phosphide. Appl. Phys. Lett. **83**, Article Number: 1.1596730 (2003)
178. W. Shi, M. Leigh, J. Zong, S. Jiang, Single-frequency terahertz source pumped by Q-switched fiber lasers based on difference-frequency generation in GaSe crystal. Opt. Lett. **32**(8), 949–951 (2007)
179. E.R. Brown, K.A. McIntosh, K.B. Nichols, C.L. Dennis, Photomixing up to 3.8 THz in low-temperature-grown GaAs. Appl. Phys. Lett. **66**, Article Number: 1.113519 (1998)
180. T. Tanabe, K. Suto, J. Nishizawa, T.K.K. Saito, Frequency-tunable high-power terahertz wave generation from GaP. J. Appl. Phys. **93**(8), Article Number: 1.1560573 (2003)
181. A. Nahata, A.S. Weling, T.F. Heinz, A wideband coherent terahertz spectroscopy system using optical rectification and electro-optic sampling. Appl. Phys. Lett. **69**, Article Number: 1.117511 (1998)
182. C. Janke, M. Först, M. Nagel, H. Kurtz, A. Bartels, Asynchronous optical sampling for high-speed characterization of integrated resonant terahertz sensors. Opt. Lett. **30**, 1405–1407 (2005)
183. A. Bartels, A. Thoma, C. Janke, T. Dekorsy, A. Dreyhaupt, S. Winnerl, M. Helm, High resolution THz spectrometer with kHz scan rates. Opt. Express **14**, 430–437 (2006)
184. A. Bartels, R. Cerna, C. Kistner, A. Thoma, F. Hudert, C. Janke, T. Dekorsy, Ultrafast time-domain spectroscopy based on high-speed asynchronous optical sampling. Rev. Sci. Instrum. **78**(3), Article Number: 035107 (2007)
185. S. Hadjiloucas, G.C. Walker, J.W. Bowen, V.M. Becerra, A. Zafiropoulos, R.K.H. Galväo, High signal to noise ratio THz spectroscopy with ASOPS and signal processing schemes for mapping and controlling molecular and bulk relaxation processes. J. Phys. Conf. Ser. **183**, Article Number: 012003 (2009)
186. G.C. Walker, *Modelling the Propagation of Terahertz Radiation in Biological Tissue*, (Ph.D. Thesis) (Centre of Medical Imaging Research, University of Leeds, 2003)
187. B. Knoll, F. Keilmann, Near-field probing of vibrational absorption for chemical microscopy. Nature **399**, 134–137 (1999)
188. B. Knoll, F. Keilmann, Enhanced dielectric contrast in scattering-type scanning near-field optical microscopy. Opt. Commun. **182**, 321–328 (2000)
189. R. Hillenbrand, F. Keilmann, Complex Optical Constants on a Subwavelength Scale. Phys. Rev. Lett. **85**(14), 3029–3032 (2000)
190. I.S. Averbukh, B.M. Chernobrod, O.A. Sedletsky, Y. Prior, Coherent near field optical microscopy. Opt. Commun. **174**, 33–41 (2000)
191. R. Hillenbrand, T. Taubner, F. Keilmann, Phonon-enhanced light-matter interaction at the nanometre scale. Nature **418**, 159–162 (2002)
192. S.J. Oh, J.Y. Kang, I.H. Maeng, J.-S. Suh, Y.-M. Huh, S.J. Haam, J.-H. Son, Nanoparticle-enabled terahertz imaging for cancer diagnosis. Opt. Express **17**(5), 3469–3475 (2009)
193. J.-H. Lee, Y.-W. Jun, S.-I. Yeon, J.-S. Shin, J.W. Cheon, Dual-mode nanoparticle probes for high-performance magnetic resonance and fluorescence imaging of neuroblastom. Angew. Chem. Int. **45**(48), 8160–8162 (2006)

194. W. Cai, K. Chen, Z.-B. Li, S.S. Gambhir, X. Chen, Dual-function probe for PET and near-infrared fluorescence imaging of tumor vasculature. J. Nucl. Med. **48**(11), 1862–1870 (2007)
195. K. Chen, Z.-B. Li, H. Wang, W. Cai, X. Chen, Dual-modality optical and positron emission tomography imaging of vascular endothelial growth factor receptor on tumor vasculature using quantum dots. Eur. J. Nucl. Med. Mol. Imaging **35**(12), 2235–2244 (2008)
196. E.S. Kawasaki, A. Player, Nanotechnology, nanomedicine, and the development of new, effective therapies for cancer. Nanomed. Nanotechnol. Biol. Med. **1**, 101–109 (2005)
197. A.P. Alivisatos, W. Gu, C. Larabell, Quantum dots as cellular probes. Annu. Rev. Biomed. Eng. **7**, 55–76 (2005)
198. W.C.W. Chan, D.J. Maxwell, X. Gao, R.E. Bailey, M. Han, S. Nie, Luminescent quantum dots for multiplexed biological detection and imaging. Curr. Opin. Biotechnol. **13**, 40–46 (2002)
199. X. Michalet, F.F. Pinaud, L.A. Bentolila, J.M. Tsay, S. Doose, J.J. Li, G. Sundaresan, A.M. Wu, S.S. Gambhir, S. Weiss, Quantum dots for live cells, in vivo imaging, and diagnostics. Science **307**(5709), 538–544 (2005)
200. W. Jifang, R. Jicun, Luminescent quantum dots: a very attractive and promising tool in biomedicine. Curr. Med. Chem. **13**, 897–909 (2006)
201. F. Keilmann, C. Gohle, R. Holzwarth, Time-domain mid-infrared frequency-comb spectrometer. Opt. Lett. **29**, 1542–1544 (2004)
202. A. Schliesser, M. Brehm, F. Keilmann, D.W. van der Weide, Frequency-comb infrared spectrometer for rapid, remote chemical sensing. Opt. Express **13**(22), 9029–9038 (2005)
203. A.P. Alivisatos, Semiconductor clusters, nanocrystals, and quantum dots. Science **271**(22), 933–937 (1996)
204. S.K. Shin, H.-J. Yoon, Y.J. Jung, J.W. Park, Nanoscale controlled self-assembled monolayers and quantum dots. Curr. Opin. Chem. Biol. **10**(5), 423–429 (2006)
205. A.L. Rogach, A. Eychmüller, S.G. Hickey, S.V. Kershaw, Infrared-emitting colloidal nanocrystals: synthesis, assembly, spectroscopy, and applications. Small **3**(4), 536–557 (2007)
206. M. Bruchez Jr., M. Moronne, P. Gin, S. Weiss, A.P. Alivisatos, Semiconductor nanocrystals as fluorescent biological labels. Science **281**, pp. 2013–2016 (1998)
207. X. Gao, L. Yang, J.A. Petros, F.F. Marshall, J.W. Simons, S. Nie, In vivo molecular and cellular imaging with quantum dots. Curr. Opin. Biotechnol. **16**, 63–72 (2005)
208. A. Fu, W. Gu, C. Larabell, A.P. Alivisatos, Semiconductor nanocrystals for biological imaging. Curr. Opin. Neural Biol. **15**, 568–575 (2005)
209. R. Hardman, A toxicologic review of quantum dots: toxicity depends on physicochemical and environmental factors. Environ. Health Perspect. **114**(2), 165–172 (2006)
210. U. Resch-Genger, M. Grabolle, S. Cavaliere-Jaricot, R. Nitschke, T. Nann, Quantum dots versus organic dyes as fluorescent labels. Nat. Methods **5**, 763–775 (2008)
211. S. Pandya, J. Yu, D. Parker, Engineering emissive europium and terbium complexes for molecular imaging and sensing. Dalton Trans. **23**, 2757–2766 (2006)
212. L.R. Medeiros, L.B. Freitas, D.D. Rosa, F.R. Silva, L.T. Birtencourt, M.I. Edelweiss, M.I. Rosa, Accuracy of magnetic resonance imaging in ovarian tumor: a systematic quantitative review. Am. J. Obstet. Gynecol. **204**(1), 67–69 (2011)
213. J.P. McCarthy, R. Weissleder, Multifunctional magnetic nanoparticles for targeted imaging and therapy. Adv. Drug Deliv. Rev. **60**(11), 1241–1251 (2008)
214. J.M. Yang, J.W. Lee, J.Y. Kang, S.J. Oh, H.-J. Ko, J.-H. Son, K.G. Lee, J.-S. Suh, Y.-M. Huh, S.J. Haam, Smart drug-loaded polymer gold nanoshells for systemic and localized therapy of human epithelial cancer. Adv. Mater. **21**(43), 4339–4342 (2009)
215. A.S. Arbab, L.A. Bashaw, B.R. Miller, E.K. Jordan, B.K. Lewis, H. Kalish, J.A. Frank, Characterization of biophysical and metabolic properties of cells labeled with superparamagnetic iron oxide nanoparticles and transfection agent for cellular MR imaging. Radiology **229**(3), 838–846 (2003)
216. P.T.C. So, *Two-photon Fluorescence Light Microscopy* (Macmillan Publishers Ltd, Encyclopedia of Life Sciences, 2002)
217. S.W. Botchway, A.W. Parker, R.H. Bisby, A.G. Crisostomo, Real-time cellular uptake of serotonin using fluorescence lifetime imaging with two-photon excitation. Microsc. Res. Tech. **71**, 267–273 (2008)

218. S.W. Botchway, K. Scherer, S. Hook, C.D. Stubbs, E. Weston, R.H. Bisby, A.W. Parker, A series of flexible design adaptations to the Nikon E-C1 and E-C2 confocal microscope systems for UV, multiphoton and FLIM imaging. J. Microsc. **258**, 68–78 (2015)
219. B.J. Gaffney, Electron Spin Resonance of Biomolecules. Rev. Cell Biol. Mol. Med. (2006). doi:10.1002/3527600906.mcb.200300104
220. P.P. Borbat, A.J. Costa-Filho, K.A. Earle, J.K. Moscicki, J.H. Freed, Electron spin resonance in studies of membranes and proteins. Science **291**, 266–269 (2001)
221. B.F. Spencer, W.F. Smith, M.T. Hibberd, P. Dawson, M. Beck, A. Bartels, I. Guiney, C.J. Humphreys, D.M. Graham, Terahertz cyclotron resonance spectroscopy of an AlGaN/GaN heterostructure using a high-field pulsed magnet and an asynchronous optical sampling technique. Appl. Phys. Lett. **108**, Article Number: 1.4948582 (2016)
222. D. Marsh, Electron spin resonance: spin labels, *Membrane Spectroscopy* (Springer, 1981)
223. E.A. Nanni, A.B. Barnes, R.G. Griffin, R.J. Temkin, THz dynamic nuclear polarization NMR. IEEE Trans. Terahertz Sci. Technol. **1**, 145–163 (2011)
224. A. Abragam, M. Goldman, Principles of dynamic nuclear polarisation. Rep. Prog. Phys. **41**(3), 395–467 (1978)
225. F. Conti, *Fisiología Médica*, 1st edn. (McGraw-Hill, New York, USA, 2015)
226. X.-X. Yin, B.W.-H. Ng, J. He, Y. Zhang, D. Abbott, Accurate image analysis of the retina using hessian matrix and binarisation of thresholded entropy with application of texture mapping. PloS one **9**(4), Article Number: e95943 (2014)
227. S. Irshad, X.X. Yin, L.Q. Li, U. Salman, Automatic Optic Disk Segmentation in Presence of Disk Blurring. Int. Symp. Vis. Comput. 13–23 (2016)
228. K.M. Twietmeyer, R.A. Chipman, Optimization of mueller matrix polarimeters in the presence of error sources. Opt. Express **16**(15), 11589–11603 (2008)
229. S.A. Burns, A.E. Elsner, M.B. Mellem-Kairala, R.B. Simmons, Improved contrast of subretinal structures using polarization analysis. Investig. Ophthalmol. Vis. Sci. **44**(9), 4061–4068 (2003)
230. M.B. Mellem-Kairala, A.E. Elsner, A. Weber, R.B. Simmons, S.A. Burns, Improved contrast of peripapillary hyperpigmentation using polarization analysis. Investig. Ophthalmol. Vis. Sci. **46**(3), 1099–1106 (2005)
231. A.E. Elsner, A. Weber, M.C. Cheney, D.A. VanNasdale, M. Miura, Imaging polarimetry in patients with neovascular age-related macular degeneration. J. Opt. Soc. Am. A **24**(5), 1468–1480 (2007)
232. D. Huang, E.A. Swanson, C.P. Lin, J.S. Schuman, W.G. Stinson, W. Chang, M.R. Hee, T. Flotte, K. Gregory, C.A. Puliafito, et al., Optical coherence tomography. Science **254**(5035), 1178–1181 (1991)
233. C. Salvini, D. Massi, A. Cappetti, M. Stante, P. Cappugi, P. Fabbri, P. Carli, Application of optical coherence tomography in non-invasive characterization of skin vascular lesions. Skin Res. Technol. **14**(1), 89–92 (2007)
234. I.K. Jang, B.E. Bouma, D.H. Kang, S.J. Park, S.W. Park, K.B. Seung, K.B. Choi, M. Shishkov, K. Schlendorf, E. Pomerantsev, S.L. Houser, H.T. Aretz, G.J. Tearney, Visualization of coronary atherosclerotic plaques in patients using optical coherence tomography: comparison with intravascular ultrasound. J. Am. Coll. Cardiol. **39**(4), 604–609 (2002)
235. M.R. Hee, J.A. Izatt, E.A. Swanson, D. Huang, J.S. Schuman, C.P. Lin, J.G. Fujimoto, Optical coherence tomography of the human retina. Arch. Ophthalmol. **113**(3), 325–332 (1995)
236. C.A. Puliafito, M.R. Hee, C.P. Lin, E. Reichel, J.S. Schuman, J.S. Duker, J.A. Izatt, E.A. Swanson, J.G. Fujimoto, Imaging of macular diseases with optical coherence tomography. Ophthalmology **102**(2), 217–229 (1995)
237. M. Wojtkowski, A. Kowalczyk, R. Leitgeb, A.F. Fercher, Full range complex spectral optical coherence tomography technique in eye imaging. Opt. Lett. **27**(16), 1415–1417 (2002)
238. J.M. Schmitt, Optical Coherence Tomography (OCT): A Review. IEEE J. Sel. Top. Quantum Electron. **5**(4), 1205–1215 (1999)
239. A.F. Fercher, W. Drexler, C.K. Hitzenberger, T. Lasser, Optical coherence tomography-principles and applications. Rep. Prog. Phys. **66**, 239–303 (2003)

240. R.C. Youngquist, S. Carr, D.E.N. Davies, Optical coherence domain reflectometry: A new optical evaluation technique. Opt. Lett. **12**(3), 158–160 (1987)
241. M.A. Hussain, A. Bhuiyan, A. Turpin, A.D. Luu, R.T. Smith et al. Automatic identification of pathology distorted retinal layer boundaries using SD-OCT imaging. IEEE Trans. Biomed. Eng. **PP**(99) (2016). doi:10.1109/TBME.2016.2619120
242. A.M. Zysk, F.T. Nguyen, A.L. Oldenburg, D.L. Marks, S.A. Boppart, Optical coherence tomography: a review of clinical development from bench to bedside. J. Biomed. Opt. **12**(5). Article Number: 051403 (2007)
243. H.G. Bezerra, M.A. Costa, G. Guagliumi, A.M. Rollins, D.I. Simon, Intracoronary optical coherence tomography: a comprehensive review. JACC: Cardiovasc. Interv. **2**(11), 1035–1046 (2009)
244. W. Drexler, U. Morgner, R.K. Ghanta, F.X. Kärtner, J.S. Schuman, J.G. Fujimoto, Ultrahigh-resolution optical coherence tomography. J. Biomed. Opt. **7**(4), 502–507 (2001)
245. U. Morgner, W. Drexler, F.X. Kärtner, X.D. Li, C. Pitris, E.P. Ippen, J.G. Fujimoto, Spectroscopic optical coherence tomography. Opt. Lett. **25**(2), 111–113 (2000)
246. T.E. Carlo, A. Romano, N.K. Waheed, J.S. Duker, A review of optical coherence tomography angiography (OCTA). Int. J. Retin. Vitreous **1**(1), 1–15 (2015)
247. R.F. Spaide, J.G. Fujimoto, N.K. Waheed, Optical coherence tomography angiography. Retina **35**(11), 2161–2162 (2015)
248. I. Grulkowski, I. Gorczynska, M. Szkulmowski, D. Szlag, A. Szkulmowska, R.A. Leitgeb, A. Kowalczyk, M. Wojtkowski, Scanning protocols dedicated to smart velocity ranging in spectral OCT. Opt. Express **17**(26), 23736–23754 (2009)
249. A. Mariampillai, B.A. Standish, E.H. Moriyama, M. Khurana, N.R. Munce et al., Speckle variance detection of microvasculature using swept-source optical coherence tomography. Opt. Lett. **33**(13), 1530–1532 (2008)
250. C. Blatter, T. Klein, B. Grajciar, T. Schmoll, W. Wieser, R. Andre, R. Huber, R.A. Leitgeb, Ultrahighspeed non-invasive widefield angiography. J. Biomed. Opt. **17**(7). Article Number: 070505 (2012)
251. A. Mariampillai, B.A. Standish, E.H. Moriyama, M. Khurana, N.R. Munce et al., Speckle variance detection of microvasculature using swept-source optical coherence tomography. Opt. Express **33**(13), 1530–1532 (2008)
252. X.J. Wang, T.E. Milner, J.S. Nelson, Characterization of fluid flow velocity by optical Doppler tomography. Opt. Lett. **20**(11), 1337–1339 (1995)
253. Y. Zhao, K.M. Brecke, H. Ren, Z. Ding, J.S. Nelson, Z. Chen, Three-dimensional reconstruction of in vivo blood vessels in human skin using phase-resolved optical Doppler tomography. IEEE J. Sel. Top. Quantum Electron. **7**(6), 931–935 (2001)
254. S. Makita, Y. Hong, M. Yamanari, T. Yatagai, Y. Yasuno, Optical coherence angiography. Opt. Express **14**(17), 7821–7840 (2006)
255. D.Y. Kim, J. Fingler, J.S. Werner, D.M. Schwartz, S.E. Fraser, R.J. Zawadzki, In vivo volumetric imaging of human retinal circulation with phase-variance optical coherence tomography. Biomed. Opt. Express **2**(6), 1504–1513 (2011)
256. D.M. Schwartz, J. Fingler, D.Y. Kim, R.J. Zawadzki, L.S. Morse, S.S. Park, S.E. Fraser, J.S. Werner, Phase-variance optical coherence tomography: a technique for noninvasive angiography. Ophthalmology **121**(1), 180–187 (2014)
257. M. Akiba, K.P. Chan, N. Tanno, Full-field optical coherence tomography by two-dimensional heterodyne detection with a pair of CCD cameras. Opt. Lett. **28**(10), 816–818 (2003)
258. Z. Chen, M. Liu, M. Minneman, L. Ginner, E. Hoover, H. Sattmann, M. Bonesi, W. Drexler, R.A. Leitgeb, Phase-stable swept source OCT angiography in human skin using an akinetic source. Biomed. Opt. Express **7**(8), 3032–3048 (2016)
259. F.E.W. Schmidt, M.E. Fry, E.M.C. Hillman, J.C. Hebden, D.T. Delpy, A 32-channel time-resolved instrument for medical optical tomography. Rev. Sci. Instrum. **71**(1), 256–265 (1999)
260. M.E. Fermann, I. Hartl, Ultrafast fibre lasers. Nat. Photonics **7**, 868–874 (2013)
261. F. Couny, F. Benabid, Optical frequency comb generation in gas-filled hollow core photonic crystal fibres. J. Opt. A Pure Appl. Opt. **11**(10). Article Number: 103002 (2009)

262. D. Strickland, G. Mourou, Compression of amplified chirped optical pulses. Opt. Commun. **56**(3), 447–449 (1985)
263. P. Maine, D. Strickland, P. Bado, M. Pessot, G. Mourou, Generation of ultrahigh peak power pulses by chirped pulse amplification. IEEE J. Quantum Electron. **24**(2), 398–403 (1988)
264. S.R. Deans, *The Radon Transform and Some of Its Applications* (Dover Publications Inc., 2007)
265. E.M.C. Hillman, J.C. Hebden, F.E.W. Schmidt, S.R. Arridge, M. Schweiger, H. Dehghani, D.T. Delpy, Calibration techniques and datatype extraction for time-resolved optical tomography. Rev. Sci. Instrum. **71**(9), 3415–3427 (2000)
266. J.C. Hebden, H. Veenstra, H. Dehghani, E.M.C. Hillman, M. Schweiger, S.R. Arridge, D.T. Delpy, Three-dimensional time-resolved optical tomography of a conical breast phantom. Appl. Opt. **40**(19), 3278–3287 (2001)
267. T. Teng, M. Lefley, D. Claremont, Use of two-dimensional matched filters for estimating a length of blood vessels newly created in angiogenesis process. Med. Biol. Eng. Comput. **40**(1), 2–13 (2002)
268. A.M. Mendonça, A. Campilho, Segmentation of retinal blood vessels by combining the detection of centerlines and morphological reconstruction. IEEE Trans. Med. Imaging **25**(9), 1200–1213 (2003)
269. S. Hammond, J. Wells, D. Marcus, L. Prisant, Ophthalmoscopic findings in malignant hypertension. J. Clin. Hypertens. **8**(3), 221–223 (2006)
270. A. Ghorbanihaghjo, A. Javadzadeh, H. Argani, N. Nezami, N. Rashtchizadeh, M. Rafeey, M. Rohbaninoubar, B. Rahimi-Ardabili, Lipoprotein(a), homocysteine, and retinal arteriosclerosis. Mol. Vis. **14**, 1692–1697 (2008)
271. J.S. Patrick, E. Marshall, *Ophthalmic Photography: Retinal Photography, Angiography, and Electronic Imaging*, 2nd edn. (Tyler Butterworth-Heinemann Medical, Chicago, Illinois, USA, 2011)
272. M. Bhargava, T.Y. Wong, Current concepts in hypertensive retinopathy. Retin. Phys. **10**(11/2013), 43–54 (2013)
273. G. Liew, J.J. Wang, Retinal Vascular Signs: A Window to the Heart? Revista Espanola de Cardiología **64**(6), 515–521 (2011)
274. R. Galvão, S. Hadjiloucas, A. Zafiropoulos, G. Walker, J. Bowen, R. Dudley, Optimization of apodization functions in thz transient spectrometry. Opt. Lett. **32**(20), 3008–3010 (2007)
275. J.W. Bowen, S. Hadjiloucas, G.C. Walker, H.W. Huebers, J. Schubert, Interferometric Technique for Measuring Terahertz Antenna Phase Patterns. IEEE Sens. J. **13**(1), 100–110 (2013)
276. N. Wiener, *Extrapolation and Smoothing of Stationary Time Series, Wiley* (U.S.A, New York, 1949)
277. I. Jolliffe, *Principal Component Analysis* (Springer-Verlag, U.S.A, New York, 1986)
278. J. Hertz, A. Krogh, R. Palmer, *Introduction to the Theory of Neural Computation* (Addison-Wesley, California, U.S.A, 1989)
279. J.N. Kapur, H.K. Kesavan, *Entropy Optimization Principles with Applications* (Academic Press, Boston, 1992)
280. E. Özarslan, P.J. Basser, T.M. Shepherd, P.E. Thelwall, B.C. Vemuri, S. Blackband, Observation of anomalous diffusion in excised tissue by characterizing the diffusion-time dependence of the MR signal. J. Magn. Reson. **183**(2), 315–323 (2006)
281. K. Bennett, K. Schmainda, R. Bennett, D. Rowe, H. Lu, J. Hyde, Characterization of continuously distributed cortical water diffusion rates with a stretched-exponential model. Magn. Reson. Med. **50**(4), 727–734 (2003)
282. P. Sen, M. Hürlimann, T. de Swiet, Debye-porod law of diffraction for diffusion in porous media. Phys. Rev. B: Condens. Matter **51**(1), 601–604 (1995)
283. L. Richard, M.O. Abdullah, D. Baleanu, X. Zhou, Anomalous diffusion expressed through fractional order differential operators in the bloch-torrey equation. J. Magn. Reson. **190**, 255–270 (2008)
284. T.H. Jochimsen, A. Schöfer, R. Bammer, M.E. Moseley, Efficient simulation of magnetic resonance imaging with bloch-torrey equations using intra-voxel magnetization gradients. J. Magn. Reson. **180**(1), 29–38 (2006)

285. X. Zhou, Q. Gao, O. Abdullah, R.L. Magin, Studies of anomalous diffusion in the human brain using fractional order calculus. Magn. Reson. Med. **63**(3), 562–569 (2010)
286. J.-L. Battagliaa, O. Cois, L. Puigsegur, A. Oustaloup, Solving an inverse heat conduction problem using a non-integer identified model. Int. J. Heat Mass Transf. **44**, 2671–2680 (2001)
287. M. Aoun, R. Malti, F. Levron, A. Oustaloup, Numerical Simulations of Fractional Systems: An Overview of Existing Methods and Improvements. Nonlinear Dyn. **38**, 117–131 (2004)
288. R. Malti, X. Moreau, F. Khemane, A. Oustaloup, Stability and resonance conditions of elementary fractional transfer functions. Automatica **47**, 2462–2467 (2011)
289. S. Victor, R. Malti, H. Garnier, A. Oustaloup, Parameter and differentiation order estimation in fractional models. Automatica **49**, 926–935 (2013)
290. Z. Wang, Fast algorithms for the discrete W transform and for the discrete fourier transform. IEEE Trans. Acoust. Speech Signal Process. ASSP **32**, 803–816 (1984)
291. Y. Arai, T. Agui, M. Nakajima, A fast DCT-SQ scheme for images. IEICE Trans. **E-71**(11), 1095–1097 (1988)
292. E. Feig, S. Winograd, Fast algorithms for the discrete cosine transform. IEEE Trans. Signal Process. **40**(9), 2174–2193 (1992)
293. K. Wahid, V. Dimitrov, G. Jullien, W. Badawy, Error-free computation of daubechies wavelets for image compression applications. Electron. Lett. **39**(5), 428–429 (2003)
294. J.F. Canny, A computational approach to edge detection. IEEE Trans. Pattern Anal. Mach. Intell. **8**(6), 679–698 (1986)
295. R. Deriche, Using Canny's criteria to derive a recursively implemented optimal edge detector. Int. J. Comput. Vis. **1**(2), 167–187 (1987)
296. M. Heath, S. Sarkar, T. Sanocki, K. Bowyer, Comparison of edge detectors: a methodology and initial study. Comput. Vis. Image Underst. **69**(1), 38–54 (1998)
297. D. Marr, E. Hidreth, Theory of edge detection. Proc. R. Soc. Lond. B **207**, 301–328 (1982)
298. J.S. Lim, *Two-Dimensional Signal and Image Processing* (Prentice-Hall, Englewood Clis, NJ, 1990)
299. B. Mathieu, P. Melchior, A. Oustaloup, C. Ceyral, Fractional differentiation for edge detection. Sig. Process. **83**, 2421–2432 (2003)
300. J.N.S. Matthews, D.G. Altman, M.J. Campbell, P. Royston, Analysis of serial measurements in medical research. Br. Med. J. **300**, 230–235 (1990)
301. P.M.J. Van den Hof, P.S.C. Heuberger, J. Bokor, System identification with generalized orthonormal basis functions. Automatica **31**, 1821–1834 (1995)
302. R. Malti, M. Aoun, F. Levron, and A. Oustaloup, Unified construction of fractional generalized orthogonal bases, in *Fractional Differentiation and its Applications, U-Books*, (2005), pp. 87–102
303. R. Malti, P. Melchior, P. Lanusse, A. Oustaloup, Towards an object oriented CRONE Toolbox for fractional differential systems, in *18th IFAC World Congress IFAC Proceedings*, vol. 44, pp. 10830–10835 (2011)
304. S.G. Mallat, *A Wavelet Tour of Signal Processing* (Academic Press, CA, San Diego, 1999)
305. I. Daubechies, *Ten Lectures on Wavelets* (Society for Industrial and Applied Mathematics, Philadelphia, USA, 1992)
306. A. Jensen, A. La Cour-Harbo, *Ripples in Mathematics: The Discrete Wavelet Transform* (Springer Verlag, Berlin, Germany, 2001)
307. S. Hadjiloucas, R. Galvão, V. Becerra, J. Bowen, R. Martini, M. Brucherseifer- et al., Comparison of state space and ARX models of a waveguide's THz transient response after optimal wavelet filtering. IEEE Trans. Microw. Theory Tech. MTT **52**(10), 2409–2419 (2004)
308. B. Ferguson, D. Abbott, Denoising techniques for terahertz responses of biological samples. Microelectron. J. **32**(12), 943–953 (2001)
309. S. Qian, D. Chen, *Joint Time-Frequency Analysis-Methods and Applications* (Prentice Hall PTR, New Jersey, 1996)
310. M. Vetterli, J. Kovacevic, *Wavelets and Subband Coding* (Prentice-Hall PTR, New Jersey, USA, 1995)

311. P.P. Vaidyanathan, *Wavelets and Filter Banks* (Wellesley-Cambridge Press, Wellesley, USA, 1996)
312. P.P. Vaidyanathan, *Multirate Systems and Filter Banks* (Prentice Hall Inc, New Jersey, USA, 1993)
313. K. Ramchandran, M. Vetterli, C. Herley, Wavelets, subband coding, and best bases. Proc. IEEE **84**(4), 541–560 (1998)
314. P. Moulin, M. Anitescu, K. Kortanek, F. Potra, The role of linear semi-infinite programming in signal-adapted QMF bank design. IEEE Trans. Signal Process. **45**(9), 2160–2174 (1997)
315. J. Tuqun, P.P. Vaidyanathan, A state-space approach to the design of globally optimal FIR energy compaction filters. IEEE Trans. Signal Process. **48**(10), 2822–2838 (2000)
316. M. Unser, On the optimality of ideal filters for pyramid and wavelet signal approximation. IEEE Trans. Signal Process. **41**(12), 3591–3596 (1993)
317. H.M. Paiva, M.N. Marins, R.K.H. Galvão, J.P.L.M. Paiva, On the space of orthonormal wavelets: additional constrains to ensure two vanishing moments. IEEE Signal Process. Lett. **16**(2), 101–104 (2009)
318. H.M. Paiva, R.K.H. Galvão, Optimized orthonormal wavelet filters with improved frequency separation. Digit. Signal Proc. **22**(4), 622–627 (2012)
319. Y. Kim, Wavelet power spectrum estimation for high-resolution terahertz time-domain spectroscopy. J. Opt. Soc. Korea **15**(1), 103–108 (2011)
320. P. Moulin, Wavelet thresholding techniques for power spectrum estimation. IEEE Trans. Signal Process. **42**(11), 126–136 (1994)
321. H. Stephani, J. Jonuscheit, C. Robine, B. Heise, Automatically detecting peaks in terahertz time-domain spectroscopy, in *Proceeding of The 20th International Conference on Pattern Recognition*, ed. by J.E. Guerrero. IEEE Computer Society Conference Publishing Services (2010), pp. 4468–4471
322. M. Otsuka, J. Nishizawa, J. Shibata, M. Ito, Quantitative evaluation of mefenamic acid polymorphs by terahertz-chemometrics. J. Pharm. Sci. **99**(9), 4048–4053 (2010)
323. H. Wu, E.J. Heilweil, A.S. Hussain, M.A. Khan, Process analytical technology (pat): Quantification approaches in terahertz spectroscopy for pharmaceutical application. J. Pharm. Sci. **97**(2), 970–984 (2008)
324. D. Zimdars, J.A. Valdmanis, J.S. White, G. Stuk, S. Williamson, W.P. Winfree et al., Technology and applications of terahertz imaging non-destructive examination: inspection of space shuttle sprayed on foam insulation, in *AIP Conference Proceedings*, eds. by T. Bulik, B. Rudak, G. Madejski, vol. 760, issue no. 1. (American Institute of Physics, USA, 2005), pp. 570–577
325. R.P. Cogdill, R.N. Forcht, Y.C. Shen, P.F. Taday, J.R. Creekmore, C.A. Anderson- et al., Comparison of terahertz pulse imaging and near-infrared spectroscopy for rapid, non-destructive analysis of tablet coating thickness and uniformity. J. Pharm. Innov. **2**(1–2), 29–36 (2007)
326. J. Stolarek, Improving energy compaction of a wavelet transform using genetic algorithm and fast neural network. Arch. Control Sci. **20**(4), 417–433 (2010)
327. I. Dinov, J. Boscardin, M. Mega, E. Sowell, A. Toga, A wavelet-based statistical analysis of FMRI data: I. motivation and data distribution modeling. Neuroinformatics **3**(4), 319–342 (2005)
328. J. Weaver, Y. Xu, D. Healy, L. Cromwell, Filtering noise from images with wavelet transforms. Magn. Reson. Med. **21**(2), 288–295 (1991)
329. M. Alexander, R. Baumgartner, A. Summers, C. Windischberger, M. Klarhoefer, E. Moser, R. Somorjai, A wavelet-based method for improving signal-to-noise ratio and contrast in MR images magnetic resonance imaging. Magn. Reson. Med. **18**(2), 169–180 (2000)
330. C.S. Anand, J.S. Sahambi, Wavelet domain non-linear filtering for MRI denoising magnetic resonance imaging. Magn. Reson. Imaging **28**(6), 842–861 (2010)
331. R.D. Nowak, Wavelet-based rician noise removal for magnetic resonance imaging. IEEE Trans. Image Process. **8**(10), 1408–1419 (1999)
332. A. Pižurica, W. Philips, I. Lemahieu, M. Acheroy, A versatile wavelet domain noise filtration technique for medical imaging. IEEE Trans. Med. Imaging **22**(3), 323–331 (2003)

333. S. Zaroubi, G. Goelman, Complex denoising of MR data via wavelet analysis: application for functional MRI magnetic resonance imaging. Magn. Reson. Imaging **18**(1), 59–68 (2000)
334. R. Wirestam, A. Bibic, J. Lätt, S. Brockstedt, F. Ståhlberg, Denoising of complex MRI data by wavelet-domain filtering: application to high-b-value diffusion-weighted imaging. Magn. Reson. Med. **56**(5), 1114–1120 (2006)
335. U.E. Ruttimann, M. Unser, R.R. Rawlings, D. Rio, N.F. Ramsey, V.S. Mattay, D.W. Hommer, J.A. Frank, D.R. Weinberger, Statistical analysis of functional MRI data in the wavelet domain. IEEE Trans. Med. Imaging **17**(2), 142–154 (1998)
336. A. Pižurica, A. Wink, E. Vansteenkiste, W. Philips, J.B. Roerdink, A review of wavelet denoising in MRI and ultrasound brain imaging. Med. Imaging Rev. **2**(2), 247–260 (2006)
337. E. Zarahn, G.K. Aguirre, M. D'Esposito, Empirical analyses of BOLD fMRI statistics. I. spatially unsmoothed data collected under null-hypothesis conditions. Neuroimage **5**(3), 179–197 (1997)
338. G.K. Aguirre, E. Zarahn, M. D'Esposito, Empirical analyses of BOLD fMRI statistics. ii. spatially smoothed data collected under null-hypothesis and experimental conditions. Neuroimage **5**(3), 199–212 (1997)
339. S. Wang, B. Ferguson, D. Abbott, X.-C. Zhang, T-ray imaging and tomography. J. Biol. Phys. **29**(2–3), 247–256 (2003)
340. H. Wang, L. Dong, J. O'Daniel, R. Mohan, A. Garden, K. Ang- et al., Validation of an accelerated 'demons' algorithm for deformable image registration in radiation therapy. Phys. Med. Biol. **50**(12), 2887–2905 (2005)
341. K.J. Worsley, S. Marrett, P. Neelin, A.C. Evans, Searching scale space for activation in PET images. Hum. Brain Mapp. **4**(1), 74–90 (1996)
342. S. Honale, V. Kapse, A review of methods for blood vessel segmentation in retinal images. Int. J. Eng. Res. Technol. **1**(10), 1–6 (2012)
343. P. Kovesi, Phase preserving denoising of images, in *Proceeding of The Australian Pattern Recognition Society Conference: DICTA* (1999), pp. 212–217
344. S. Fischer, F. Sroubek, L. Perrinet, R. Redondo, G. Cristobal, Selfinvertible 2D log-Gabor wavelets. Int. J. Comput. Vis. **75**(2), 231–246 (2007)
345. D. Pandey, X. Yin, H. Wang, Y. Zhang, Accurate vessel segmentation using maximum entropy incorporating line detection and phase preserved denoising. Comput. Vis. Image Underst. **155**, 162–172 (2016)
346. I. Delakis, O. Hammad, R.I. Kitney, Wavelet-based de-noising algorithm for images acquired with parallel magnetic resonance imaging (MRI). Phys. Med. Biol. **52**(13), 3741–3751 (2007)
347. G. Piella, A general framework for multiresolution image fusion: from pixels to regions. Inf. Fusion **4**(4), 259–280 (2003)
348. E. Morris, L. Liberman, *Pattern Classification and Scene Analysis* (John Wiley and Sons Inc, New York, NY, 1973)
349. J. Shawe-Taylor, N. Cristianini, *Kernel Methods for Pattern Analysis* (Cambridge University Press, Cambridge, UK, 2004)
350. Siuly, X.-X. Yin, S. Hadjiloucas, and Y. Zhang, Classification of THz pulse signals using two-dimensional cross-correlation feature extraction and non-linear classifiers. IEEE Trans. Signal Process. **127**, 64–82 92016)
351. H. Stephani, B. Heise, K. Wiesauer, S. Katzletz, D. Molter, J. Jonuscheid et al., A feature set for enhanced automatic segmentation of hyperspectral terahertz images, in *Proceedings of the 2011 Irish Machine Vision and Image Processing Conference*, eds. by O. Ghita, D. Molloy, R. Sadleir. (IEEE Computer Society Conference Publishing Services, (USA), 2011), pp. 117–122
352. Q. Fu, L.M. Cheng, F. Liu, Terahertz time-domain spectroscopy analysis with wave atoms transform, in *Proceedings of the 2011 Asia-Pacific Signal and Information Processing Association*, vol. 2013, issue no. 1. (IEEE Computer Society Conference Publishing Services, (USA), 2011). Article Number: APSIPA137
353. H.M. Paiva, R.K.H. Galvão, Wavelet-packet identification of dynamic systems in frequency sub-bands. Signal Process. **86**(8), 2001–2008 (2006)

354. X.-X. Yin, B.M. Fischer, B.W.-H Ng, D. Abbott, H.M. Paiva, R.K.H. Galvão, S. Hadjiloucas, G.C. Walker, J.W. Bowen, Classification of lactose and mandelic acid THz spectra using subspace and wavelet-packet algorithms, in *Microelectronics: Design, Technology, and Packaging III*, eds. by A.J. Hariz, V.K. Varadan. Proceedings of SPIE, vol. 6798 (SPIE, Bellingham, WA, 2008). Article Number: 679814
355. L. Zhang, H. Zhong, D.-C. Zhu, J. Zuo, C. Zhang, Feature extraction without phase error for THz reflective spectroscopy. Arch. Control Sci. **55**(1), 127–132 (2011)
356. C. Davatzikos, Why voxel-based morphometric analysis should be used with great caution when characterizing group differences. Neuroimage **23**(1), 17–20 (2004)
357. K.A. Norman, S.M. Polyn, G.J. Detre, J.V. Haxby, Beyond mind-reading: multi-voxel pattern analysis of fMRI data. Trends Cogn. Sci. **10**(9), 230–242 (2006)
358. Y.A. Tolias, S.M. Panas, A fuzzy vessel tracking algorithm for retinal images based on fuzzy clustering. IEEE Trans. Med. Imaging **17**(2), 263–273 (1998)
359. K. Akyol, B. Şen, Ş. Bayır, Automatic detection of optic disc in retinal image by using keypoint detection, texture analysis, and visual dictionary techniques. Comput. Math. Methods Med. Article Number: 6814791 (2016)
360. E. Ricci, R. Perfetti, Retinal blood vessel segmentation using line operators and support vector classification. IEEE Trans. Med. Imaging **26**(10), 1357–1365 (2007)
361. G. Azzopardia, N. Strisciuglioa, M. Ventob, N. Petkova, Trainable COSFIRE filters for vessel delineation with application to retinal images. Med. Image Anal. **19**(1), 46–57 (2015)
362. J. Richiardi, M. Gschwind, S. Simioni, J.-M. Annoni, B. Greco, P. Hagmann, M. Schluep, P. Vuilleumier, D. Van-De, Classifying minimallydisabled multiple sclerosis patients from resting-state functional connectivity. NeuroImage **62**(3), 2021–2033 (2012)
363. J.V. Haxby, M.I. Gobbini, M.L. Furey, A. Ishai, J.L. Schouten, P. Pietrini, Distributed and overlapping representations of faces and objects in ventral temporal cortex. Science **293**(5539), 2425–2430 (2001)
364. R. Ryniec, P. Zagrajek, N. Palka, Terahertz frequency domain spectroscopy identification system based on decision trees. Acta Phys. Pol. A **122**(5), 891–895 (2012)
365. Z. Xu, J. Tu, J. Li, Y. Pi, Research on micro-feature extraction algorithm of target based on terahertz radar. EURASIP J. Wirel. Commun. Netw. **2013**(77), 1–9 (2013)
366. G. Hieftje, R. Bystroff, R. Lim, Application of correlation analysis for signal-to-noise enhancement in flame spectrometry: use of correlation in determination of rhodium by atomic fluorescence. Anal. Chem. **45**(2), 253–258 (1973)
367. S. Dutta, A. Chatterjee, S. Munshi, Correlation techniques and least square support vector machine combine for frequency domain based ECG beat classification. Med. Eng. Phys. **32**(10), 1161–1169 (2010)
368. Siuly, Y. Li, P. Wen, Modified CC-LR algorithm with three diverse feature sets for motor imagery tasks classification in EEG based brain computer interface. Comput. Methods Programs Biomed. **113**(3), 767–780 (2014)
369. R. De Veaux, P. Velleman, D. Bock, *Intro Stats*, 3rd edn. (Pearson Addison Wesley, Boston, 2008)
370. S. Siuly, E. Kabir, H. Wang, Y. Zhang, Improving the separability of motor imagery EEG signals using a cross correlation-based least square support vector machine for brain computer interface. Comput. Math. Methods Med. **20**(4), 526–538 (2012)
371. M.D. Pickles, M. Lowry, P. Gibbs, Pretreatment prognostic value of dynamic contrast-enhanced magnetic resonance imaging vascular, texture, shape, and size parameters compared with traditional survival indicators obtained from locally advanced breast cancer patients. Invest. Radiol. **51**(3), 177–185 (2016)
372. D. Woolf, A. Padhani, N. Taylor, A. Gogbashian, S. Li, M. Beresford, M. Ah-See, J. Stirling, D. Collins, A. Makris, Assessing response in breast cancer with dynamic contrast-enhanced magnetic resonance imaging: are signal intensity-time curves adequate? Breast Cancer Res. Treat. **147**(2), 335–343 (2014)
373. X. Yang, M. Knopp, Quantifying tumor vascular heterogeneity with dynamic contrast-enhanced magnetic resonance imaging: a review. J. Biomed. Biotechnol. Article ID 732848(2011)

374. A. Jackson, J. O'Connor, G. Parker, G. Jayson, Imaging tumor vascular heterogeneity and angiogenesis using dynamic contrast-enhanced magnetic resonance imaging. Clin. Cancer Res. **13**(12), 3449–3459 (2007)
375. N. Just, Improving tumour heterogeneity MRI assessment with histograms. Br. J. Cancer **111**(12), 2205–2213 (2014)
376. M. Asselin, J. O'Connor, R. Boellaard, N. Thacker, A. Jackson, Quantifying heterogeneity in human tumours using MRI and PET. Eur. J. Cancer **48**(4), 447–455 (2012)
377. F. Davnall, C.S.P. Yip, G. Ljungqvist, M. Selmi, F. Ng, B. Sanghera- et al., Assessment of tumor heterogeneity: an emerging imaging tool for clinical practice? Insights Imaging **3**(6), 573–589 (2012)
378. L. Alic, W. Niessen, J. Veenland, Quantification of heterogeneity as a biomarker in tumor imaging: a systematic review. PloS one **9**(10), Article Number: e110300 (2014)
379. S.A. Waugh, C.A. Purdie, L.B. Jordan, S. Vinnicombe, R.A. Lerski, P. Martin, A.M. Thompson, Magnetic resonance imaging texture analysis classification of primary breast cancer. J. Biomed. Biotechnol. **26**(2), 322–330 (2016)
380. B. Chaudhury, M. Zhou, D.B. Goldgof, L.O. Hall, R.A. Gatenby, R.J. Gillies, B.K. Patel, R.J. Weinfurtner, J.S. Drukteinis, Heterogeneity in intratumoral regions with rapid gadolinium washout correlates with estrogen receptor status and nodal metastasis. J. Magn. Reson. Imaging **42**(5), 1421–1430 (2015)
381. C. Gallego-Ortiz, A.L. Martel, Improving the accuracy of computer-aided diagnosis for breast MR imaging by differentiating between mass and nonmass lesions. Radiology **278**(3), 679–688 (2016)
382. A. Ahmed, P. Gibbs, M. Pickles, L. Turnbull, Texture analysis in assessment and prediction of chemotherapy response in breast cancer. J. Magn. Reson. Imaging **38**(1), 89–101 (2013)
383. R. Haralick, K. Shanmugam, I. Dinstein, Textural features for image classification. IEEE Trans. Syst. Man Cybern. **3**(6), 610–621 (1973)
384. J.R. Teruel, M.G. Heldahl, P.E. Goa, M. Pickles, S. Lundgren, T.F. Bathen, P. Gibbs, Dynamic contrast-enhanced MRI texture analysis for pretreatment prediction of clinical and pathological response to neoadjuvant chemotherapy in patients with locally advanced breast cancer. J. Magn. Reson. Imaging **27**(8), 887–896 (2014)
385. X.X. Yin, B.W.-H. Ng, K. Ramamohanarao, D. Abbott, Tensor based sparse decomposition of 3D shape for visual detection of mirror symmetry. Comput. Methods Programs Biomed. **108**(2), 629–643 (2012)
386. M.J. Fox, P. Gibbs, M.D. Pickles, Minkowski functionals: An MRI texture analysis tool for determination of the aggressiveness of breast cancer. J. Magn. Reson. Imaging **43**(4), 903–910 (2016)
387. H. Boehm, C. Fink, U. Attenberger, C. Becker, J. Behr, M. Reiser, Automated classification of normal and pathologic pulmonary tissue by topological texture features extracted from multi-detector CT in 3D. Eur. Radiol. **18**(12), 2745–2755 (2008)
388. H. Boehm, T. Schneider, S. Buhmann-Kirchhoff, T. Schlossbauer, D. Rjosk-Dendorfer, S. Britsch, M. Reiser, Automated classification of breast parenchymal density: topologic analysis of x-ray attenuation patterns depicted with digital mammography. Am. J. Roentgenol. **191**(6), W275–W282 (2008)
389. H. Boehm, T. Fischer, D. Riosk, S. Britsch, M. Reiser, Application of the minkowski-functionals for automated pattern classification of breast parenchyma depicted by digital mammography, in *Proceeding of SPIE on Medical Imaging 2008: Computer-Aided Diagnosis, Pts 1 and 2*, eds. by M.L. Giger, N. Karssemeijer, vol. 6915 (SPIE Digital Library, Bellingham, 2008), Art No 691522
390. M. Nagarajan, M. Huber, T. Schlossbauer, G. Leinsinger, A. Krol, A. Wismuller, Classification of small lesions in dynamic breast MRI: eliminating the need for precise lesion segmentation through spatiotemporal analysis of contrast enhancement. Mach. Vis. Appl. **24**(7), 1371–1381 (2013)
391. T. Larkin, H. Canuto, M. Kettunen, T. Booth, D. Hu, A. Krishnan, S. Bohndiek et al., Analysis of image heterogeneity using 2D minkowski functionals detects tumor responses to treatment. Magn. Reson. Med. **71**(1), 402–410 (2014)

392. H. Canuto, C. McLachlan, M. Kettunen, M. Velic, A. Krishnan, A. Neves, M. de Backer, D. Hu, M. Hobson, K. Brindle, Characterization of image heterogeneity using 2D minkowski functionals increases the sensitivity of detection of a targeted MRI contrast agent. Magn. Reson. Med. **61**(5), 1218–1224 (2009)
393. H. Krim, T. Gentimis, H. Chintakunta, Discovering the whole by the coarse: a topological paradigm for data analysis. IEEE Signal Process. Mag. **33**(2), 95–104 (2016)
394. J. Ernst, M.K. Singh, V. Ramesh, Discrete texture traces: topological representation of geometric context. Proc. IEEE Conf. Comput. Vis. Pattern Recognit. (CVPR) **71**(1), 422–429 (2012)
395. P. Saveliev, A graph, non-tree representation of the topology of a gray scale image, in *Proceedings IS&T/SPIE Electronic Imaging*, vol. 7870, pp. O1–O19 (2011)
396. P. Skraba, M. Ovsjanikov, F. Chazal, L. Guibas, Persistence based segmentation of deformable shapes, in *Proceeding of IEEE Computer Society Conference on Computer Vision and Pattern Recognition Workshops (CVPRW)*, (2010), pp. 45–52
397. M. Vejdemo-Johansson, F.T. Pokorny, P. Skraba, D. Kragic, Cohomological learning of periodic motion. Appl. Algebra Eng. Commun. Comput. **26**(1), 5–26 (2015)
398. M.C. Kale, J.D. Fleig, N. İmal, Assessment of feasibility to use computer aided texture analysis based tool for parametric images of suspicious lesions in DCE-MR mammography. Comput. Math. Methods Med. **23** Article Number: 872676 (2013)
399. J. Wang, F. Kato, N. Oyama-Manabe, R. Li, Y. Cui, K.K. Tha, H. Yamashita, K. Kudo, H. Shirato, Identifying triple-negative breast cancer using background parenchymal enhancement heterogeneity on dynamic contrast-enhanced MRI: a pilot radiomics study. PloS one **10**(11), Article Number: e0143308 (2015)
400. J. Wang, X. Wang, M. Xia, X. Liao, A. Evans, Y. He, GRETNA: a graph theoretical network analysis toolbox for imaging connectomics. Frontiers in Human Neuroscience 9. Article Number: 386 (2015)
401. N. Michoux, S.V. den Broeck, L. Lacoste, L. Fellah, C. Galant, M. Berlière, I. Leconte, Texture analysis on MR images helps predicting non-response to NAC in breast cancer. BMC Cancer **15**(574) (2015). doi:10.1186/s12885-015-1563-8
402. R. Conners, M. Trivedi, C. Harlow, Segmentation of a high-resolution urban scene using texture operators. Comput. Vis. Graph. Image Process. **25**(3), 273–310 (1984)
403. M.A. Mazurowski, J. Zhang, L.J. Grimm, S.C. Yoon, J.I. Silber, Radiogenomic analysis of breast cancer: Luminal B molecular subtype is associated with enhancement dynamics at MR imaging. Radiology **273**(2), 365–372 (2014)
404. L.J. Grimm, J. Zhang, M.A. Mazurowski, Computational approach to radiogenomics of breast cancer: Luminal A and luminal B molecular subtypes are associated with imaging features on routine breast MRI extracted using computer vision algorithms. J. Magn. Reson. Imaging **42**(4), 902–907 (2015)
405. E.J. Sutton, J.H. Oh, B.Z. Dashevsky, H. Veeraraghavan, A.P. Apte, S.B. Thakur et al., Breast cancer subtype intertumor heterogeneity: MRI-based features predict results of a genomic assay. J. Magn. Reson. Imaging **42**(5), 1398–1406 (2015)
406. I. Daubechies, E. Roussos, S. Takerkart, M. Benharrosh, C. Golden, K. D'Ardenne, W. Richter, J.D. Cohen, J. Haxby, Independent component analysis for brain fMRI does not select for independence. Proc. Natl. Acad. Sci. **106**(26), 10415–10422 (2009)
407. M.D. Greicius, K. Supekar, V. Menon, R.F. Dougherty, Resting-state functional connectivity reflects structural connectivity in the default mode network. Cereb. Cortex **19**, 72–78 (2009)
408. J.D. Power, A.L. Cohen, S.M. Nelson, G.S. Wig, K.A. Barnes, J.A. Church, A.C. Vogel, T.O. Laumann, F.M. Miezin, B.L. Schlaggar, S.E. Petersen, Functional network organization of the human brain. Neuron **72**(4), 665–678 (2011)
409. E. Bullmore, O. Sporns, Complex brain networks: graph theoretical analysis of structural and functional systems. Nat. Rev. Neurosci. **10**, 186–198 (2009)
410. M. Rubinov, O. Sporns, Complex network measures of brain connectivity: Uses and interpretations. NeuroImage **52**(3), 1059–1069 (2010)

411. G. Caldarelli, *Scale-Free Networks Complex Webs in Nature and Technology* (Oxford University Press, Oxford, New York, 2007)
412. M. Newman, *Networks: An Introduction* (Oxford University Press, Oxford, New York, 2009)
413. O. Sporns, Graph theory methods for the analysis of neural connectivity patterns, in *Neuroscience Databases: A Practical Guide*, ed. by R.Kötter. (Springer, New York, 2003), pp. 169–183
414. H. Onias, A. Viol, F. Palhano-Fontes, K. Andrade, M. Sturzbecher, G. Viswanathan, D. de Araujo, Brain complex network analysis by means of resting state fMRI and graph analysis: Will it be helpful in clinical epilepsy? Epilepsy Behav. **38**, 71–80 (2014)
415. V. Latora, S. Marchiori, Efficient behavior of small-world networks. Phys. Rev. Lett. **87**(19), 198701–1–198701–4 (2001)
416. A. Fornito, A. Zalesky, E. Bullmore, *Fundamentals of Brian Network Analysis* (Elsevier, London, UK, 2016)
417. Y. He, A. Dagher, Z. Chen, A. Charil, A. Zijdenbos, K. Worsley, A. Evanscorresponding, Impaired small-world efficiency in structural cortical networks in multiple sclerosis associated with white matter lesion load. Brain **132**(12), 3366–3379 (2009)
418. D. Watts, S. Strogatz, Collective dynamics of 'small-world' networks. Nature **393**, 440–442 (1998)
419. L. da F. Costa, F.A. Rodrigues, A.S. Cristino, Complex networks: the key to systems biology. Genetics Mol. Biol. **31**(3), 591–601 (2008)
420. P. Hagmann, L. Cammoun, X. Gigandet, R. Meuli, C.J. Honey, V.J. Wedeen, O. Sporns, Mapping the structural core of human cerebral cortex. Plos Biol. **6**(7), Article Number: e0060159 (2008)
421. B. Zhang, L. Zhang, L. Zhang, F. Karray, Retinal vessel extraction by matched filter with first-order derivative of gaussian. Comput. Biol. Med. **40**(4), 438–445 (2010)
422. G. Luo, C. Opas, M. Shankar, Detection and measurement of retinal vessels in fundus images using amplitude modified second-order Gaussian filter. IEEE Trans. Biomed. Eng. **49**(2), 168–172 (2008)
423. A.F. Frangi, W.J. Niessen, K.L. Vincken, M.A. Viergever, Multiscale vessel enhancement filtering, in *Proceedings of the Third International Conference on Medical Image Computing and Computer-Assisted Intervention—MICCAI 1998*. Lecture Notes in Computer Science, vol. 1496, pp. 130–137 (1998)
424. M. Palomera, Pérez, M. Martinez Perez, H. Benítez Pérez, J. Ortega Arjona, Parallel multiscale feature extraction and region growing: application in retinal blood vessel detection. IEEE Trans. Inf. Technol. Biomed. **14**(2), 500–506 (2010)
425. Y. Wang, G. Ji, P. Lin, E. Trucco, Retinal vessel segmentation using multiwavelet kernels and multiscale hierarchical decomposition. Pattern Recognit. **46**(8), 2117–2133 (2013)
426. P. Feng, Y. Pan, B. Wei, W. Jin, D. Mi, Enhancing retinal image by the contourlet transform. Pattern Recognit. Lett. **28**, 516–522 (2007)
427. J. Soares, M. Cree, Retinal vessel segmentation using the 2D Gabor wavelet and supervised classification. IEEE Trans. Inf Technol. Biomed. **25**(9), 1214–1222 (2006)
428. G. Zaaopardi, N. Petkov, Trainable COSFIRE filters for keypoint detection and pattern recognition. IEEE Trans. Pattern Anal. Mach. Intell. **35**(2), 490–503 (2013)
429. W.H. Spencer, *Ophthalmic Pathology: An Atlas and Textbook* (Elsevier-Health Sciences Division, Philadelphia, PA, 1996)
430. U.T. Nguyen, A. Bhuiyana, A. Park, K. Ramamohanaraoa, An effective retinal blood vessel segmentation method using multi-scale line detection. Pattern Recognit. **46**(3), 703–715 (2013)
431. A. Bhuiyan, R. Kawasaki, E. Lamoureux, R. Kotagiri, T.Y. Wong, Retinal artery-vein caliber grading using colour fundus imaging. Comput. Methods Programs Biomed. **111**(1), 104–114 (2013)
432. Y. Kanagasingam, A. Bhuiyan, M.D. Abramoff, R.T. Smith, L. Goldschmidt, T.Y. Wong, Progress on retinal image analysis for age related macular degeneration. Prog. Retin. Eye Res. **38**, 20–42 (2014)

433. S. Kirkpatrick, C.D. Gelatt Jr., M.P. Vecchi, Optimization by simmulated annealing. Science **220**(1), 671–680 (1983)
434. M. Fraz, P. Remagnino, A. Hoppem, B. Uyyanonvara, A. Rudnicka, C. Owen, S. Barman, Blood vessel segmentation methodologies in retinal images-a survey. Comput. Methods Programs Biomed. **108**(1), 407–433 (2012)
435. J. Schürmann, *Pattern Classification: A Unified View of Statistical and Neural Approaches* (John Wiley and Sons Inc, New York, USA, 1996)
436. R. Pan, S. Zhao, J. Shen, Terahertz spectra applications in identification of illicit drugs using support vector machines, in *Proceeding of 2010 Symposium on Security Detection and Information Processing*, eds. by M. Li, D. Yu. vol. 7 (Elsevier Ltd., (Netherlands), 2010), pp. 15–21
437. H. Selvaraj, S.T. Selvi, D. Selvathi, L. Gewali, Brain MRI slices classification using least squares support vector machine. Int. J. Intell. Comput. Med. Sci. Image Process. **1**(1), 21–33 (2007)
438. J. Dukart, K. Mueller, H. Barthel, A. Villringer, O. Sabri, M.L. Schroeter, Meta-analysis based SVM classification enables accurate detection of alzheimer's disease across different clinical centers using FDG-PET and MRI. Psychiatry Res. Neuroimaging **212**(3), 230–236 (2013)
439. D. Singh, K. Kaur, Classification of abnormalities in brain MRI images using GLCM, PCA and SVM. Int. J. Eng. Adv. Technol. **1**(6), 243–248 (2012)
440. E.I. Zacharaki, S. Wang, S. Chawla, D.S. Yoo, R. Wolf, E.R. Melhem, C. Davatzikos, Classification of brain tumor type and grade using MRI texture and shape in a machine learning scheme. Magn. Reson. Med. **62**(2), 1609–1618 (2009)
441. N. Zhang, S. Ruan, S. Lebonvallet, Q. Liao, Y. Zhu, Multi-kernel SVM based classification for brain tumor segmentation of MRI multi-sequence, in *16th IEEE International Conference on Image Processing* (2009), pp. 3373–3376
442. A. Ortiz, J.M. Gérriz, J. Ramírez, F. Martínez-Murcia, LVQ-SVM based CAD tool applied to structural MRI for the diagnosis of the alzheimer's disease. Pattern Recognit. Lett. **34**(14), 1725–1733 (2013)
443. H.-I. Suk, D. Shen, Deep learning-based feature representation for AD/MCI classification. Med. Image Comput. Comput. Assist. Interv. **8150**, 583–590 (2013)
444. C. Aguilar, E. Westman, J.-S. Muehlboeck, P. Mecocci, B. Vellas, M. Tsolaki, I. Kloszewska, H. Soininen, S. Lovestone, C. Spenger, A. Simmons, L.-O. Wahlund, Different multivariate techniques for automated classification of MRI data in alzheimer's disease and mild cognitive impairment. Psychiatry Res. Neuroimaging **212**(2), 89–98 (2013)
445. A. Akselrod-Ballin, M. Galun, M.J. Gomori, R. Basri, A. Brandt, Atlas guided identification of brain structures by combining 3D segmentation and SVM classification. Med. Image Comput. Comput. Assist. Interv. **4191**, 209–216 (2006)
446. S. Ozer, D.L. Langer, X. Liu, M.A. Haider, T.H. van der Kwast, A.J. Evans, Y. Yang, M.N. Wernick, I.S. Yetik, Supervised and unsupervised methods for prostate cancer segmentation with multispectral MRI. Med. Phys. **37**(4), 1873–1883 (2010)
447. X.-X. Yin, S. Hadjiloucasb, J. He, Y. Zhang, Y. Wang, D. Zhang, Application of complex extreme learning machine to multiclass classification problems with high dimensionality: A THz spectra classification problem. Digit. Signal Proc. **40**, 40–52 (2015)
448. G.B. Huang, H. Zhou, X. Ding, R. Zhang, Extreme learning machine for regression and multiclass classification. IEEE Trans. Syst. Man Cybern. B Cybern. **42**(2), 513–529 (2011)
449. G.-B. Huang, D. Wang, Y. Lan, Extreme learning machines: a survey. Int. J. Mach. Learn. Cybern. **2**(2), 107–122 (2011)
450. C.J.C. Burges, A tutorial on support vector machines for pattern recognition. Data Min. Knowl. Disc. **2**, 121–167 (1998)
451. V. Vapnik, *The Nature of Statistical Learning Theory* (Springer-Verlag, New York, USA, 1995)
452. N. Cristianini, J. Shawe-Taylor, *An Introduction to Support Vector Machines and Other Kernel Based Methods* (Cambridge University Press, Cambridge, UK, 2000)

453. K.R. Muller, S. Mika, G. Ratsch, K. Tsuda, B. Schölkopf, An introduction to kernel-based learning algorithms. IEEE Trans. Neural Netw. **12**(2), 181–201 (2001)
454. B. Schölkopf, A. Smola, *Learning with Kernels Support Vector Machines, Regularization, Optimization, and Beyond* (MIT Press, Cambridge, MA, 2002)
455. M.A. Hearst, Trends controversies: Support vector machines. IEEE Intell. Syst. **13**(4), 18–28 (1998)
456. T.M. Cover, Geometrical and statistical properties of systems of linear inequalities with applications in pattern recognition. IEEE Trans. Electron. Comput. **14**, 326–334 (1965)
457. G.-B. Huang, H. Zhou, X. Ding, R. Zhang, Extreme learning machine for regression and multiclass classification. IEEE Trans. Syst. Man Cybern. B Cybern. **42**(2), 513–529 (2012)
458. P. Bouboulis, K. Slavakis, S. Theodoridis, Adaptive learning in complex reproducing kernel hilbert spaces employing wirtinger's subgradients. IEEE Trans. Neural Netw. Learn. Syst. **2**(99), 260–276 (2012)
459. F.A. Tobar, A. Kuh, D.P. Mandic, A novel augmented complex valued kernel LMS, in *Proceeding of the 7th IEEE Sensor Array and Multichannel Workshop 2012* (IEEE Computer Society Conference Publishing Services, (USA), 2012), pp. 473–476
460. A. El-Gindy, G.M. Hadad, Nonparametric bayes error estimation using unclassified samples. J. AOAC Int. **95**(3), 609–623 (2012)
461. M.E. Van-Valkenburg, In memoriam: Hendrik W. Bode (1905–1982). IEEE Trans. Autom. Control **AC-29**(3), 193–194 (1984)
462. S. Le-Cessie, J. Van-Houwelingen, Ridge estimators in logistic regression. Appl. Stat. **41**(1), 191–201 (1992)
463. F. Zahid, G. Tutz, Ridge estimation for multinomial logit models with symmetric side constraints. Comput. Stat. **28**(3), 1017–1034 (2013)
464. M. Wiggins, A. Saad, B. Litt, G. Vachtsevanos, Evolving a bayesian classifier for ECG-based age classification in medical applications. Appl. Soft Comput. **8**(1), 599–608 (2011)
465. M. Nuss, Chemistry is right for t-rays. IEEE Circuits Devices **12**(2), 25–30 (1996)
466. W. Chaovalitwongse, Y. Fan, R. Sachdeo, On the time series k-nearest neighbor classification of abnormal brain activity. IEEE Trans. Syst. Man Cybern. Part A: Syst. Hum. **37**(6), 1005–1016 (2007)
467. B. Efron, Estimating the error rate of a prediction rule: improvement on cross-validation. J. Am. Stat. Assoc. **78**(382), 316–331 (1983)
468. Siuly, E. Kabir, H. Wang, Y. Zhang, Exploring sampling in the detection of multicategory EEG signals. Comput. Math. Methods Med. Article Number: 576437 (2015)
469. L. Patnaik, O. Manyamb, Epileptic EEG detection using neural networks and post-classification. Comput. Methods Programs Biomed. **9**(1), 100–109 (2008)
470. L. Fraiwan, K. Lweesy, N. Khasawneh, M. Fraiwan, H. Wenz, H. Dickhaus, Classification of sleep stages using multi-wavelet time frequency entropy and LDA. Methods Inf. Med. **49**(3), 230–237 (2010)
471. L. Eadie, C.B. Reid, A. Fitzgerald, V. Wallace, Optimizing multi-dimensional terahertz imaging analysis for colon cancer diagnosis. Expert Syst. Appl. **40**(6), 2043–2050 (2013)
472. J. Jensen, *Introductory Digital Image Processing-A Remote Sensing Perspective* (Prentice Hall Inc, Upper Saddle River, New Jersey, 1996)
473. M.A. Brun, F. Formanek, A. Yasuda, M. Sekine, N. Ando, Y. Eishii, Terahertz imaging applied to cancer diagnosis. Phys. Med. Biol. **55**(16), 4615–4623 (2010)
474. M.W. Ayech, D. Ziou, Terahertz image segmentation based on k-harmonic-means clustering and statistical feature extraction modeling, in *Proceeding of 21st IEEE International Conference on Pattern Recognition* (IEEE Computer Society Conference Publishing Services, (USA), 2012), pp. 222–225
475. M.W. Ayech, D. Ziou, Segmentation of terahertz imaging using k-means clustering based on ranked set sampling. Expert Syst. Appl. **42**(6), 2959–2974 (2015)
476. M.W. Ayech, D. Ziou, Automated feature weighting and random pixel sampling in k-means clustering for terahertz image segmentation. IEEE Comput. Vis. Pattern Recognit. 35–40 (2015)

477. E. Leiss Holzinger, K. Wiesauer, H. Stephani, B. Heise, D. Stifter, B. Kriechbaumer et al., Imaging of the inner structure of cave bear teeth by novel non-destructive techniques. Palaeontologia electronica **18**(1), Art No. 18.1.1T, (2015)
478. M. Brito, E. Chavez, A. Quiroz, J. Yukich, Connectivity of the mutual k-nearest-neighbor graph in clustering and outlier detection. Probab. Lett. **35**, 33–42 (1997)
479. E. Berry, J.W. Handley, A.J. Fitzgerald, W.J. Merchant, R.D. Boyle, N.N. Zinov'ev- et al., Multispectral classification techniques for terahertz pulsed imaging: an example in histopathology. Med. Eng. Phys. **26**(5), 423–430 (2004)
480. P. Bankhead, C.N. Scholfield, J.G. McGeown, T.M. Curtis, Fast retinal vessel detection and measurement using wavelets and edge location refinement. PLoS one **7**(3), art. no. e32435, (2012)
481. J. Staal, M.D. Abramoff, M. Niemeijer, M.A. Viergever, B. van Ginneken, Ridge-based vessel segmentation in color images of the retina. IEEE Trans. Med. Imaging **23**(4), 501–509 (2004)
482. P. Choukikar, A.K. Patel, R.S. Mishra, Segmenting the optic disc in retinal images using bihistogram equalization and thresholding the connected regions. Int. J. Emerg. Technol. Adv. Eng. **4**(6), 933–942 (2014)
483. K. Yaseen, A. Tariq, M.U. Akram, A comparison and evaluation of computerized methods for OD localization and detection in retinal images. Int. J. Futur. Comput. Commun. **2**(6), 613–616 (2013)
484. A. Aquino, M.E. Gegúndez-Arias, D. Marín, Detecting the optic disc boundary in digital fundus images using morphological, edge detection, and feature extraction techniques. IEEE Trans. Med. Imaging **29**(11), 1860–1869 (2010)
485. A. Usman, S.A. Khitran, M.U. Akram, Y. Nadeem, A robust algorithm for optic disc segmentation from colored fundus images, in *Proceeding of ICIAR, Part II*, eds. by A. Campilho, M. Kamel. LNCS 8815 (Springer International Publishing, (Switzerland), 2014), pp. 303–310
486. D. Relan, T. MacGillivray, L. Ballerini, E. Trucco, Retinal vessel classification: sorting arteries and veins, in *Proceeding of 35th Annual International Conference of the IEEE EMBS*, vol. 2013, pp. 7396–7399 (2013)
487. M. Saez, S. González, Vázquez, M. González Penedo, M. Barceló, M. Pena Seijo, G. Coll de Tuero, A. Pose Reino, Development of an automated system to classify retinal vessels into arteries and veins. Comput. Methods Programs Biomed. **108**(1), 367–376 (2012)
488. D. Ortiz, M. Cubides, A. Suárez, M. Zequera, Q.J., J. Gómez, N. Arroyo, Support system for the preventive diagnosis of hypertensive retinopathy, in *Proceeding of 32nd Annual International Conference of the IEEE EMBS*, vol. 2010, pp. 7396–7399 (2010)
489. R. Estrada, M.J. Allingham, P.S. Mettu, S.W. Cousins, C. Tomasi, S. Farsiu, Retinal artery-vein classification via topology estimation. Comput. Methods Programs Biomed. **34**(12), 2518–2534 (2015)
490. C. Herweh, P.A. Ringleb, G. Rauch, S. Gerry, L. Behrens, M. Mählenbruch et al., Performance of e-ASPECTS software in comparison to that of stroke physicians on assessing CT scans of acute ischemic stroke patients. Int. J. Stroke **11**(4), 438–445 (2016)
491. S. Nagel, D. Sinha, D. Day, W. Reith, R. Chapot, P. Papanagiotou et al., 'e-ASPECTS software is non-inferior to neuroradiologists in applying the ASPECT score to computed tomography scans of acute ischemic stroke patients. Int. J. Stroke (2016). (In Press)
492. D.G. Altman, J.M. Bland, Measurement in medicine: the analysis of method comparison studies. J. R. Stat. Soc. D (The Statistician) **32**, 307–317 (1983)
493. A.M. Euser, F.W. Dekker, S. le Cessie, A practical approach to Bland-Altman plots and variation coefficients for log transformed variables. J. Clin. Epidemiol. **61**, 978–982 (2008)
494. D.R. Matthews, J.P. Hosker, An unbiased, flexible computer programme for glucose clamping, with graphics and running statistics. Diabetologia **27**, 308–309 (1984)
495. M. De Luca, C.F. Beckmann, N. De Stefano, P.M. Matthews, S.M. Smith, fMRI resting state networks define distinct modes of long-distance interactions in the human brain. NeuroImage **29**, 1359–1367 (2006)
496. S. Orel, M.D. Schnall, C.M. Powell, M.G. Hochman, L.J. Solin, B.L. Fowble- et al., Staging of suspected breast-cancer-effect of MR imaging and MR-guided imaging and biopsy. Radiology **196**(1), 115–122 (1995)

497. D. Saslow, C. Boetes, W. Burke, S. Harms, M.O. Leach, C.D. Lehman- et al., American cancer society guidelines for breast screening with MRI as an adjunct to mammography. CA Cancer J. Clin. **57**(2), 75–89 (2007)
498. B. Szabó, P. Aspelin, M. Wiberg, B. Bone, Dynamic MR imaging of the breast - analysis of kinetic and morphologic diagnostic criteria. Acta Radiol. **44**(4), 379–386 (2003)
499. C.W. Piccoli, Contrast-enhanced breast MRI: factors affecting sensitivity and specificity. Eur. Radiol. **7**(Suppl. 5), S281–S288 (1997)
500. K. Nie, J.-H. Chen, H.J. Yu, Y. Chu, O. Nalcioglu, M.-Y. Su, Quantitative analysis of lesion morphology and texture features for diagnostic prediction in breast MRI. Acta Radiol. **15**(12), 1513–1525 (2008)
501. B.K. Szabó, P. Aspelin, M.K. Wiberg, Neural network approach to the segmentation and classification of dynamic magnetic resonance images of the breast: comparison with empiric and quantitative kinetic parameters. Acta Radiol. **11**(12), 1344–1354 (2004)
502. T. Twellmann, A. Meyer Baese, O. Lange, S. Foo, T.W. Nattkemper, Model-free visualization of suspicious lesions in breast MRI based on supervised and unsupervised learning. Eng. Appl. Artif. Intell. **21**(2), 129–140 (2008)
503. W. Chen, M.L. Giger, U. Bick, G.M. Newstead, Automatic identification and classification of characteristic kinetic curves of breast lesion on DCE-MRI. Acta Radiol. **33**(8), 2878–2887 (2006)
504. C.E. McLaren, W.-P. Chen, K. Nie, M.-Y. Su, Prediction of malignant breast lesions from mri features: a comparison of artificial neural network and logistic regression techniques. Acta Radiol. **16**(7), 842–851 (2009)
505. L.A. Meinel, A.H. Stolpen, K.S. Berbaum, L.L. Fajardo, J.M. Reinhardt, Breast MRI lesion classification: improved performance of human readers with a backpropagation neural network computer-aided (CAD) system. J. Magn. Reson. Imaging **25**(1), 89–95 (2007)
506. A. Penn, S. Thompson, R. Brem, C. Lehman, P. Weatherall, M. Schnall- et al., Morphologic blooming in breast MRI as a characterization of margin for discriminating benign from malignant lesions. Acta Radiol. **13**(11), 1344–1354 (2006)
507. P. Gibbs, L.W. Turnbull, Texture analysis of contast-enhanced MR images of the breast. Magn. Reson. Med. **50**(1), 92–98 (2003)
508. H. Degani, V. Gusis, D. Weinstein, S. Fields, S. Strano, Mapping pathophysiological features of breast tumors by MRI at high spatial resolution. Nat. Med. **3**(7), 780–782 (1997)
509. D. Weinstein, S. Strano, P. Cohen, S. Fields, J.M. Gomori, H. Degani, Breast fibroadenoma: mapping of pathophysiologic features with three-time-point, contrast-enhanced MR imaging-pilot study. Radiology **210**(1), 233–240 (1999)
510. E.A.M. Hauth, H. Jaeger, S. Maderwald, A. Muhler, R. Kimmig, M. Forsting, Quantitative 2- and 3-dimensional analysis of pharmacokinetic model-derived variables for breast lesions in dynamic, contrast-enhanced MR mammography. Eur. J. Radiol. **66**(6), 300–308 (2008)
511. J. Pan, B.E. Dogan, S. Carkaci, L. Santiago, E. Arribas, S.B. Cantor- et al., Comparing performance of the CADstream and thedynaCAD breast MRI CAD systems. J. Digit. Imaging **26**(5), 971–976 (2013)
512. F. Keyvanfard, M.A. Shoorehdeli, M. Teshnehlab, K. Nie, M.-Y. Su, Feasibility of high temporal resolution breast DCE-MRI using compressed sensing theory. Neural Comput. Appl. **22**(1), 35–45 (2013)
513. T. Helbich, Contrast-enhanced magnetic resonance imaging of the breast. Eur. J. Radiol. **34**(3), 208–219 (2000)
514. C.E. Beckman, S.M. Smith, Tensorial extensions of independent component analysis for multi-subject FMRI analysis. NeuroImage **25**(1), 294–311 (2005)
515. Y. Lee, Y. Lin, G. Wahba, Multicategory support vector machines: theory and application to the classification of microarray data and satellite radiance data. J. Am. Stat. Assoc. **99**(465), 67–82 (2004)
516. J. Weston, C. Watkins, *Multi-Class Support Vector Machines* (Department of Computer Science, Royal Holloway, Unviersity of London, London, U.K., 1998)

517. I. Tsochantaridis, T. Hofmann, T. Joachims, Y. Altun, Support vector machine learning for interdependent and structured output spaces, in *Proceedings of the 21st International Conference on Machine Learning* (2004), pp. 104–111
518. E.J. Bayro Corrochano, N. Arana Daniel, Clifford support vector machines for classification, regression, and recurrence. IEEE Trans. Neural Netw. **21**(11), 1731–1746 (2010)
519. E. Hitzer, Angles between subspaces computed in clifford algebra. Proc. Int. Conf. Numer. Anal. Appl. Math. **1281**, 1476–1479 (2010)
520. C. Doran, A. Lasenby, *Geometric Algebra for Physicists* (Cambridge University Press, Cambridge, UK, 2003)
521. L. Dorst, D. Fontijne, S. Mann, *Geometric Algebra for Computer Science: An Object-oriented Approach to Geometry* (Morgan Kaufmann, Burlington, MA, 2007)
522. L. Dorst, Tutorial: structure-preserving representation of euclidean motions through conformal geometric algebra computing. IEEE Comput. Graph. Appl. **22**(3), 24–31 (2002)
523. L. Dorst, Tutorial: Structure-preserving representation of euclidean motions through conformal geometric algebra computing (2010), pp. 35–52
524. L. Dorst, The representation of rigid body motions in the conformal model of geometric algebra, in *Human Motion*, ed. by B. Rosenhahn, R. Klette, D. Metaxas (Springer, The Netherlands, Dordrecht, 2008), pp. 507–529
525. S. Mann, L. Dorst, T. Bouma, The making of a geometric algebra package in matlab, in *Research Report CS-99-27* (University of Waterloo, 1999)
526. E. Hodneland, A. Lundervold, J. Rørvik, A. Munthe-Kaas, Normalized gradient fields for nonlinear motion correction of DCE-MRI time series. Comput. Med. Imaging Graph. **38**(3), 202–210 (2014)
527. N. Michoux, J.P. Vallée, A. Pechère-Bertschi, X. Montet, L. Buehler, B.E. Van Beers, Analysis of contrast-enhanced MR images to assess renal function. Magma **19**(4), 167–179 (2006)
528. J. Tokuda, H. Mamata, R.R. Gill, N. Hata, R. Kikinis, R.F.P. Jr et al., Impact of nonrigid motion correction technique on pixel-wise pharmacokinetic analysis of free-breathing pulmonary dynamic contrast-enhanced MR imaging. J. Magn. Reson. Imaging **33**(4), 968–973 (2011)
529. J.P.B. O'Connor, A. Jackson, G.J.M. Parker, G.C. Jayson, DCE-MRI biomarkers in the clinical evaluation of antiangiogenic and vascular disrupting agents. Br. J. Cancer **96**, 189–195 (2007)
530. D. Zikic, S. Sourbron, X.X. Feng, H.J. Michaely, A. Khamene, N. Navab, Automatic alignment of renal DCE-MRI image series for improvement of quantitative tracer kinetic studies, in *Proceedings of the SPIE*, eds. by J.M. Reinhardt, J.P.W. Pluim, vol. 6914 (SPIE, (USA), 2008). (Art. No. 691432)
531. D. Rueckert, L.I. Sonoda, C. Hayes, D.L.G. Hill, M.O. Leach, D.J. Hawkes, Nonrigid registration using free-form deformations: application to breast mr images. IEEE Trans. Med. Imaging **18**(8), 712–721 (1999)
532. T. Rohlfing, C.R. Maurer, W.G. O'Dell, J. Zhong, Modeling liver motion and deformation during the respiratory cycle using intensity-based nonrigid registration of gated MR images. Med. Phys. **31**(3), 427–432 (2004)
533. Y. Yim, H. Hong, Y.G. Shin, Deformable lung registration between exhale andinhale ct scans using active cells in a combined gradient force approach. Med. Phys. **37**(8), 4307–4017 (2010)
534. G. Janssens, L. Jacques, J.O. de Xivry, X. Geets, B. Macq, Diffeomorphic registra-tion of images with variable contrast enhancement. Int. J. Biomed. Imaging **2011**(3), Art. No. 891585 (2011)
535. T. Mansi, X. Pennec, M. Sermesant, H. Delingette, N. Ayache, Logdemons revisited: consistent regularisation and incompressibility constraint for soft tissue track-ing in medical images, in *Proceedings of Medical Image Computing and Computer-Assisted Intervention—MICCAI 2010*, eds. by T. Jiang, N. Navab, J. Pluim, M. Viergever. LNCS6362 (Springer-Verlag, Berlin, Heidelberg, 2010), pp. 652–659
536. J. Modersitzki, FLIRT with rigidity-image registration with a local non-rigidity penalty. Int. J. Comput. Vis. **76**(2), 153–163 (2007)
537. A.D. Merrem, F.G. Zöllner, M. Reich, A. Lundervold, J. Rorvik, L.R. Schad, A variational approach to image registration in dynamic contrast-enhanced MRI of the human kidney. Magn. Reson. Imaging **31**(5), 771–777 (2013)

538. V.S. Lee, H. Rusinek, M.E. Noz, P. Lee, M. Raghavan, E.L. Kramer, Dynamic three dimensional MR renography for the measurement of single kidney function: initial experience. Radiology **227**(1), 289–294 (2003)
539. T. Song, V.L. Lee, H. Rusinek, M. Kaur, A.F. Laine, Automatic 4-D registration in dynamic MR renography based on over-complete dyadic wavelet and fourier transforms, in *Proceedings of the 8th International Conference on Medical Image Computing and Computer-Assisted Intervention*, eds. by J. Duncan, G. Gerig. LNCS3750 (Part II) (Springer-Verlag, Berlin, Heidelberg, 2005), pp. 205–213
540. G.A. Buonaccorsi, J.P. O'Connor, A. Caunce, C. Roberts, S. Cheung, Y. Watson et al., Tracer kinetic model-driven registration for dynamic contrast-enhanced MRI timeseries data. Magn. Reson. Med. **58**(5), 1010–1019 (2007)
541. G.A. Buonaccorsi, C. Roberts, S. Cheung, Y. Watson, J.P. O'Connor, K. Davies- et al., Comparison of the performance of tracer kinetic model-driven registration for dynamic contrast enhanced MRI using different models of contrast enhancement. Acad. Radiol. **13**(9), 1112–1123 (2006)
542. Y. Sun, J. Moura, C. Ho, Subpixel registration in renal perfusion MR image sequence. Proc. IEEE Int. Symp. Biomed. Imaging: Nano to Macro **1**, 700–703 (2004)
543. F.G. Zöllner, R. Sance, P. Rogelj, M.J. Ledesma-Carbayo, J. Rørvik, A. Santos- et al., Assessment of 3D DCE-MRI of the kidneys using non-rigid image registration and segmentation of voxel time courses. Comput. Med. Imaging Graph. **33**(3), 171–181 (2008)
544. H.J. Johnson, G.E. Christensen, Consistent landmark and intensity-based image registration. IEEE Trans. Med. Imaging **21**(5), 450–461 (2002)
545. T. Rohlfing, C.R. Maurer Jr., D.A. Bluemke, M.A. Jacobs, Volume-preserving nonrigid registration of MR breast images using free-form deformation with an incompressibility constraint. IEEE Trans. Med. Imaging **22**(6), 730–741 (2003)
546. D. Loeckx, F. Maes, D. Vandermeulen, P. Suetens, Nonrigid image registration using free-form deformations with a local rigidity constraint, in *Proceedings of Medical Image Computing and Computer-Assisted Intervention - MICCAI 2004*, eds. by C. Barillot, D. Haynor, J. Falcao e Cunha, P. Hellier. LNCS3216, (Springer-Verlag, Berlin, Heidelberg, 2004), pp. 639–646
547. S.Schäfera., U. Preimb, S. Glaßera, B. Preima, K.D. Tönniesa, Local similarity measures for lesion registration in DCE-MRI of the breast. Ann. BMVA **2011**(3),1–13 (2011)
548. S. Glaßer, S. Schäfer, S. Oeltze, U. Preim, K. Tönnies, B. Preim, A visual analytics approach to diagnosis of breast DCE-MRI data. Comput. Graph. **34**(5), 602–611 (2010)
549. F.G. Zöllner, R. Sance, P. Rogelj, M.J. Ledesma-Carbayo, J. Rørvik, A. Santos- et al., Assessment of 3D DCE-MRI of the kidneys using non-rigid image registration and segmentation of voxel time courses. Comput. Med. Imaging Graph. **33**(1), 171–181 (2009)
550. M. Bhushan, J.A. Schnabel, L. Risser, M.P. Heinrich, J.M. Brady, M. Jenkinson, Motion correction and parameter estimation in DCE-MRI sequences: application to colorectal cancer, in *Proceedings of Medical Image Computing and Computer-Assisted Intervention—MICCAI 2011*, eds. by G. Fichtinger, A. Martel, T. Peters. LNCS6891 (Part I), (Springer-Verlag, Berlin, Heidelberg, 2011), pp. 476–483
551. W. Lin, J. Guo, M.A. Rosen, H.K. Song, Respiratory motion-compensated radial dynamic contrast-enhanced (DCE)-MRI of chest and abdominal lesions. Magn. Reson. Med. **60**(5), 1135–1146 (2008)
552. J.B. Antoine Maintz, M.A. Viergever, A survey of medical image registration. Comput. Surv. **24**(4), 325–376 (1992)
553. A.N. Kumar, K.W. Short, D.W. Piston, A motion correction framework for time series sequences in microscopy images. Microsc. Microanal. **19**(2), 433–450 (2013)
554. L. Zhukov, K. Museth, D. Breen, R. Whitakery, A.H. Barr, Level set modeling and segmentation of DT-MRI brain data. J. Electron. Imaging **12**(1), 125–133 (2003)
555. T.F. Chan, L.A. Vese, Active contours without edges. IEEE Trans. Image Process. **10**(2), 266–277 (2001)
556. J. Andersson, C. Hutton, R.T.J. Ashburner, K. Friston, Modelling geometric distortions in EPI time series. NeuroImage **13**(5), 903–919 (2001)

557. M.A.O. Vasilescu, D. Terzopoulos, Multilinear analysis of image ensembles: Tensorfaces, in *Proceeding of the European Conference on Computer Vision* (2002), pp. 447–460
558. T. Kolda, B.W. Bader, Tensor decompositions and applications. SIAM Rev. **51**(3), 455–500 (2009)
559. T. Hazan, S. Polak, A. Shashua, Sparse image coding using a 3D non-negative tensor factorization, in *Proceeding of the Tenth IEEE International Conference on Computer Vision*, vol. 1, pp. 50–57 (2005)
560. G. Bartzokis, P.H. Lu, J. Mintz, Human brain myelination and amyloid beta deposition in alzheimer's disease. Alzheimer's & Dementia **3**(2), 122–125 (2007)
561. D.F. Plusquellic, K. Siegrist, E.J. Heilweil, O. Esenturk, Applications of terahertz spectroscopy in biosystems. ChemPhysChem **8**(7), 2412–2431 (2007)
562. S.J. Oh, J. Choi, I. Maeng, J.Y. Park, K. Lee, Y.M. Huh et al., Molecular imaging with terahertz waves. Opt. Express **19**(5), 4009–4016 (2011)
563. D. Tao, X. Li, X. Wu, W. Hu, S. Maybank, Supervised tensor learning. Knowl. Inf. Syst. **13**(1), 1–42 (2007)
564. M. Signoretto, L. Lathauwer, J. Suykens, A kernel based framework to tensorial data analysis. Neural Netw. **24**(8), 861–874 (2011)
565. L. He, X. Kong, P.S. Yu, A.B. Ragin, Z. Hao, X. Yang, DuSK: A dual structure-preserving kernel for supervised tensor learning with applications to neuroimages, in *Proceedings of SIAM International Conference on Data Mining 2014, SDM 2014*, vol. 1. Society for Industrial and Applied Mathematics Publications, (Philadelphia, United Stages, 2014), pp. 127–135
566. X. Han, Y. Zhong, L. He, P.S. Yu, L.Zhang, The unsupervised hierarchical convolutional sparse auto-encoder for neuroimaging data classification, in *Proceedings of 8th International Conference on Brain Informatics and Health*, vol. 9250 (Springer Verlag, (London, United Kingdom), 2015), pp. 156–166
567. C. Habeck, Y. Stern, Alzheimer's Disease Neuroimaging Initiative, Multivariate data analysis for neuroimaging data: Overview and application to alzheimer's disease. Cell Biochem. Biophys. **58**(2), 53–67 (2010)
568. D.Y. Tsao, W.A. Freiwald, T.A. Knutsen, J.B. Mandeville, R.B.H. Tootell, Faces and objects in macaque cerebral cortex. Nat. Neurosci. **6**, 989–995 (2003)
569. T.A. Carlson, P. Schrater, S. He, Patterns of activity in the categorical representations of objects. J. Cogn. Neurosci. **15**(5), 704–717 (2003)
570. S. Bray, C. Chang, F. Hoeft, Applications of multivariate pattern classifi cation analyses in developmental neuroimaging of healthy and clinical populations. Front. Hum. Neurosci. **3**(32), 1–12 (2009)
571. J. Cummings, M.S. Mega, *Neuropsychiatry Behav. Neurosci.* (Oxford University Press, Oxford, New York, 2003)
572. W.C. Drevets, Neuroimaging studies of mood disorders. Biol. Psychiatry **48**(8), 813–829 (2000)
573. C.H.-Y. Fu, J. Mourao-Miranda, S.G. Costafreda, A. Khanna, A.F. Marquand, S.C.-R. Williams, M.J. Brammer, Neuroimaging studies of mood disorders. Biol. Psychiatry **63**(7), 656–662 (2008)
574. B. Cao, X. Kong, P.S. Yu, A review of heterogeneous data mining for brain disorder identification. Brain Inf. **2**(4), 253–264 (2015)
575. I. Davidson, S. Gilpin, O. Carmichael, P. Walker, Network discovery via constrained tensor analysis of fMRI data, in *KDD'13, Proceedings of the 19th ACM SIGKDD International Conference on Knowledge Discovery and Data Mining* (2013), pp. 194–202
576. S. Vega-Pons, F.B. Kessler, P. Avesani, Network discovery via constrained tensor analysis of fMRI data, in *2013 International Workshop on Pattern Recognition in Neuroimaging (PRNI)* (2013), pp. 136–139
577. B. Jie, D. Zhang, C.-Y. Wee, D. Shen, Topological graph kernel on multiple thresholded functional connectivity networks for mild cognitive impairment classification. Hum. Brain Mapp. **35**(7), 2876–2897 (2014)

578. N. Shervashidze, P. Schweitzer, E. van Leeuwen, K. Mehlhorn, K. Borgwardt, Weisfeiler-lehman graph kernels. J. Mach. Learn. Res. **12**, 2539–2561 (2011)
579. S.N. Vishwanathan, N.N. Schraudolph, R. Kondor, K.M. Borgwardt, Graph kernels. J. Mach. Learn. Res. **11**, 1201–1242 (2010)
580. K.M. Borgwardt, C.S. Ong, S. Schönauer, S.V.N. Vishwanathan, A.J. Smola, H.-P. Kriegel, Protein function prediction via graph kernels. Bioinformatics **21**(Suppl. 1), i47–i56 (2005)
581. T. Gärtner, P. Flach, S. Wrobel, Hardness results and efficient alternatives, in *Proceedings of Sixteenth Annual Conference on Computational Learning Theory and Seventh Kernel Workshop*. LNAI 2777, (Speringer-Verlag, (Berlin, Heidelberg), 2003), pp. 129–143
582. H. Kashima, K. Tsuda, A. Inokuchi, Marginalized kernels between labeled graphs, in *Proceedings of the 20th International Conference on Machine Learning (ICML)* (2003)
583. T. Horváth, T.G. Gärtner, S. Wrobel, Cyclic pattern kernels for predictive graph mining, in *Proceedings of the ACM SIGKDD Conference on Knowledge Discovery and Data Mining* (2004), pp. 158–167
584. N. Shervashidze, K.M. Borgwardt, Fast subtree kernels on graphs, in *Proceedings of the Conference on Advances in Neural Information Processing Systems*, eds. by Y. Bengio, D. Schuurmans, J. Lafferty, C.K.I. Williams, A. Culotta (Curran, 2009), pp. 1660–1668
585. G. Camps-Valls, N. Shervashidze, K. Borgwardt, Spatiospectral remote sensing image classification with graph kernels. IEEE Geosci. Remote Sens. Lett. **7**, 741–745 (2010)
586. Q. Yu, E.B. Erhardt, J. Sui, Y. Du, H. He, D. Hjelm, M.S. Cetin, S. Rachakonda, R.L. Miller, G. Pearlson, V.D. Calhoun, Assessing dynamic brain graphs of time-varying connectivity in fMRI data: application to healthy controls and patients with schizophrenia. NeuroImage **107**, 345–355 (2015)
587. K.M. Borgwardt, H.-P. Kriegel, Shortest-path kernels on graphs, in *Proceeding ICDM'05 Proceedings of the Fifth IEEE International Conference on Data Mining* (2005), pp. 74–81
588. F. Pereira, T. Mitchell, M. Botvinick, Machine learning classifiers and fMRI: a tutorial overview. Neuroimage **45**(1, Subppl), S199–S209 (2008)
589. J. Richiardi, S. Achard, H. Bunke, D.V.D. Ville, Machine learning with brain graphs: predictive modeling approaches for functional imaging in systems neuroscience. IEEE Signal Process. Mag. **30**(3), 58–70 (2013)
590. N.U.F. Dosenbach, B. Nardos, A.L. Cohen, D.A. Fair, J.D. Power, J.A. Church et al., Machine learning with brain graphs: predictive modeling approaches for functional imaging in systems neuroscience. Science **329**(5997), 1358–1361 (2010)
591. N.K. Logothetis, J. Pauls, M. Augath, T. Trinath, A. Oeltermann, Neurophysiological investigation of the basis of the fMRI signal. Nature **412**, 150–157 (2001)
592. N.K. Logothetis, B.A. Wandell, Interpreting the BOLD signal. Annu. Rev. Physiol. **66**, 735–769 (2004)
593. N.K. Logothetis, J. Pfeuffer, On the nature of the BOLD fMRI contrast mechanism. Magn. Reson. Imaging **22**, 1517–1531 (2004)
594. N.K. Logothetis, What we can do and what we cannot do with fMRI. Nature **453**, 869–878 (2008)
595. N.K. Logothetis, The neural basis of the blood-oxygen-level-dependent functional magnetic resonance imaging signal. Philos. Trans. R. Soc. B **357**, 1003–1037 (2002)
596. B. Haider, A. Duque, A.R. Hasenstaub, D.A. McCormick, Neocortical network activity in vivo is generated through a dynamic balance of excitation and inhibition. J. Neurosci. **26**, 4535–4545 (2006)
597. B. Krekelberg, G.M. Boynton, R.J. van Wezel, Adaptation: from single cells to BOLD signals. Trends Neurosci. **29**, 250–256 (2006)
598. A. Viswanathan, R.D. Freeman, Neurometabolic coupling in cerebral cortex reflects synaptic more than spiking activity. Nat. Neurosci. **10**, 1308–1312 (2007)
599. R.J. Douglas, K.A. Martin, Neuronal circuits of the neocortex. Annu. Rev. Neurosci. **27**, 419–451 (2004)
600. A. Vedaldi, V.G.M. Varma, A. Zisserman, Multiple kernels for object detection, in *2009 IEEE 12th International Conference on Computer Vision (ICCV)* (2009), pp. 606–613

601. A. Vedaldi, A. Zisserman, Efficient additive kernels via explicit feature maps. IEEE Trans. Pattern Anal. Mach. Intell. **34**, 480–492 (2012)
602. K. Simonyan, A. Vedaldi, A. Zisserman, Learning local feature descriptors using convex optimisation. IEEE Trans. Pattern Anal. Mach. Intell. **36**, 1573–1585 (2014)
603. J. Revaud, P. Weinzaepfel, Z. Harchaoui, C. Schmid, Deepmatching: hierarchical deformable dense matching. Int. J. Comput. Vision **120**(3), 300–323 (2016)
604. A.W. Harley, An interactive node-link visualization of convolutional neural networks, in *International Symposium on Visual Computing* (2015), pp. 867–877
605. B. Fulkerson, A. Vedaldi, S. Soatto, Class segmentation and object localization with superpixel neighborhoods, in *2009 IEEE 12th International Conference on Computer Vision (ICCV)* (2009), pp. 670–677
606. M.C.S. Maji, I. Kokkinos, A. Vedaldi, Deep filter banks for texture recognition, description, and segmentation. Int. J. Comput. Vision **118**, 65–94 (2016)
607. R.-R. Jorge, B.-C. Eduardo, Medical image segmentation, volume representation and registration using spheres in the geometric algebra framework. Pattern Recognit. **40**(1), 171–188 (2007)
608. G. Cybenko, Approximation by superposition of a sigmoidal function. Math. Control Signals Syst. **2**(4), 303–314 (1989)
609. K. Hornik, Multilayer feedforward networks are universal approximators. Neural Netw. **2**(5), 359–366 (1989)
610. K. Tachibana, E. Hitzer, Tutorial note on GA neural networks, in *Proceeding of The 3rd International Conference on Applied Geometric Algebras in Computer Science and Engineering* (2008), pp. 1–20
611. E. Bayro Corrochano, S. Buchholz, Geometric neural networks, visual and motor signal neurocomputation, in *Algebraic Frames for the Perception-Action Cycle*, eds. by G. Sommer, Y.Y. Zeevi, vol. 1315 (Springer-Verlag, Heidelberg, New York, 2005), pp. 379–394
612. Y. Bengio, Learning deep architectures for AI. Found. Trends Mach. Learn. **2**(1), 1–127 (2009)
613. G.E. Hinton, S. Osindero, Y. Teh, A fast learning algorithm for deep belief nets. Neural Comput. **18**(7), 1527–1554 (2006)
614. G.E. Hinton, R. Salakhutdinov, Reducing the dimensionality of data with neural networks. Science **313**(5786), 504–507 (2006)
615. Y. Bengio, Y. LeCun, Scaling learning algorithms towards AI, in *Large Scale Kernel Machines*, ed. by L. Bottou, O. Chapelle, D. DeCoste, J. Weston (MIT Press, Cambridge, MA, 2007)
616. Y. Bengio, P. Lamblin, D. Popovici, H. Larochelle, Greedy layer-wise training of deep networks, in *Advances in Neural Information Processing Systems*, eds. by J.P.B. Schälkopf, T. Hoffman, vol. 19 (MIT Press, Cambridge, MA, 2007), pp. 153–160
617. H. Larochelle, D. Erhan, A. Courville, J. Bergstra, Y. Bengio, An empirical evaluation of deep architectures on problems with many factors of variation, in *Proceedings of the Twenty-fourth International Conference on Machine Learning*, ed. by Z. Ghahramani (Canada, ACM, Montreal (Qc), 2007), pp. 473–480
618. H. Lee, R. Grosse, R. Ranganath, A.Y. Ng, Convolutional deep belief networks for scalable unsupervised learning of hierarchical representations, in *Proceedings of the Twenty-sixth International Conference on Machine Learning*, ed. by L. Bottou, M. Littman (Canada, ACM, Montreal (Qc), 2009), pp. 609–616
619. M. Ranzato, Y.-L. Boureau, Y. LeCun, Sparse feature learning for deep belief networks, in *Advances in Neural Information Processing Systems*, eds. by J. Platt, D. Koller, Y. Singer, S. Roweis, vol. 20 (MIT Press, Cambridge, MA, 2008), pp. 1185–1192
620. R. Salakhutdinov, G.E. Hinton, Using deep belief nets to learn covariance kernels for gaussian processes, in *Advances in Neural Information Processing Systems*, eds. by J. Platt, D. Koller, Y. Singer, S. Roweis, vol. 20 (MIT Press, Cambridge, MA, 2008), pp. 1249–1256
621. S. Osindero, G.E. Hinton, Modeling image patches with a directed hierarchy of markov random field, in *Advances in Neural Information Processing Systems*, eds. by J. Platt, D. Koller, Y. Singer, S. Roweis, vol. 20 (MIT Press, Cambridge, MA, 2008), pp. 1249–1256

622. M. Ranzato, F. Huang, Y. Boureau, Y. LeCun, Unsupervised learning of invariant feature hierarchies with applications to object recognition, in *Proceedings of the Computer Vision and Pattern Recognition Conference* (IEEE Press, 2007), pp. 1–8
623. I. Levner, *Data Driven Object Segmentation*, Ph.D. Thesis, (Department of Computer Science, University of Alberta, Edmonton, Canada, 2008)
624. L. Breiman, J.H. Friedman, R.A. Olshen, C.J. Stone, *Classif. Regres. Trees* (Wadsworth International Group, Belmont, CA, 1984)
625. D.E. Rumelhart, G.E. Hinton, R.J. Williams, Learning representations by back-propagating errors. Nature **323**, 533–536 (1986)
626. G. Taylor, G.E. Hinton, S. Roweis, Modeling human motion using binary latent variables, in *Advances in Neural Information Processing Systems*, eds. by J.P.B. Schölkopf, T. Hoffman, vol. 19 (MIT Press, Cambridge, MA, 2007), pp. 1345–1352
627. G.E. Hinton, Products of experts, in *Proceedings of the Ninth International Conference on Artificial Neural Networks*, vol. 1, pp. 1–6 (1999)
628. J. Baxter, A bayesian/information theoretic model of learning via multiple task sampling. Mach. Learn. **28**(1), 7–40 (1997)
629. N. Intrator, S. Edelman, How to make a low-dimensional representation suitable for diverse tasks. Connect. Sci. (Spec. Issue Transf. Neural Netw.) **8**, 205–224 (1996)
630. S. Thrun, Is learning the n-th thing any easier than learning the first?, in *Human Motion*, eds. by D. Touretzky, M. Mozer, M. Hasselmo, vol. 8 (MIT Press, Cambridge, MA, 1996), pp. 640–646
631. R. Raina, A. Battle, H. Lee, B. Packer, A.Y. Ng, Self-taught learning: transfer learning from unlabeled data, in *Proceedings of the Twenty-fourth International Conference on Machine Learning*, ed. by Z. Ghahramani (Canada, ACM, Montreal (Qc), 2007), pp. 759–766
632. R. Collobert, J. Weston, A unified architecture for natural language processing: Deep neural networks with multitask learning, in *Proceedings of the Twenty-fourth International Conference on Machine Learning*, ed. by W.W. Cohen, A. McCallum, S.T. Roweis (Canada, ACM, Montreal (Qc), 2008), pp. 160–167
633. H. Bourlard, Y. Kamp, Auto-association by multilayer perceptrons and singular value decomposition. Biol. Cybern. **59**(4), 291–294 (1988)
634. P. Vincent, H. Larochelle, Y. Bengio, P.-A. Manzagol, Extracting and composing robust features with denoising autoencoders, in *Proceedings of the Twenty-fifth International Conference on Machine Learning*, ed. by W.W. Cohen, A. McCallum, S.T. Roweis (Canada, ACM, Montreal (Qc), 2008), pp. 1096–1103
635. Y. Freund, R.E. Schapire, Experiments with a new boosting algorithm, in *Machine Learning: Proceedings of Thirteenth International Conference* (ACM, USA, 1999), pp. 148–156
636. D.H. Wolpert, Stacked generalization. Neural Netw. **5**, 241–249 (1992)
637. L. Breiman, J.H. Friedman, R.A. Olshen, C.J. Stone, *Classification and Regression Trees* (Wadsworth International Group, Belmont, CA, 1984)
638. L. Rokach, O. Maimon, Top-down induction of decision trees classifiers-a survey. IEEE Trans. Syst. Man Cybern. Part C Appl. Rev. **35**(4), 476–487 (2005)
639. A. Khazaee, A. Ebrahimzadeh, A. Babajani-Feremi, Application of pattern recognition and graph theoretical approaches to analysis of brain network in Alzheimer's disease. J. Med. Imaging Health Inf. **5**(6), 1145–1155 (2015)
640. W.M. Wells, W.L. Grimson, R. Kikinis, F.A. Jolesz, Adaptive segmentation of MRI data. IEEE Trans. Med. Imaging **15**(4), 429–442 (1996)
641. S.P. Lloyd, Least squares quantization in PCM. IEEE Trans. Inf. Theory **28**(2), 129–137 (1982)
642. P.S. Bradley, U. Fayyad, Refining initial points for K-means clustering, in *Proceedings 15th International Conference Machine Learning* (1998), pp. 91–99
643. O. Irsoy, O.T. Yildiz, E. Alpaydin, Soft decision trees, in *Proceeding of 21nd International Conference on Pattern Recognition* (2012), pp. 1819–1822
644. O. Irsoy, O.T. Yildiz, E. Alpaydin, Budding trees, in *Proceeding of 22nd International Conference on Pattern Recognition* (2014), pp. 3582–3587

645. Y. Yoo, T. Brosch, A. Traboulsee, B.K.-B. Li, R. Tam, Deep learning of image features from unlabeled data for multiple sclerosis lesion segmentation, in *Proceeding of MLMI 2014*, eds. by G. Wu et al., vol. 8679 (Springer International Publishing, Switzerland, 2014), pp. 117–124
646. R. Kafieh, H. Rabbani, S. Kermani, A review of algorithms for segmentation of optical coherence tomography from retina. J. Med. Signals Sens. **3**(1), 45–60 (2013)
647. R.K.H. Galvão, J.P. Matsuura, J.R. Colombo Jr., S. Hadjiloucas, Detecting compositional changes in dielectric materials simulated by three-dimensional RC network models. IEEE Trans. Dielectr. Electr. Insul. **24**(2), 1141–1152 (2017)

Index

X. Yin et al., *Pattern Classification of Medical Images: Computer Aided Diagnosis*, Health Information Science, DOI 10.1007/978-3-319-57027-3

Printed in the United States
By Bookmasters